Pass
CNOR®!

Pass CNOR®!

Nancymarie Phillips, BA, BSN, PhD, RN, MEd, RNFA, CNOR(E)
Department of Perioperative Education
Director and Professor Emeritus
Perioperative Nursing, Registered Nurse First Assistants,
Surgical Technology
Lakeland Community College
Kirtland, Ohio

Anita Hornacky, BS, RN, CST, CNOR
Surgical Pharmacology Instructor
Lakeland Community College
Kirtland, Ohio

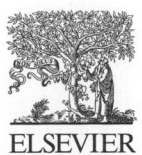

ELSEVIER

3251 Riverport Lane
St. Louis, Missouri 63043

PASS CNOR®!
FIRST EDITION

ISBN: 978-0-323-58197-4

Notices

Knowledge and best practice in this field are constantly changing. As new research and experience broaden our understanding, changes in research methods, professional practices, or medical treatment may become necessary.

Practitioners and researchers must always rely on their own experience and knowledge in evaluating and using any information, methods, compounds, or experiments described herein. In using such information or methods they should be mindful of their own safety and the safety of others, including parties for whom they have a professional responsibility.

With respect to any drug or pharmaceutical products identified, readers are advised to check the most current information provided (i) on procedures featured or (ii) by the manufacturer of each product to be administered, to verify the recommended dose or formula, the method and duration of administration, and contraindications. It is the responsibility of the practitioners, relying on their own experience and knowledge of the patient, to make diagnoses, to determine dosages and the best treatment for each individual patient, and to take all appropriate safety precautions.

To the fullest extent of the law, neither the Publisher nor the authors, contributors, or editors assume any liability for any injury and/or damage to persons or property as a matter of products' liability, negligence or otherwise, or from any use or operation of any methods, products, instructions, or ideas contained in the material herein.

Library of Congress Control Number: 2019941295

Content Strategist: Sandra Clark
Content Development Manager: Lisa Newton
Senior Content Development Specialist: Laura Selkirk
Publishing Services Manager: Shereen Jameel
Production Manager: Nadhiya Sekar
Design Direction: Ryan Cook

Printed in the United states
Last digit is the print number: 9 8 7 6 5 4 3 2 1

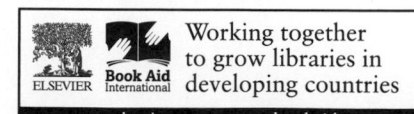

This book is dedicated to the perioperative nurses who have built the profession before our time and the perioperative nurses who will continue the building after we have gone.

Preface

Pass CNOR®! is designed to guide the perioperative nurse in preparation for taking the CNOR examination. The content of this text is derived from the AORN *Guidelines for Perioperative Practice* (2019), *Rothrock's Care of the Patient in Surgery*, 16th edition, and Phillips's *Berry and Kohn's Operating Room Technique*, 14th edition. The material included is geared toward certification-level knowledge, not basic perioperative nursing. This book is not intended to be a comprehensive text on perioperative nursing. The outline format is directed at salient knowledge that is easily resourced and validated in the three references used.

The structure of the format begins with important issues associated with professional perioperative nursing, including certification itself. The text progresses into baseline elements that include hand hygiene, appropriate attire, sterile and aseptic techniques, and the perioperative environment. Perioperative safety is defined and precedes the progressive chapters of patient care throughout the phases of surgical care. *Surgical Pharmacology and Anesthesia* is a separate chapter to describe the commonly used drugs and medications used in the operating room.

A chapter about surgical instruments and equipment provides a review of certification-level knowledge expected of perioperative nurses in all surgical environments. Another chapter describes activities and items used in multiple surgical procedures in a collection of specialized topics.

Finally, a user-friendly section includes a practice examination with answers and rationales.

Reviewers

Dee A. Boner, BSN, MSN, CNOR
Principal IT Trainer
eStar Training – OpTime/Anesthesia Periop
Vanderbilt University Medical Center
Nashville, Tennessee

Jay Bowers, BSN, RN, CNOR, TNCC
Clinical Coordinator and Educator for Bariatric, Trauma,
Surg-Onc, Peds, General, Plastics, and OMS
Perioperative Services
West Virginia Healthcare
Morgantown, West Virginia

Amy Jocelyn Broadhurst, BS, BSN, RN, CNOR, CBN
OR Staff Nurse
Operating Room
Christiana Care Wilmington Hospital
Wilmington, Delaware

Theresa Criscitelli, EdD, RN, CNOR
AVP Administration
Perioperative and Procedural Services
New York University – Winthrop Hospital
Mineola, New York

Holly S. Ervine, MSN, RN, CNOR
Surgical Services Professional Educator, Nursing
Organizational Learning
WellStar Health System
Atlanta, Georgia

Nancy E. Fellows, MSN, MPA, RN, CNOR
Sr. Clinical Education Consultant
Advanced Sterilization Products
Irvine, California

Laurie M. Gronowski, BSN, RN, CNOR
Staff Nurse
Beachwood ASC
Cleveland Clinic
Beachwood, Ohio

Candice Kiskadden, MSN, RN, CNOR
Instructor of Nursing
RN-BSN Program
Mercyhurst University
Erie, Pennsylvania

Susan Lynch, BSN, MSN, PhD, RN, CSSM, CNOR
Associate Director of Surgical Services
Penn Medicine, Chester County Hospital
West Chester, Pennsylvania

Angela Mercer, MSN, RN, CNOR
Staff Nurse
Perioperative Services
Christiana Care Health System
Newark, Delaware

Cynthia Ann Toale, BSN, RN, CNOR
Retired, Associate Unit Nursing Director,
Operating Room
UPMC Hamot
Erie, Pennsylvania

Susanna S. Walsh, BSN, RN, RNFA, CSSM, CNOR
Perioperative Manager
Operating Room
Vanderbilt University Medical Center
Nashville, Tennessee

Contents

Pass
CNOR®!

CHAPTER 1

Professional Issues and Accountability in Perioperative Nursing

Professional perioperative nurses follow an evidence-based set of standards and practices that provide safe and efficient patient care before, during, and after surgical intervention. The perioperative registered nurse (RN) demonstrates the knowledge and skill that embodies proficiency and competence. Certification as a perioperative nurse (CNOR) is the credential attained by the qualified, experienced RN who has surpassed basic entry-level practice with distinction.

What Is CNOR Certification?

CNOR is not an acronym. It stands for certified perioperative nurse. Perioperative nursing is not only relegated to intraoperative patient care but encompasses nursing care within the whole of the surgical patient environment. The specialty credential CNOR is recognized and sanctioned by the National Commission for Certifying Agencies (NCCA), the American Board for Specialty Nursing Certification (ABSNC), and the American Nurses Credentialing Center (ANCC). The Competency & Credentialing Institute (CCI) is accredited by NCCA and maintains this recognition by compliance with high standards of program excellence.

CNOR certification is a specialized credential that is maintained by professional development and continued integration of applied scientific inquiry. Best practices are supported by remaining current in knowledge and collegial leadership, and meeting desired patient care outcomes.

Who Is Eligible for CNOR Certification?

Potential candidates for CNOR certification are licensed RNs (without restrictions) who currently practice patient care in the perioperative environment where invasive surgical procedures are performed and have 2400 hours (2 years) of perioperative nursing practice. Direct intraoperative patient care of 1200 hours is incorporated into the eligibility requirement. Confirmation of eligibility will be audited by CCI. CCI will validate employment history and licensure status. The potential candidate will be notified of eligibility status by CCI. More information about eligibility can be found online at https://www.cc-institute.org.

What Are the Benefits of CNOR Certification?

Perioperative nurses with the credential CNOR represent the high standards of professional patient care valued by patients and employers alike. The recognition by staff and coworkers serves as an example of professional achievement. The facility is recognized by providing nursing excellence for ANCC Magnet Status compliance. CNOR certification validates personal satisfaction and professional competency in patient care. Additional benefits of CNOR certification are:
1. recognition of competency in perioperative nursing,
2. professional pride in exceeding expectations of baseline knowledge,
3. most employing facilities prefer certified RNs.
   a. Some facilities provide career advancement and promotions based on certification credentials.
   b. Some facilities offer a bonus for certification and recertification.
   c. Some facilities offer fee reimbursement for a passing examination score.

Maintaining the CNOR Credential

The CNOR credential is valid for 5 years. Eligibility for recertification includes current CNOR and unrestricted licensure as an RN. The recertification candidate is required to be employed full or part time in perioperative nursing as an educator, administrator, researcher, or clinical practice for a minimum of 500 hours during the 5-year certification cycle. A minimum of 250 hours of the 500 hours must be in the intraoperative patient care area. The certification 5-year cycle is designated by CCI as January to December per certified year.

One option is recertification by retaking and passing the CNOR examination. Alternatively, during the active certification period, the perioperative nurse has the opportunity to accrue credit for professional activities toward the goal of recertification by contact hours or points. Complete documentation of each contact hour is required in the formal certificate of attendance or transcript if audited by CCI.

1. Recertification by 125 approved contact hours
   a. Contact hours are approved by the providers listed on the CCI website (https://www.cc-institute.org). The total must include 75 contact hours in perioperative nursing topics.
   b. Academic credits toward a degree at a formal college or university up to 62.5 (50%) contact hours. A grade of C or better is required. The recertifying perioperative nurse does not need to be enrolled in a formal program to apply the following ANCC contact hour calculations:
      1) One semester hour equals 15 contact hours.
      2) One quarter hour equals 10 contact hours.
   c. Continuing medical education (CME) units up to 65.5 contact hours. CME hours are available online and are sometimes presented in the workplace by medical equipment companies or physicians. One CME equals 1 contact hour.
2. Recertification by points (Table 1.1): Recertification can be accomplished by professional educational activities that have a point value assigned by CCI. A total of 300 points is required for recertification. Some categories have limits for the number of points allowed. If audited by CCI, the appropriate written documentation is required.
3. Extension of recertification period
   a. Application for a 1-year recertification extension can be made twice in a 10-year period by contacting CCI. This covers two 5-year certification cycles.
   b. Application is required during the year of expiration.
   c. The extension is good for only 1 year and requires the applicant to continue to accrue contact hours or other recertification methods during this time period.
   d. Audits may be done for quality-assurance purposes.
   e. Recertification application can be submitted at any time during the extension year.
4. Retirement and emeritus options
   a. Emeritus status is a credential applied for at retirement.
   b. One-time fee and does not need to be renewed once granted by CCI.
   c. The emeritus credential application can be made by a retiring CNOR in good standing. The fee is not dependent on AORN membership.
   d. The CNOR emeritus credential designator is CNOR(E).

Preparing for the CNOR Examination

The first step in preparing for the CNOR examination is determining eligibility and readiness to test. CCI has prepared a CNOR Readiness Survey available for download on the CCI website (https://www.cc-institute.org) for the purpose of self-assessment. This survey serves as a snapshot of current perioperative practice and issues for evaluating strengths and areas for improvement. Using this tool is helpful when deciding a focused path for study.

The beginning of the survey affirms licensure and employment status. Subsequent sections look at

TABLE 1.1   Point Calculations for Recertification

Educational Activity Performed	Calculation	Maximum Number of Points Accumulated During 5-Year Recertification Period
Present continuing education	1 contact hour = 2 points 1 CME credit = 2 points	100 points = 50 contact hours 50 points = 25 CME credits
Academic study in a degree program	1 semester hour = 15 points 1 quarter hour = 10 points	Unlimited when it advances perioperative nursing career (BSN, MSN, DNP, also MBA)
Teaching a perioperative course	Each class = 30 points	Maximum 150 points
Presentation	60 minutes = 10 points	Maximum 150 points
Serve on board or committee	National/international = 30 points per year Local or facility = 15 points per year	Maximum 150 points
Precepting and Mentoring (Orienting)	Mentoring one person = 25 points	Maximum 100 points Only four different persons/employees
Volunteer for CCI test development committee	Job analysis = 40 points Item writer = 30 points Cut score/standard setting = 30 points Item review = 20 points Form review = 15 points PIN = 15 points	Maximum 100 points

CCI, Competency & Credentialing Institute; *CME,* continuing medical education; *PIN,* problem identification notification.

individual practice content. Experiential evaluation of current perioperative practice is broken down into target resource categories, such as preoperative patient care activities, intraoperative patient care activities, postoperative patient care activities, professional issues, on-site facility affiliations, and source material. Some study materials suggested are the current editions of AORN *Guidelines for Perioperative Practice, CNOR Exam Prep* by CCI, *Alexander's Care of the Patient in Surgery*, and *Berry & Kohn's Operating Room Technique*. CCI offers CNOR prep webinars. AORN offers workshops for CNOR certification preparation.

Additional questions discuss providing adequate study time and experienced resource persons for guidance as the process ensues. The CNOR Readiness Survey can help the potential certification candidate identify barriers that can cause a testing delay and better establish realistic timelines to ensure success. The survey allows the potential candidate an opportunity to self-measure each of the nine content areas on the examination by perceived levels of competence. These content areas are listed on the survey with the percentage of questions per topic appearing on the test.

1. Preoperative assessment and diagnosis: 12%
2. Develop an individualized plan of care and identify expected outcomes: 10%
3. Intraoperative activities: 27%
4. Communication: 10%
5. Transfer of care: 6%
6. Cleaning, disinfecting, packaging, sterilization, and transporting and storing instruments and supplies: 9%
7. Emergency situations: 11%
8. Management of personnel, services, and materials: 6%
9. Professional accountability: 9%

What Is the Best Way to Learn?

Every person learns and recalls information differently. Many things have a direct influence on the preparation for certification testing. Certification-level knowledge is an extraction from experience, observation of colleagues, and learning from new experiences. The following list may help guide potential CNOR candidates organize and prepare for the certification examination.

1. **Learning styles and how to use them:** Everyone's learning style is different. Determining a learning style that works is a first step in assimilating knowledge. Most adults learn by association. They see or experience a surgical procedure or process and are not always aware of the amount of knowledge retained. Much of the necessary content is already known, but not completely organized.

    Internal organization strategies can help. Start by finding the learning style that best stimulates recall of knowledge and identification of any missing facets. Seven learning styles are presented here to assist in aligning thought processes in preparation for effective study. These styles can be used in tandem with each other or in solitary form.

    a. **Visual learning:** Utilization of pictures and images. Look at pictures of incisions, surgical procedures, skin preps, patient positioning, and devices used in the operating room (OR). Images, in combination with other visual resources, can help connect previous experiences with newly integrated information. Videos can be used in this way also. Creating flowcharts or diagrams using images is useful. Sometimes making flash cards is a portable visual tool.

    b. **Kinesthetic or physical learning:** Utilization of daily work tasks such as actually performing patient positioning, skin preps, scrubbing, and other aseptic techniques can help stimulate details associated with patient care standards and reinforce associative memory.

    c. **Auditory learning:** Utilization of recorded lectures or dialogue during surgical procedures is beneficial for many adults. In the auditory learner, hearing descriptions by the surgeon and vocalizing counts, medications, and data during time-out periods structures mental images of necessary knowledge. Reading into a voice recorder is a useful method for listening to material when performing other tasks of daily living.

    d. **Verbal learning:** Utilization of oral repetition is useful for some adult learners. Reading out loud, reciting specific facts in list form, verbally spelling complex or new terms can trigger memorization. In some circumstances, mentoring others and orally teaching orientees or students causes recall of subliminal memory. This is helpful when questions are asked of the teacher by new learners.

    e. **Analytic learning:** Utilization of highly structured lists or algorithms helps organize key points. Creating systems from smallest elements to the total picture leads to solid understanding. Another approach is to examine a concept and break it down into smaller individual components. Associative memory is often triggered by building or dissecting a particular area of study. The analytic process incorporates many combinations of learning styles.

    f. **Group learning:** Utilization of study groups with other nurses, who have different learning styles, offers a variety of methods for approaching perioperative topics. A combination of visual, verbal, and auditory discussions can provide clarity by associating a global view of the subject matter. Working with team members, while providing patient care during a case, is a form of kinesthetic learning by physical activity.

    g. **Solo learning:** Utilization of private time for self-study allows multimodal learning approaches in any order. Working alone, without interacting with others, affords the opportunity to speak out loud to gather and organize information.

2. **Test-taking tips:** Determine your learning style(s) and put it to work.
   a. **Form a manageable mindset** by setting a few limits such as a reasonable time frame for completion and develop incremental study periods. For example, knowing that the examination will be taken in 3 months, you establish 2 hours every other day as reasonable study periods.
      1) **Allow time for adequate sleep.** Evaluate whether preferences include being a morning or night person.
      2) **Do not skip meals.** Avoid excessive snacks. Studying after a large meal can diminish energy and cause drowsiness. Drink plenty of water.
      3) **Incorporate routine breaks.** Get up and walk away from the study material.
   b. **Select an environment with minimal distraction.** Good lighting and a comfortable place to sit and spread out study materials should be planned. A multiplug electric outlet nearby is useful if electronic devices or a computer will be used. Some candidates like music or television playing in the background; others like absolute silence. Cell phones should be set on silent or completely turned off if possible.
   c. **Keep study supplies on hand.** These items may include paper, pens, pencils (plain lead and/or colored), scissors, paperclips, a stapler, notebooks, or file folders. Highlighters and sticky note pads are helpful for marking areas in texts and documents. A USB flash drive can be used to store study articles electronically if a computer is used.
   d. **Identify specific topics of focus.** Make lists or outlines in terms that you can understand. Color-code areas of study to organize specific subjects. Some nurses find it useful to start on areas that are most problematic and work on the concept in increments. Drawing pictures in the study notes can help reinforce memory.
   e. **Create mnemonics** using the first letter of each item in a list to create a phrase. Personal mnemonics can be created or commonly used ones can be found online via search engines using key terms such as "medical mnemonics."
      1) **Example of a mnemonic phrase:** "On Old Olympus Tiny Top A Fin And German Viewed Some Hops." The first letter in each word stands for the first letter of each cranial nerve.
      2) **Example of a mnemonic real word** (a real word created from each first letter of items in a list): *SAMPLE*. This mnemonic word can be used for assessing the patient's history as in **S**igns and *symptoms*, **A**llergies, **M**edications, **P**ast medical history, **L**ast meal, **E**vents leading to illness.
   f. **Take advantage of practice examinations.** CCI has a few downloadable sample questions on its website (https://www.cc-institute.org). Another option is for study groups to generate their own sets of questions. Each person in the group should create 5 to 10 questions to share. Divide the study material into sections such as medications, patient positioning, preoperative patient interview questions, time out content, or sterile technique.

Design of the CNOR Examination

1. The CNOR examination measures certification-level knowledge over minimal competency.
   a. Critical thinking employs cognitive action verbs like the following examples:
      1) *Application* of knowledge
      2) *Assimilation* of learned experiences
      3) *Differentiation* of questionable actions
      4) *Organization* of practice behaviors
      5) *Evaluation* of desired outcomes
   b. Clinical competency and professional judgment are assessed.
      1) Selection of answers defines the level of comprehensive knowledge.
      2) Patient advocacy is incorporated.
      3) Ethics influence each action.
2. Anatomy of the CNOR examination
   a. A total of 200 questions covering nine domains of perioperative nursing
      1) Computerized. No computer experience is necessary. Instructions and short tutorial are available at the time of testing.
      2) Multiple-choice questions with four selections as answers. No multiple answer combinations (i.e., no "none of the above" or "all of the above" selections) are included.
      3) Only one correct answer. The other selections may look plausible but are not correct.
      4) The test is scored based on 185 of the 200 questions. Of the total 200 questions, 15 questions are pretest questions and are not counted in the final score.
   b. 3 hours and 45 minutes is allotted to complete the examination
      1) The candidate is able to mark questions to return to for additional review.
      2) If the minimum passing parameter of 620 is met, the entirety of the test is to be completed. The computer does not shut off when the minimum has been met. Possible scores range from 200 to 800. Passage or failure is reported to the candidate when the test is completed.
      3) Nothing can be brought into the testing center. No cell phones or personal items. Security is monitored by staff of the center and video surveillance.
         a) A secure locked personal locker is provided.
         b) The testing center will provide scratch paper and pencils.
         c) Ear plugs are available on request. Personal ear plugs are not permitted.

4) Security breaches can cause removal from the examination.
   a) Suspected cheating noted by staff or video surveillance
   b) Disruptive behavior
   c) Use of methods to copy or communicate test questions
   d) Falsification of personal identification when taking the test
   e) Video evidence will be sent to CCI and reviewed by the testing agency
5) Additional considerations include:
   a) If the test is not scheduled with the testing agency during the testing window, the testing fee is forfeited and reapplication with new fee is required.
   b) Tardiness in excess of 15 minutes for appointed test time is considered absence and the test fee is forfeited.
   c) CCI has a program "Take Two" wherein a candidate can sign up for two opportunities to test at the time of initial examination application in the event of not passing the first time without additional full cost. This is open to first-time applicants only for a discounted fee. The 3-month testing window within the 12-month application period applies. Extensions for the 12-month period are not available.
   d) Potential first-time candidates who do not avail themselves of the "Take Two" option are subject to the full fee for a second registration if the test is not passed during the first sitting.
   e) The "Take Two" option is not available for recertification.
   f) A different examination is administered for each sitting.
   g) A fee is charged for change of testing dates with the testing center and is nonrefundable.
6) Use of the CNOR credential after successful examination passage
   a) CNOR is not an acronym for specific words; it signifies certification as a perioperative nurse.
   b) CNOR is a trademarked credential and may only be used after verification of examination passage by CCI.
   c) CNOR is valid for 5 years and expires on December 31 of the certification period.
   d) CNOR can be revoked by CCI for falsification of information, revocation or probation of nursing licensure, breach of confidentiality, or outstanding debt to CCI. An appeals process is available.

Approaches for CNOR Testing

1. A period of 3 months is allotted between scheduling the examination and actually taking the test. This time period is referred to as the testing window.

2. Three months is adequate time to review the nine domains tested during the CNOR examination.
3. Divide the material into smaller study segments to avoid cramming at the last minute.
4. Methods of answering the questions include:
   a. Read the question and attempt to supply the answer without reading the choices first.
   b. Read the question followed by reading the answer choices. Mentally eliminate the choices that do not answer the question.
   c. Mark the question for review at the end of the test if the answer does not feel obvious. This is a timed test and the review must be done before the time runs out. Do not linger over questions for extended periods.
   d. Use the test to take a test. Sometimes proceeding through the testing process can stimulate recall for an uncertain question. It can help to mentally repeat the question in words that are most familiar.
   e. Remember that the practices at the employing facility may differ from the current published best practices. The questions are based on current best practices published by the AORN *Guidelines for Perioperative Practice.*
   f. Do not overthink the question. Read through the question at face value. Do not add facts or surmise details not provided in the question. Do not add words or meanings that are not there.
   g. Trigger terms such as "first action," "best option," or "initial" point to specific answers.
   h. Rarely is it necessary to change an answer. Do not second-guess the initial answer selected. Often test takers change the answer only to find out later that they erased a correct choice. An old saying "Chance favors the educated mind" rings true here. Usually the first answer selected is correct.
   i. Do not leave any questions blank. They will be counted as wrong answers. Use an educated guess, but only as a last resort. That guess could be correct and often is.
   j. Wearing a watch can be useful because this is a timed test. Some facilities do not permit watches because they could be used as cheating devices. The testing room usually has a wall clock. Time can be measured by the number of questions answered in half the allotted time. For example, 100 questions should be answered within 90 minutes.

Preparing for the Day of Testing

1. Get a good night's sleep.
   a. For some individuals, 6 to 8 hours is adequate.
   b. Avoid sleeping medication or alcohol. These can alter the quality of sleep and leave the user groggy in the morning.
   c. Cramming all night will be exhausting and detract from mental clarity.
2. A morning testing time might be advisable over late afternoon, when anxiety can build and cause undue stress. Some people feel fatigue later in the day.

3. Eat a breakfast that contains some protein and carbohydrates.
   a. Eating only carbohydrates can cause an insulin surge that can feel physically draining.
   b. Avoid excessive caffeine intake to avoid feeling jittery.
4. Arrive at the testing center at least 20 minutes early.
   a. Be sure to know the center's location and parking availability.
   b. A trial drive by the day before the test can allay the risk of getting lost or being late for the testing appointment.
   c. The early arrival provides time for a restroom visit and a quick drink of water.
5. Dress sensibly and comfortably. No need for high fashion. Layers may be advisable to manage the temperature inside the testing area.
6. Bring a government-issued identification card with a signature.
   a. A driver's license or military identification cards are examples of appropriate identification.
   b. Some centers require two forms of identification.
   c. Some centers will accept a photo ID work badge as the second form.
   d. Instructions concerning identification requirements will be given when registering for the test.
7. Think positively.
   a. Taking the examination with an attitude of impending doom is self-defeating and can affect the outcome.
   b. Believe that a passing score is attainable and definitely an identified goal.
8. Be aware that other professionals use the same testing center for specialized examinations.
   a. Some of the other people will finish their tests at various times.
   b. This should not influence the rate of perceived time required to complete the CNOR examination.

Professional Standards and Accountability

Professional perioperative nurses have an obligation to provide safe and efficient patient care. By following evidence-based practice, standards, and guidelines established by organizations at the national level, the patient's outcome demonstrates the nurse's dedication to meeting the ethical responsibility of care.

Other nationally recognized organizations expand on regulatory standards for the environment, equipment, and generalized safety and are controlled by governmental law. Certification-level knowledge includes knowing where the standards, guidelines, and identified best practices originated.

Standards of Nursing Care

Standards of nursing care are defined and developed by recognized professional organizations to guide nurses in providing patient care. Examples of professional nursing organizations and specialty credentialing include the following:

1. **ANA** (American Nurses Association; https://www.nursingworld.org) provides professional nursing standards.
   a. **ANCC** (American Nurses Credentialing Center; https://www.nursingworld.org/ancc) sets the standard for nursing education programs.
   b. Magnet recognition for hospitals to recognize high-quality nursing processes and patient care is promoted by ANA.
2. **AORN**
   a. **AORN** (Association of Perioperative Registered Nurses; https://www.aorn.org) supports perioperative nursing through development of perioperative nursing education, standards, guidelines, and leadership.
   b. **AST** (Association of Surgical Technologists; https://www.ast.org) was originally affiliated with AORN. AST is now a separate organization that sets the standard for surgical technology.
      1) NBSTSA (National Board of Surgical Technology and Surgical Assisting; https://www.nbstsa.org) is the preferred certifying body for surgical technologists.
      2) ARC-STSA (Accreditation Review Council on Education in Surgical Technology and Surgical Assisting; http://www.arcstsa.org) is the accrediting organization for surgical technology programs.
3. **NCCA** (National Commission for Certifying Agencies; https://www.credentialingexcellence.org/ncca) sets the standard for professional certifying organizations to ensure the health, safety, and welfare of the public.
4. **ABSNC** (American Board for Specialty Nursing Certification; http://www.nursingcertification.org) is the organization that accredits nursing certification bodies.
5. **CCI** (Competency and Credentialing Institute; https://www.cc-institute.org) is the organization that provides certification opportunities for perioperative nurses, both staff and management.

Regulatory Organizations Associated With Governmental Control

1. **OSHA** (Occupational Safety and Health Administration; https://www.osha.gov) assures safe and healthy working conditions by setting and enforcing standards. It offers education, specialty training, and compliance assistance. OSHA is part of the Division of Labor.
2. **FDA** (US Food and Drug Administration; https://www.fda.gov) is part of the Department of Health and Human Services (HHS); it controls and monitors the safety and efficacy of drugs, medical supplies, food, and other consumer products.
   a. **CDRH** (Center for Devices and Radiological Health; http://www.cdrh.us) is under the FDA and regulates all radiation-emitting electronic products including lasers.

3. **CMS** (Centers for Medicare and Medicaid Services; https://www.cms.gov) is the branch of the HHS that regulates Medicare, Medicaid, and the health insurance industry. CMS developed a "no pay list" for preventable events that harm patients and will not be financially reimbursed.
4. **HIPAA** (Health Insurance Portability and Accountability Act; https://www.hhs.gov/hipaa/index.html) is a law under the HHS and not a separate organization. This act was designed to ensure privacy of patient health-related information by federal enforcement.
5. **AHRQ** (Agency for Healthcare Research and Quality; https://www.ahrq.gov) develops clinical practice guidelines based on research, professional judgment, safety, and efficacy. Performance can be measured by using AHRQ research.
6. **CDC** (Centers for Disease Control and Prevention; https://www.cdc.gov) provides scientific research about disease etiology and spread. The CDC responds to emergencies and uses research data to provide timely intervention and protection internationally.
   a. **NIOSH** (National Institute for Occupational Safety and Health; https://www.cdc.gov/niosh) generates research that tracks work-related disease, exposure, and illness. The research is translated into safety practices aimed at creating occupational safety for the present and the future. This branch of the CDC was established as a research group through the Occupational Safety Act of 1970.
7. **EPA** (Environmental Protection Agency; https://www.epa.gov) implements congressional law about the environment and ecosystems by establishing regulations and national standards. The EPA has the authority to enforce the regulations.
8. **NIH** (National Institutes of Health; https://www.nih.gov) is a part of the HHS and is the largest biomedical research organization in the world. Research at the NIH is directed at enhancing health, life, and reducing disease and injury in all environments. The NIH promotes the highest level of scientific inquiry and social accountability during the investigative research process.
9. **WHO** (World Health Organization; https://www.who.int/en) is an international organization that works with governments all over the world to promote and support the highest level of health for all populations. WHO fights both infectious (flu and HIV) and noncommunicable (coronary and cancer) diseases. The WHO globally assists mothers and infants, and ensures the safety of air, water, and food. Medications and vaccines are distributed in more than 150 countries worldwide.

Nonprofit Organizations That Set Standards Followed by Professional Associations

1. **NFPA** (National Fire Protection Association; https://www.nfpa.org) develops fire safety codes through research, education, and advocacy.
2. **TJC** (The Joint Commission; https://www.jointcommission.org) is a certifying and accrediting organization for facilities that provide healthcare services to the public. They set the National Patient Safety Goals (NPSG). Performance standards are monitored and evaluated by TJC.
3. **NQF** (National Quality Forum; http://www.qualityforum.org) is an organization that measures and sets standards to make health care safer, enhance value of care, and improve outcomes. NQF works with key public and private sector leaders to prioritize factors affecting healthcare policy.
4. **AAMI** (Association for the Advancement of Medical Instrumentation; http://www.aami.org) is comprised of professionals with the mission of developing, managing, and supporting healthcare technology. The medical device industry relies on the consensus of AAMI regarding technologic instruments, aseptic processing, and sterilization.
5. **ANSI** (American National Standards Institute; https://www.ansi.org) was formed to establish guidelines for equipment and potentially toxic materials. ANSI provides accreditation for manufacturers who comply with national standards and competency for use of specialized equipment.
6. **APIC** (Association for Professionals in Infection Control and Epidemiology; https://apic.org) promotes best practices to prevent infection. APIC collects and analyzes data about infection risk and control. The interpretation of the data helps to generate interventions for implementation by patient care workers.
7. **ECRI** (ECRI Institute; https://www.ecri.org) was formerly known as the Emergency Care Research Institute. The nonprofit ECRI was formed to organize objective independent research for examining medical procedures, devices, drugs, and processes without bias to improve patient care. The US government has designated ECRI as a patient safety organization, although not under governmental control. Researchers in the organization have no financial interest in any medical organization to maintain objectivity.
8. **ACGIH** (American Conference of Governmental Industrial Hygienists; https://www.acgih.org) is a research organization that collects and analyzes data concerning industrial and occupational health and safety.
9. **IHI-NPSF** (Institute for Healthcare Improvement: National Patient Safety Foundation [1996]; http://www.ihi.org) is a not-for-profit organization founded by the **AMA** (American Medical Association).

Communicating the Nursing Process
(Fig. 1.1)
Reviewing the Nursing Process

1. **Assessment** begins with identifying the patient using at least two methods: confirmed name (ask patient to say or spell name as appropriate) and birth date (month, day, and year). Confirm the planned surgical procedure and surgical site. Patient should verbalize the planned procedure and possibly point to the site as appropriate.

    The nurse should also look at the surgical site to observe confirmatory marking with the surgeon's initials. Data concerning identification and surgical procedure should be compared with the surgical consent form. Confirm that the patient has given informed consent for the surgeon to perform the surgical procedure. A parent or guardian may accompany a minor child or incompetent adult and contribute to the assessment process.

    a. Physiologic data

    1) Perform objective observation of patient's overall appearance and mobility. Note any skin redness, previous scars, or unusual appearance. Listen for speech and breathing sounds as dialogue takes place. Note any smells, such as unusual breath or body odor.

    2) During the discussion the nurse can touch patient's skin, possibly feeling a wrist pulse, skin temperature, skin texture, or moisture. If shaking the patient's hand, the nurse can observe for grip.

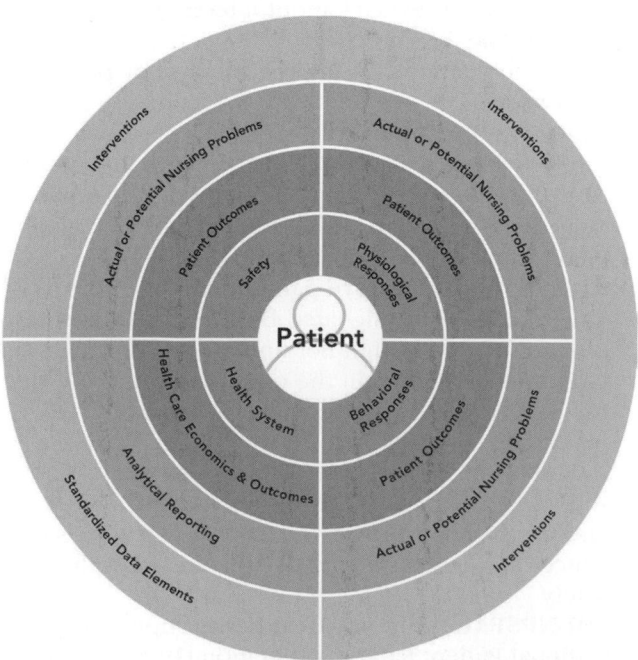

Figure 1.1 AORN Perioperative Patient Care Model. Reprinted with permission from Guidelines for Perioperative Practice. Copyright © 2018, AORN, Inc, 2170 S. Parker Road, Suite 400, Denver, CO 80231. All rights reserved.

3) Results of laboratory tests, diagnostic procedures, baseline vital signs, pain level as appropriate, and scans are reviewed.

4) Medical conditions or comorbidities should be reviewed. The patient should discuss medications and dietary herbal supplements taken routinely and on the day of surgery. Examples include diabetes, hypertension, hypercholesterolemia, or cardiac medications. Recreational drugs, medical marijuana, and alcohol should be discussed. Allergies and sensitivities should be identified and documented. The nurse should ask about known reactions when exposed to allergen.

5) Previous surgical history, prosthetics, and implants should be identified and documented. Body piercings should be removed.

6) The nurse should determine the patient's NPO status and last oral intake of food or liquids. The patient may need to void. This may be delayed if a Foley catheter will be used during the surgical procedure.

    b. Psychologic of data

    1) The nurse should objectively observe the patient's affect and behavior during the physiologic assessment process. Does the patient respond appropriately to questions? Does the patient indicate understanding of the discussion with the nurse? Is the patient confused?

    2) Does the patient speak clearly with understanding of the language? Is an interpreter needed?

    3) Is the patient crying or demonstrating restless behavior? Is the patient restrained or violent?

    4) Is the patient conscious? Is the patient's mental status caused by presurgical sedation? Does the patient have a cognitive disorder, such as autism or developmental challenge?

    c. Psychosocial data

    1) Include appropriate family and significant others as appropriate during the assessment process. Is the patient alone without a support person? Is the patient a minor who requires a parent's or guardian's consent? Is the patient a documented emancipated minor and capable to give consent?

    2) Is the patient a member of a religious community and requesting any procedure follow a religious belief system? Has the patient signed any documents concerning refusal of blood products? (Example: Jehovah's Witness)

    d. Document and transmit assessment data in an appropriate manner

    1) The assessment findings are documented in a manner that can be retrieved by the perioperative care team. Abbreviations should be avoided. Documentation can be in writing or through electronic computer software. This documentation is part of the surgical safety

checklist referred to as the Universal Protocol established by WHO.

  2) The pertinent assessment findings are communicated verbally to appropriate caregivers, such as the surgeon, anesthesia provider, circulating nurse, scrub person, and RN first assistant.

2. Nursing diagnosis

  a. Nursing diagnosis differs from medical diagnosis. Nursing diagnosis is developed by analysis of the assessment data and identification of actual and potential problems or conditions affected by the care planned and rendered by professional RNs. This analysis provides information necessary for planning nursing interventions. Medical diagnosis is determined using data derived from the physician's physical examination, laboratory tests, scans, pathology reports, and other diagnostic methods.

  b. Nursing diagnosis is expressed in professional nursing terms as described by **NANDA-I** (North American Nursing Diagnosis Association International, Inc.; http://www.nanda.org). NANDA-I nursing diagnosis strives to standardize nursing terminology to reflect evidence-based practice in professional nursing. As of 2018, there are 235 accepted nursing diagnoses described by NANDA-I. Interventions and outcomes are defined following NANDA-I nursing diagnoses through the following methods:

    1) Diagnostic information collected

    2) Characteristic signs and symptoms exhibited by the patient

    3) Associated factors that cause the diagnosis

    4) Risks that expose the patient to develop the diagnosis

  c. NANDA-I is categorized by 13 domains wherein the individual nursing diagnoses are classified.

    1) Domain 1: Health promotion

    2) Domain 2: Nutrition

    3) Domain 3: Elimination and exchange

    4) Domain 4: Activity and rest

    5) Domain 5: Perception and cognition

    6) Domain 6: Self-perception

    7) Domain 7: Role relationships

    8) Domain 8: Sexuality

    9) Domain 9: Coping and stress behavior

    10) Domain 10: Life principles

    11) Domain 11: Safety and protection

    12) Domain 12: Comfort

    13) Domain 13: Growth and development

  d. AORN developed the **PNDS** (Perioperative Nursing Data Set). The PNDS is the only accepted standardized documentation language that is specific to perioperative nursing.

    The PNDS is the first specialty language accepted by ANA's Committee on Nursing Practice Information (1999) that defines and describes patient care throughout the perioperative care experience. The PNDS system allows for standardized capture of nursing care data for use in consistent research.

    1) The primary PNDS is associated with risks to the patients.

    2) The purpose of the PNDS is to prevent a potential problem.

    3) The PNDS helps to align appropriate and effective care.

    4) The PNDS helps the nurse select patient-specific nursing diagnoses and establish the necessary interventions as the plan of care and identification of desired outcomes.

  e. Domains of the PNDS are specific to the perioperative nursing process. Four domains are used to frame the nursing diagnoses derived from the PNDS (Table 1.2).

    1) Domain 1: (D1) Safety

    2) Domain 2: (D2) Physiologic responses

    3) Domain 3-A: (D3-A) Behavioral responses: Knowledge

    Domain 3-B: (D3-B) Behavioral responses: Rights/Ethics

    4) Domain 4: (D4) Health system

  f. Domains of the PNDS mesh with the nursing process and in documentation systems use a letter system in combination with the domain that corresponds to the nursing standardized language.

    1) **A**—Assessment

    2) **Im**—Implementation

    3) **E**—Evaluation

    4) **O**—Outcome

3. Outcome identification

  a. Each of the 39 identified perioperative patient care outcomes integrates the standardized PNDS with the corresponding NANDA-I nursing diagnosis.

  b. Outcomes should be realistic, attainable, and appropriately aligned with prescribed medical treatment.

  c. Each PNDS perioperative outcome is numbered and prefixed with "O" in documentation.

  d. The patient's desired outcomes are taken into consideration during development of the plan of care.

4. Planning

  a. Patient care is planned using perioperative nursing diagnoses and identification of the desired outcomes. The PNDS identifies 93 nursing diagnoses specific to perioperative nursing.

  b. Patients are included in planning as much as possible.

5. Implementation

  a. The PNDS identifies 151 standardized perioperative interventions that are documented with a prefix "Im."

  b. Implementation of the plan of care is documented as appropriate according to facility policy.

6. Evaluation

  a. The PNDS is used to document the evaluation of the 39 standardized outcomes using the prefix "E."

TABLE 1.2   Perioperative Nursing Data Set Example in Action

Perioperative Nursing Data Set Domain	Perioperative Nursing Diagnosis	Plan	Implementation	Outcome and Evaluation
D1: Safety	Assessment reveals risk for limited mobility in moving from transport cart to operating bed	Arrange appropriate personnel and transfer device for patient moving between surfaces. Moving procedure is explained to patient.	Four personnel use a Davis roller with draw sheet to move patient between surfaces. Person at the head of bed will call the count for synchronized move.	Patient is safely moved between surfaces without injury. Skin and musculoskeletal indicators are without redness, abrasions, or pain.
D2: Physiologic responses	Assessment reveals risk for injury associated with positioning for the planned procedure	Appropriate positioning devices and pressure reduction padding will be used.	Patient is positioned using correct positioning devices and gel padding for skin pressure reduction in areas in contact with operating bed and positioning devices.	Patient positioning is performed using the correct devices and pressure reduction padding. Patient's skin and musculoskeletal integrity are intact at the conclusion of the planned surgical procedure.
D3-A: Behavioral responses of patient and family: Knowledge	Assessment reveals risk for elevated anxiety about the planned procedure	Demonstrate calm and assuring behavior during identification process with patient. Observe for site marking and patient affirmation of the planned procedure.	Speak softly in terms the patient understands and listen for verbal clues of patient understanding. Reinforce affirmation by having patient repeat knowledge of procedure and possibly point to the planned surgical site.	Patient will state the planned procedure and indicate location of the surgical site correctly. Surgical site is appropriately marked per facility policy.
D3-B: Behavioral responses of patient and family: Rights/Ethics	Assessment reveals risk for patient privacy and confidentiality	Identification of the patient and the planned procedure will be performed in a private setting, and patient records will be accessed only by authorized personnel.	Personnel conduct patient interview and assessment in a private setting observing the Health Insurance Portability and Accountability Act guidelines concerning patient confidentiality.	Patient confidentiality is maintained, and the patient demonstrates that privacy has been preserved.
D4: Health system wherein the patient care is delivered	Documentation of patient care is provided through approved institutional means	Perioperative nurses will gather and document data during patient care.	Standardized perioperative nursing language is used to document patient care.	Documentation of patient care is retrievable, analyzed for use in research, and provides data for improving patient care.

b. The AORN Perioperative Patient-Focused Model describes and reflects the entire nursing process in outcome terms identified by the nursing diagnoses. The perioperative outcomes are documented with the prefix "O."

Incorporating the PNDS

1. Documenting nursing care using the PNDS is accomplished using an alpha-numeric system.
2. Each nursing diagnosis has a numeric code that is prefaced by the appropriate domain indicator. The

PNDS has four domains extracted from the NANDA-I domains that are applicable to perioperative patient care.

3. Using the PNDS is not mandatory; however, several OR software programs have incorporated the PNDS into the patient care documentation systems for consistent collection of data.

4. AORN SYNTEGRITY™ is a system for perioperative scheduling and documentation that can be incorporated into the patient's electronic health record. The PNDS is built into the OR documentation platform.

Legal and Ethical Issues
Reviewing Legal and Ethical Concerns

1. **Doctrines of legal responsibility.** Professional practice requires caregivers to provide safety for all patients. Inherent in these doctrines is a code of practice parameters that also provides liability protection for personnel. One main point to remember is that each person on the team carries responsibility for his or her own individual or independent actions. There is no such thing as practicing under some else's license. A nurse cannot lose licensure over another person's actions. Only the board of nursing can sanction or remove a nurse's license, not a court of law.

   a. *Borrowed servant rule (aka Captain of the ship).* Previously, the *surgeon* was considered to have complete control over the OR. The surgeon only has control specific tasks related to direct supervision. Examples include first assisting activities such as suturing.

   Each person working in the OR is an employee of the facility and is expected to perform his or her duties according to facility policy, such as counting or preparing medications for the field.

   b. *Doctrine of the reasonable man.* A court of law measures the activities of the OR personnel against local and national standards in the case of an untoward event involving a patient. The question that surfaces is did the caregiver provide the same care that another caregiver with the same educational preparation would give under the same or similar circumstances. Any deviation that causes harm can be considered unreasonable.

   c. *Doctrine of* res ipsa loquitur. The Latin meaning is "The thing speaks for itself." An untoward event in the OR can be very obvious to a court of law. An example is a retained sponge or other foreign object in the patient's body after invasive surgery. The prevailing thought is if not for the surgical procedure, the object would not be inside the patient. Any unintentional retained foreign object can pose a hazard to the health of the patient.

   d. *Doctrine of respondeat superior.* An employer can be held liable for the actions of employees. If an employee takes an independent action that harms the patient, the employer can be held liable because they have the employee on the payroll and carry the responsibility for activities on the premises.

   e. *Doctrine of corporate negligence.* The employer is not only responsible for the actions of employees, but also for the policies and procedures set forth for the tasks to be accomplished. Competency monitoring, and performance evaluations of the staff and physicians are the responsibility of the employer. Only qualified personnel are acceptable for employment.

   f. *Extension doctrine.* The surgeon may perform procedures only for which the patient has given informed consent. During a planned surgical procedure, the surgeon may encounter additional pathology associated with the organ in question. An example might be a vascular attachment between adjacent organs or tumor extension. The surgeon might have to extend the procedure for the benefit of the patient's life and health. This does not include taking a nonproblematic organ like the appendix during a hysterectomy.

   g. *Assault and battery.* Assault is the threat to cause harm and battery is actually touching and harming the patient without obtaining consent. An incidental organ removal, such as an appendectomy *without* consent during cholecystectomy is an example of battery.

   h. *Invasion of privacy.* Patient records are private and my not be viewed by nonauthorized personnel. Other identifying information, such as a visible name on the surgical schedule that could be seen by passing patients and visitors is a breach of privacy. Many facilities have employees sign confidentiality agreements and have harsh penalties for looking at random patient records out of curiosity.

   i. *Abandonment.* Responsibility for patient care requires the caregiver to remain with the patient. Leaving the patient without handing over care to another caregiver of the same status is abandonment.

2. **General consent** to treat is signed when the patient enters the hospital or treatment center and agrees to be admitted. An admitting clerk processes the patient's insurance information. The existence of any advance directives, such as durable power of attorney or living will, will be assessed and documented per federal regulations. An ID bracelet may be applied in this process. The patient signs a form that allows the staff and physicians to render routine daily care. This is not informed consent but becomes part of the permanent medical record.

   a. Emergency patients may bypass the admissions process and go directly to a treatment area. Treatment may be given without consent while trying to find family or significant other, who can give consent. This applies also to someone incapacitated by drugs or alcohol and unconscious patients.

b. Minors require a parent or guardian's consent. In an emergency situation treatment can be given until consent can be obtained.

c. A minor who is a parent may give consent for his or her own child.

d. A minor is considered emancipated if living on his or her own and separate from a parent. These minors may have court documents to validate an emancipated status and may provide consent for self.

e. Illiterate patients can sign with an "X" or other distinct mark. The nurse can indicate "patient's mark" next to the patient's mark. Since illiterate patients cannot read or write, acknowledgement of understand should be obtained at the time of marking the form.

3. **Informed consent** is a process conducted between the patient (or parent/guardian) and the treating physician, anesthesia provider, or interventionalist who will be performing a specific procedure. The process includes a description of the intended procedure complete with the benefits and risks. Alternative treatment options are discussed.

   The informed consent process is documented in the patient's medical record and is sometimes confirmed by signatures of the patient, physician, and a witness. If a form is used, it becomes part of the permanent medical record. The perioperative nurse may serve as a signing witness; however, he or she is not responsible for obtaining informed consent from the patient.

4. **Advance directives and DNR** (do not resuscitate) are part of the Patient Self-Determination Act passed by Congress in 1991. This law enables the patient to participate in decision making before a procedure is performed. This process allows the patient to refuse treatment as well. Some facilities use "Allow Natural Death" (**AND**) in place of DNR terminology.

a. Advance directives include a durable power of attorney for decision making if the patient becomes incapacitated. This includes personal daily affairs and health conditions.

b. A living will enables the patient to predetermine a course of treatment and refusal of treatment if the situation becomes hopeless.

c. DNR or AND orders are issued to prevent resuscitation efforts if death is eminent and expected in select cases. On the patient care division, the DNR orders are upheld if the patient shows signs of death, such as cardiac and respiratory arrest. DNR orders may be suspended if the patient is in the OR for supportive treatment, such as placement of a central venous access.

   Vital support will be applied during the OR period, and DNR will be reinstated when the patient returns to the care division. In rare circumstances the DNR order may remain in effect during the OR procedure; however, the DNR is well documented and follows facility policies and patient and/or family wishes regarding this special situation.

Universal Protocol

Universal Protocol is a standardized method of providing safe care for every patient by specific activities geared toward reducing the risk for patient harm. TJC developed the concept of the prevention of "wrong person-wrong site-wrong procedure" scenario. The process of Universal Protocol was designed by Dr. Atul Gawande for WHO and intended for global use regardless of the size or technologic level of the perioperative environment. AORN also created a comprehensive surgical checklist to guide the process. The patient should participate as much as possible (Fig. 1.2).

1. Clear definitions of times associated with entering and leaving perioperative care include:

a. *Sign in:* arrival in room before anesthesia is administered

b. *Time out:* before skin incision when the team confirms the Universal Protocol

c. *Anesthesia start time:* anesthesia provider begins to render care

d. *Incision time:* the surgeon begins the surgical procedure

e. *Closure time:* surgeon completes the surgical procedure and the dressing is applied

f. *Anesthesia stop time:* anesthesia provider stops administering anesthesia

g. *Sign out:* patient leaves the room; document when handover of care to next appropriate caregiver (perianesthesia nurse) takes place

h. Other intraoperative times that should be documented include the following:

   1) *Tourniquet time:* Document pressure and when inflated/deflated.

   2) *Cross clamp time:* Document when clamp is applied to vessel and removed.

   3) *Pump times:* Document when the heart is stopped and the patient is on and off cardiopulmonary bypass.

   4) *Cardiopulmonary resuscitation times (CPR):* If the patient suffers a cardiac arrest during the surgical procedure and resuscitation is performed, all measures are recorded with times.

   5) *Staff relief times:* At breaks or change of shift the names and times are documented.

   6) *Vital signs:* When the perioperative nurse is monitoring a patient the vital signs and times should be recorded. Any concerns should be reported to the surgeon.

2. Use a minimum of two methods for confirming identification of the patient. Common methods include asking the patient's name and birth date. Cognitive assessment can include asking the patient to spell the last name.

COMPREHENSIVE SURGICAL CHECKLIST

Blue = World Health Organization (WHO)   Green = The Joint Commission - Universal Protocol (JC) 2013 National Patient Safety Goals   Orange = JC and WHO

PREPROCEDURE CHECK-IN	SIGN-IN	TIME-OUT	SIGN-OUT
In Holding Area	Before Induction of Anesthesia	Before Skin Incision	Before the Patient Leaves the OR
Patient/patient representative actively confirms with Registered Nurse (RN):	RN and anesthesia care provider confirm:	Initiated by designated team member All other activities to be suspended (unless a life-threatening emergency)	RN confirms:
Identity □ Yes Procedure and procedure site □ Yes Consent(s) □ Yes Site marked □ Yes □ N/A by person performing the procedure **RN confirms presence of:** History and physical □ Yes Preanesthesia assessment □ Yes Diagnostic and radiologic test results □ Yes □ N/A Blood products □ Yes □ N/A Any special equipment, devices, implants □ Yes □ N/A Include in Preprocedure check-in as per institutional custom: Beta blocker medication given (SCIP) □ Yes □N/A Venous thromboembolism prophylaxis ordered (SCIP) □ Yes □N/A Normothermia measures (SCIP) □Yes □N/A	Confirmation of: identity, procedure, procedure site and consent(s) □ Yes Site marked □ Yes □ N/A by person performing the procedure Patient allergies Yes N/A Difficult airway or aspiration risk? □ No □ Yes (preparation confirmed) Risk of blood loss (greater than 500 mL) □ Yes □ N/A # of units available _____ Anesthesia safety check completed □ Yes **Briefing:** All members of the team have discussed care plan and addressed concerns □ Yes	Introduction of team members □ Yes **All:** Confirmation of the following: identity, procedure, incision site, consent(s) □ Yes Site is marked and visible □ Yes □ N/A Relevant images properly labeled and displayed □ Yes □ N/A Any equipment concerns? **Anticipated Critical Events Surgeon:** States the following: □ Critical or nonroutine steps □ Case duration □ Anticipated blood loss **Anesthesia provider:** □ Antibiotic prophylaxis within 1 hour before incision □ Yes □N/A □ Additional concerns? **Scrub and circulating nurse:** □ Sterilization indicators have been confirmed □ Additional concerns?	Name of operative procedure Completion of sponge, sharp, and instrument counts □ Yes □ N/A Specimens identified and labeled □ Yes □ N/A Any equipment problems to be addressed? □ Yes □ N/A **To all team members:** What are the key concerns for recovery and management of this patient? _____ _____ _____ _____ _____ _____ _____ June 2013 AORN

The Joint Commission does not stipulate which team member initiates any section of the checklist except for site marking. The Joint Commission also does not stipulate where these activities occur. See the Universal Protocol for details on the Joint Commission requirements.

Figure 1.2 AORN comprehensive surgical checklist. (Reprinted with permission from AORN.org. Copyright © 2013, AORN, Inc. All rights reserved.)

3. Identify the surgical site and the intended surgical procedure. This information must coordinate with the patient's informed consent process. The person performing the procedure should be the person who does the marking. The patient (or guardian) must demonstrate understanding of the procedure and confirmation of the surgical site.

4. The team must verbalize and affirm the patient's identity, planned procedure, health conditions, such as allergies/sensitivities, presence of necessary equipment, positioning supplies, implants, and devices. Some facilities document the confirmation of sterilization indicators.

5. Validate scans, x-rays, laboratory results, blood products, preoperative medications, and any special circumstances (e.g., blood refusal).

6. Ensure documentation of accountability for counting sponges, sharps, and instruments before procedure, at the closure of a cavity within a cavity, and after the procedure.

7. All specimens must be correctly documented and labeled, and sent to the appropriate processing department. Specimens are verified at the sign-out period.

National Patient Safety Goals (NPSG)

NPSG were developed by TJC to improve healthcare safety for the consumer. Each year the patient safety goals are reviewed, evaluated, and updated. Patient safety goals are measured against the standards of care set by TJC. The full explanations and descriptions of the NPSGs can be found online at https://www.jointcommission.org.

1. Identify patients correctly using at least two methods.
2. Improve staff communication.
3. Use medications safely, especially labeling in surgery.
4. Use alarms on all equipment safely.
5. Prevent infection.
6. Identify patient safety risks.
7. Prevent mistakes in surgery.

Sentinel Event

A sentinel event is an unanticipated occurrence that causes serious harm or death to a patient. The harm can be physiologic or psychological for the patient. A sentinel event is investigated through a process known as *root cause analysis*. This investigative method reviews actions for variations in a retrospective approach to identify the cause. TJC requires that a root cause analysis be performed within 45 days and an action plan for correction established.

Professional accountability requires voluntary reporting of sentinel events and the root cause analysis to determine how the event led to an unfavorable outcome for the patient. The Patient Safety and Quality Improvement Act of 2005 encourages facilities to report incidents on a voluntary basis for more accurate documentation.

1. Reportable events
   a. Any unintentional retained object from a surgical procedure
   b. Incompatible blood transfusion that causes a hemolytic reaction
   c. Patient fall that causes death or permanent injury
   d. Medication error that causes death or permanent injury
   e. Patient suicide within 72 hours of hospitalization
   f. Patient elopement that results in suicide, homicide, or permanent injury
   g. Patient abduction from the healthcare facility
   h. Rape of a patient
   i. Infant discharged to wrong family
   j. Surgery on the wrong patient or wrong body part
   k. Maternal death during delivery
   l. Intrapartum neonate (over 2500 g) death unrelated to congenital defect
   m. Assault or other crime resulting in patient death or permanent injury
2. Nonreportable events
   a. Any "near miss"—a possible situation that resolves without meeting the criteria for a reportable sentinel event
   b. Full resolution of limb or body function within 2 weeks of the initial injury
   c. Medication error that does not result in permanent injury or death of the patient
   d. Unsuccessful suicide attempt by the patient
   e. Death or permanent injury after patient leaves against medical advice
   f. Sentinel event that has not affected the patient
   g. Hemolytic reaction with no lasting clinical effects
   h. Retained foreign object with no loss of function

Never Events

Never events are defined by CMS as preventable situations that cause harm to patients, extending length of stay and requiring additional treatments. CMS created a list of nonreimbursable care associated with patient events caused by caregiver error and injury during the care period.

1. Blood incompatibility
2. Poor control of blood glucose
3. Air embolus
4. Urinary tract infection associated with catheterization
5. Postoperative deep vein thrombosis or pulmonary embolus after hip or knee replacement
6. Fall or other trauma during care
7. Additional procedure for removal of retained foreign object in surgery
8. Pressure injury
9. Postoperative infection after orthopedic or bariatric surgery
10. Postoperative infection after coronary artery bypass surgery
11. Blood-borne infection from intravascular catheter

Professional perioperative nursing encompasses patient care, professional behaviors, and knowledge of how standards and guidelines are determined by professional and governmental organizations.

Taking the CNOR examination is a statement of proficiency, knowledge, and competence. The CNOR credential is recognized as a statement of professionalism and dedication to safe and efficient perioperative patient care.

LEARNING ACTIVITIES

1. **INSTRUCTIONS:** Complete the crossword puzzle. Use the clues to help identify the words.

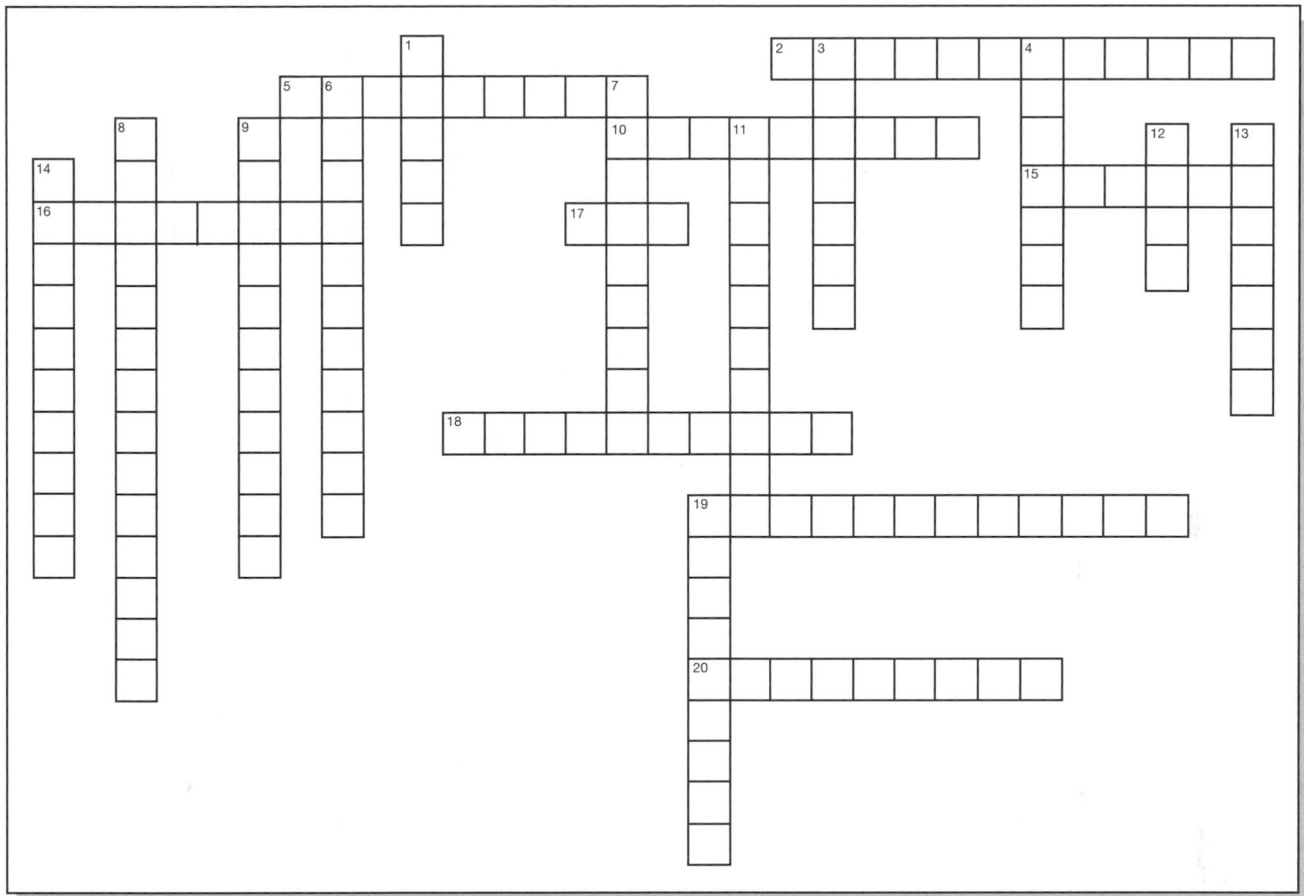

ACROSS

2. Leaving the patient unattended
5. Patient older than 65 years
10. Assessment data gathered by observing the patient
15. Process of reconciling items used during a surgical procedure
16. Tissue sample sent to pathology
17. Terminally ill patient requests no intervention
18. Assessment data gathered by listening to the patient
19. Patient care delivered by the nurse
20. Recorded treatment and validation of care throughout the perioperative care period

DOWN

1. Underage patient
3. Actually harming a patient
4. The end result of nursing intervention
6. Young patient who is responsible for self
7. Assessment of the patient's understanding
8. Use two forms of these data to confirm who the patient is
9. Patient has more than one active disease
11. Review and assessment of patient's outcome
12. Specialized perioperative nursing language
13. The threat to cause harm
14. Observational summation of the patient's condition
19. Microbial invasion that causes patient harm

II. **INSTRUCTIONS:** Complete the crossword puzzle. Use the clues to help identify the words.

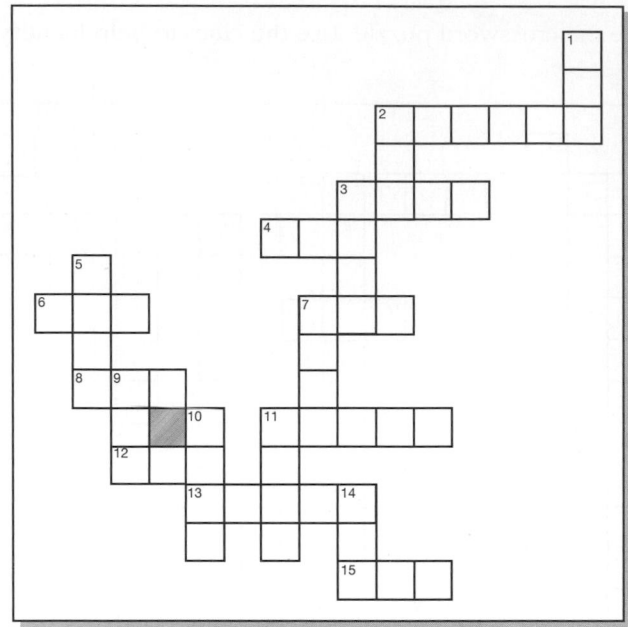

ACROSS

2. National Board of Surgical Technology and Surgical Assisting
3. Agency for Healthcare Research and Quality

4. World Health Organization
6. US Environmental Protection Agency
7. American Nurses Association

8. Competency and Credentialing Institute
11. National Institute for Occupational Safety and Health

12. Centers for Medicare and Medicaid Services
13. Healthcare Insurance Portability and Accountability Act
15. The Joint Commission

DOWN

1. US Food and Drug Administration
2. National Institutes of Health
3. Association of peri-Operative Registered Nurses

5. Association for Professionals in Infection Control and Epidemiology
7. Association for the Advancement of

Medical Instrumentation
9. Centers for Disease Control and Prevention

10. Occupational Safety and Health Administration
11. National Fire Protection Agency
14. Association of Surgical Technologists

III. **INSTRUCTIONS:** Complete the crossword puzzle. Use the clues to help identify the words.

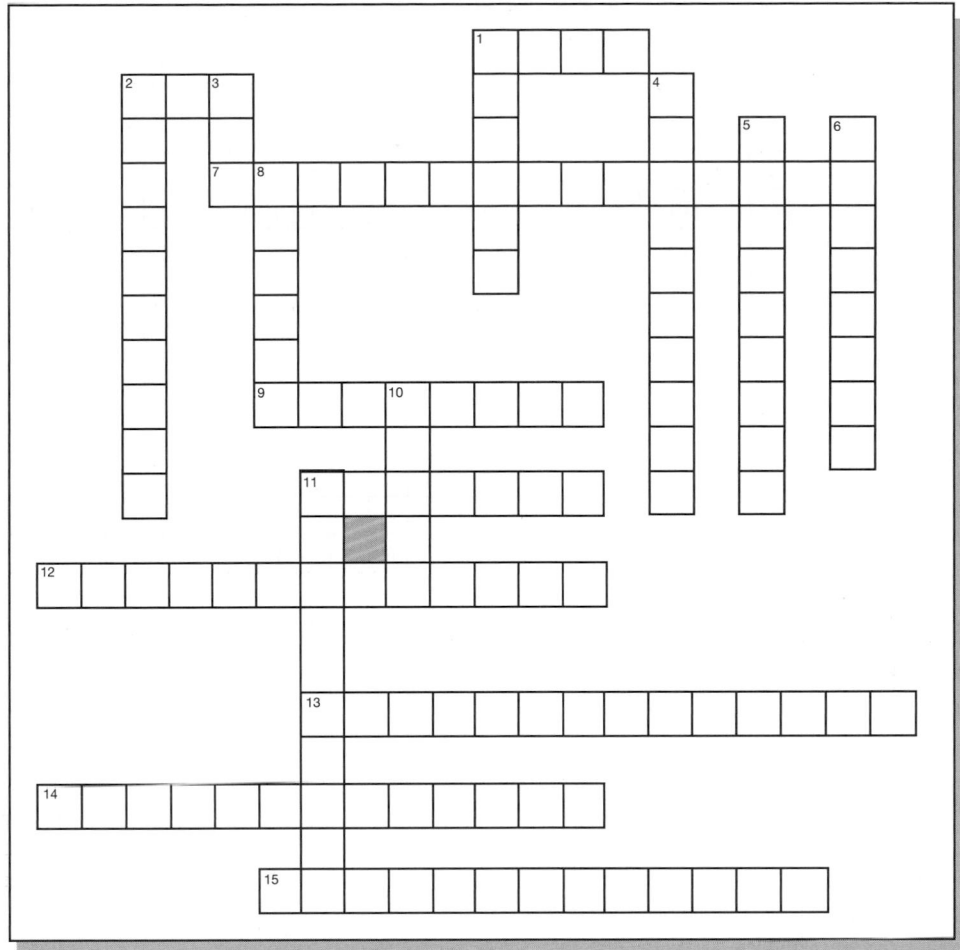

ACROSS

1. Accepted professional language of perioperative nursing
2. Allow natural death
7. Continued maintenance of a credential
9. Professional practice principle
11. Permission for an action
12. Recorded permanent citation
13. Enacting part of a plan
14. Record of activities
15. Credential earned by validation of professional knowledge and skill

DOWN

1. Facility-defined course of action
2. Evaluation of patient data
3. Do not resuscitate
4. Appraisal of an action
5. Legal accountability for actions
6. Self-designed cue for remembering
8. Practice principles of integrity
10. Source of the nursing diagnosis
11. Inherent belief of morals

LEARNING ACTIVITIES ANSWERS

I.

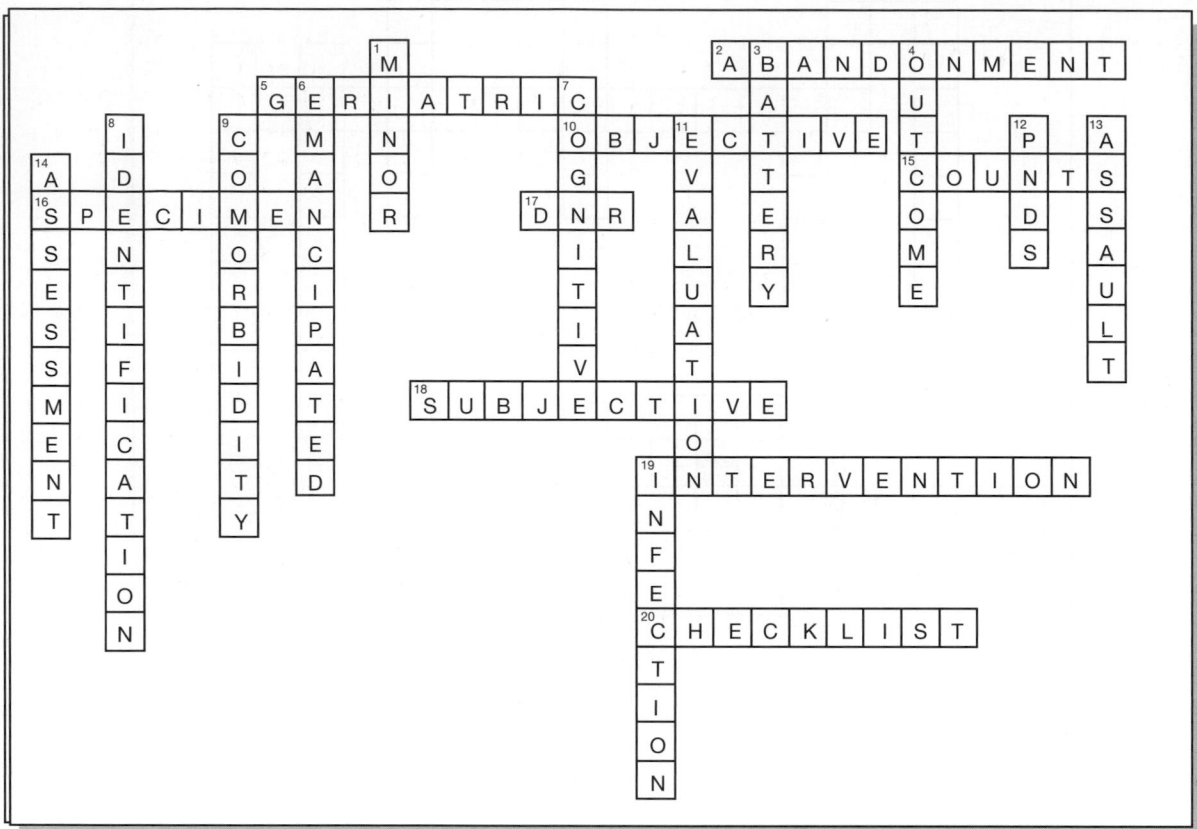

II.

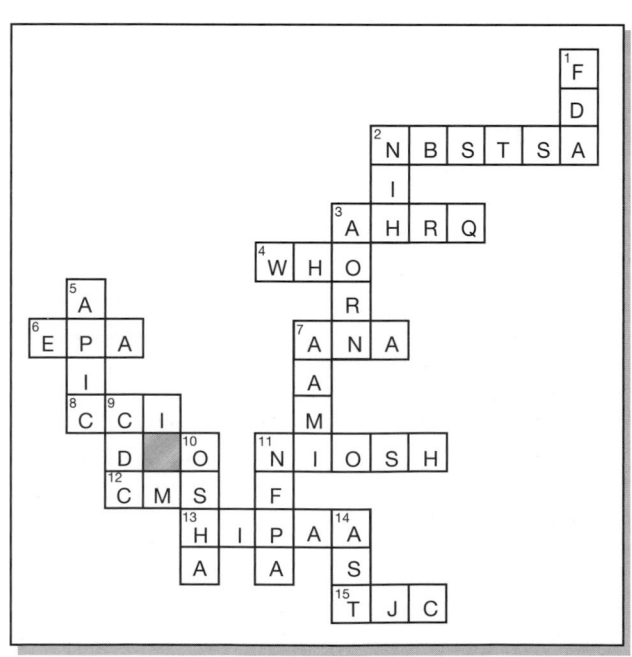

III.

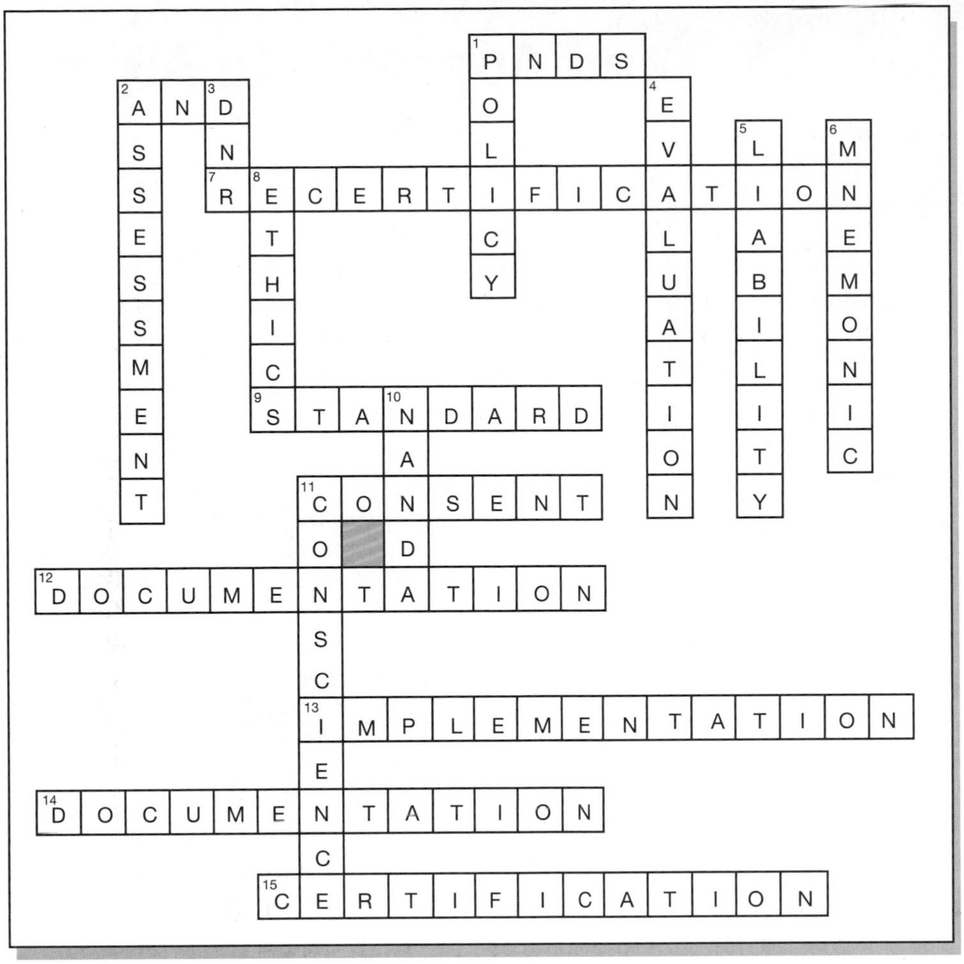
1 PNDS
1 POLICY
2 AND
2 ASSESSMENT
3 DN
4 EVALUATION
5 LIABILITY
6 MNEMONIC
7 RECERTIFICATION
8 ETHIC
9 STANDARD
10 NANDA
11 CONSENT
11 CONSCIENCE
12 DOCUMENTATION
13 IMPLEMENTATION
14 DOCUMENTATION
15 CERTIFICATION

Hand Hygiene and Appropriate Attire

The type of hand hygiene differs according to the task or technique being performed. Current recommended practices can be found in AORN's *Guidelines for Perioperative Practice.*

Hand hygiene is the first line of defense against the spread of microorganisms. The WHO set forth a campaign to make hand hygiene a priority among healthcare workers to prevent the spread of healthcare-associated infections and surgical-site infections (SSIs).

Hand hygiene performed at the correct time is effective in preventing the spread of infectious microorganisms. Gloves do not take the place of hand hygiene. Gloves are not 100% impervious.

Hand Hygiene

Hand hygiene can be broken down into three categories: handwashing, surgical hand scrub (mechanical/chemical), and hand antiseptic rubs.

1. When should hand hygiene be performed?
   a. Before and after patient contact
   b. After touching patient surroundings
   c. Before and after wearing gloves
   d. Before and after eating
   e. Before and after using the restroom
   f. When hands come in contact with blood or bodily fluids
   g. Before performing aseptic or sterile procedures
   h. If hands are visibly dirty
   i. If exposure to endospore-forming bacteria such as *Clostridium difficile*
   j. Before handling medication
2. **Handwashing** is performed using soap and water. Handwashing stations should be used for handwashing only. Other activities such as cleaning instruments may contaminate the sink and can spread microorganisms by splashing or aerosolization.

   Handwashing stations with no-touch controls reduce cross contamination by avoiding touching sink handles. Paper towel dispensers should be located next to the sink to prevent dripping. AORN's guidelines for handwashing include:
   a. Remove all jewelry on hands and wrists.
   b. Wet hands with water. Water temperature is not a factor in microbial removal (facility water temperature ranges between 70°F and 80°F). Hot water can cause dermatitis.

   c. Apply soap to cover all surfaces of the hands and wrists. Rub hands together vigorously for at least 15 seconds.
   d. Rinse thoroughly.
   e. Dry hands completely with a disposable paper towel. Turn water off with the paper towel.
   f. Facility-approved hand lotion is acceptable after handwashing to prevent skin dermatitis if not immediately applying gloves. Some hand lotions can cause degradation of the glove material.
3. **Hand hygiene** with an alcohol-based rub is permitted in the healthcare setting when hands are free from visible soil or potential exposure. Alcohol-based dispensers should be located at the point of use and must be in compliance with government regulations because they contain flammable alcohol.
   a. Education for using alcohol-based hand rubs should be product specific, including the amount of product, how to correctly cover all hand surfaces, and drying instructions. Place instructions with demonstration application next to the dispenser if possible.
   b. When applied, do not wave hands and arms to hasten the drying process. This creates air currents and disperses skin cells and microorganisms.
4. **Surgical scrubbing.** Surgical hand hygiene or scrubbing is the process to remove as many microorganisms from the skin as possible. The scrub person must wear proper attire for the restricted area, including close-fitting scrub suit (or top tucked in), head cover that encloses all hair, mask, and appropriate eyewear.

   Surgical hand hygiene can be done with a brush (mechanical) and antiseptic solution (chemical) or brushless hand rub (chemical). Brush method of scrubbing is recommended for the first scrub of the day. The surgical scrub is not a sterile procedure because skin and tap water are not sterile.
   a. Natural fingernails should be kept short, no longer than 2 mm. Nails should be in good condition without cracks. Do not wear artificial nails or extenders; they can harbor bacteria. Follow facility policy on the use of nail polish and gel polishes.
   b. Remove all jewelry from hands, wrists, and neck. Remove large or dangling earrings. Some facilities

allow small stud earrings if they are covered. Read the facility policy concerning jewelry.

c. The scrub room is adjacent to the operating room (OR) and contains deep sinks with automatic faucet sensors, and foot or knee devices to control the water. The deep sinks prevent the back splash of water onto the person scrubbing. Antiseptic hand soaps should be near the sinks.

5. **Surgical scrub with a brush.** A timed or counted brushstroke method can be used. Ten strokes per surface, or 2 to 5 minutes total. Follow manufacturer's recommendations (Fig. 2.1).

   a. Open sterile gown and gloves on separate surface away from main sterile field in the OR.

   b. Select the proper antiseptic (some facilities have all-in-one single-use brush/sponge, nail pick, and soap). Open brush package, then turn on water to a comfortable temperature.

   c. Clean underneath fingernails with the nail pick under running water. Dispose of the nail pick in the appropriate trash container. If a package contains only a brush/sponge, 2 to 3 mL of antiseptic soap is needed. Be sure to brush under nails and rinse. Use the brush with caution, it can damage skin.

   d. Keep both hands elevated above elbows; begin scrubbing with the thumb, then move to each finger, covering all four sides of the fingers.

   e. Scrub the back of the hand and palm (order does not matter), from small finger to thumb. Scrub in one direction over the wrists and up each arm in a circular motion, finishing 2 inches above the elbow. Do not scrub back down over the arms.

   f. Discard scrub sponge/brush in the appropriate trash container.

   g. Hold hands higher than the elbows, away from clothing. Rinse each hand thoroughly starting with the fingers in one direction.

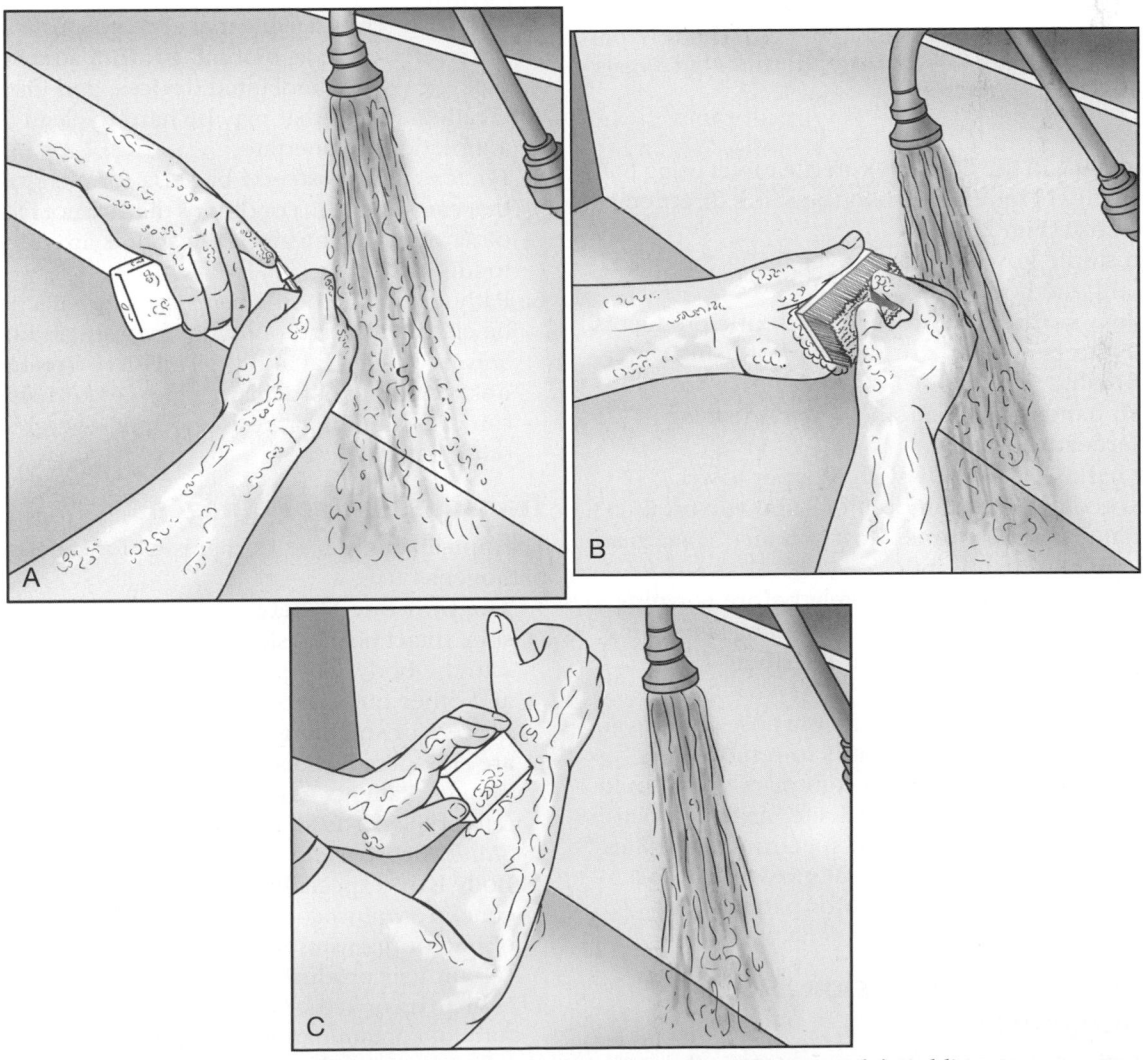

Figure 2.1 Traditional surgical scrub technique. (A) Cleaning nails with plastic nail cleaner. (B) Holding sponge perpendicular to nails facilitates thorough scrubbing of underside of nails. (C) Holding sponge lengthwise along arm covers maximum area with each stroke. (From Rothrock, J. [2019]. *Alexander's care of the patient in surgery* [16th ed.]. St. Louis, MO: Elsevier.)

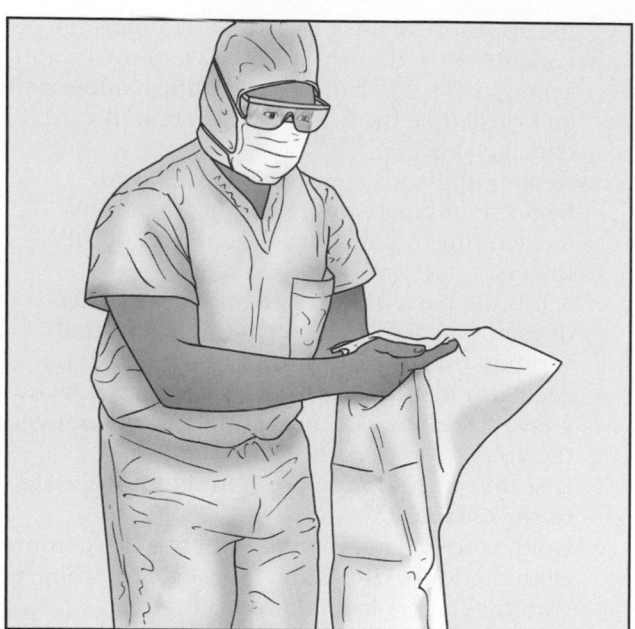

Figure 2.2 Drying hands and forearms. Fingers and hand are dried thoroughly before forearm is dried. Extending arms reduces the possibility of contaminating towel or hands. (From Rothrock, J. [2019]. *Alexander's care of the patient in surgery* [16th ed.]. St. Louis, MO: Elsevier.)

h. Dry hands in the OR with a sterile towel using half of the towel for each arm in the same direction as the scrub (Fig. 2.2).

i. Don sterile gown. Apply gloves using the closed gloving method.

6. **Brushless surgical hand rub.** Antiseptic product is rubbed into hands and arms instead of using water and a brush.

a. Wash hands with soap and water, cleaning underneath the nails.

b. Dry hands thoroughly with a paper towel.

c. Use recommended amount of hand rub product on hands and forearms. Most products contain an alcohol-based antiseptic.

d. Let the product dry completely before gowning and gloving. Do not wave arms to hasten drying. This causes air currents that distribute microorganisms.

7. **Antimicrobial skin agents.** The purpose of using an antiseptic skin cleansing agent is to remove any visible soil, lotions, or skin slough or oils that could contaminate a patient's surgical site. Antimicrobial cleansers are fast-acting, broad-spectrum antiseptics, effective in preventing microbial growth. These antiseptic agents are also used for patient skin preparation (Table 2.1).

Preventing the Transmission of Microorganisms

People or direct person-to-person contact is the main source of transmission of microorganisms in the health-care setting. Microorganisms flourish in warm, moist areas. Therefore, the body becomes a great host for resident and pathologic microorganisms to harbor. Microorganisms do not cause infection in a healthy person unless they are transferred to an area where they can reproduce. Microorganisms can be spread by contact, droplets, air, blood, and bodily fluids.

1. **Resident florae** live in certain body parts, where they assist in the function of that system. Resident florae can be found in mucus of the respiratory tract, sweat glands, gastrointestinal and reproductive tracts, and oil glands. If the microorganisms or florae multiply to an unsafe number, they can spread or migrate and become a pathogen.

2. **Pathogens** can cause infection to the host or be spread to a patient, causing an SSI. Other microorganisms such as fungi, yeast, and bacteria can live in the air and surrounding objects.

3. Each individual microorganism has its own environment in which it can flourish. For example, aerobic microorganisms need oxygen to survive. In contrast, anaerobic microorganisms can live without oxygen.

4. Bacteria secrete a slime that accumulates and forms a layer referred to as biofilm. **Biofilm** attaches to biologic tissue, implanted devices, and instruments, creating a layer that may be hard to clean or for antibiotics to penetrate.

5. *Bacillus* and *Clostridia* bacteria form endospores that can survive in conditions that are not favorable to other microorganisms. Endospores are difficult to kill.

6. Pathogenic microorganisms causing infections must be cultured to find out what they are and the mechanism for survival and transmission. Treating an unknown microorganism with standard antibiotics can cause antibiotic resistance and overgrowth of other natural flora.

Transmission of Pathogens

The human body has mechanisms for defense against pathogens.

1. **The first line of defense** is the largest organ, the skin. Intact healthy skin acts as a barrier against entry into the body. The skin of OR staff, patients, and other caregivers can cause infection by the process of shedding dead skin cells. Personnel who are shedders can disperse up to 30,000 particles per minute. Patients who are shedders have a higher rate of SSIs. The sloughed cells often contain *Staphylococcus aureus*.

2. Body hair, especially hair on top of the head, may contain *Staphylococcus*. Hair follicles harbor all kinds of microorganisms that may remain with the use of certain hair products.

3. Human error in the OR is also an outside (exogenous) form of contamination; that is, not following through with aseptic and sterile techniques. Accidental contamination of a sterile field can happen (e.g., hair on the field or a hole in a glove).

TABLE 2.1   Antimicrobial Agents for Surgical Scrubbing and Surgical-Site Preparation

Antimicrobial Agent	Action	Use and Special Considerations
Povidone iodine Concentrations: 10%, 7.5%, 2%, 0.5%	Intermediate acting/oxidation bacteria and viruses Minimal residual effect Inactivated by blood and mucus	External use Use with caution: iodine sensitivity Can be irritating to the skin Do not preheat; this can cause evaporation and concentration of the solution
Chlorhexidine gluconate Concentration: 4%	Intermediate acting/disrupts cell membrane of microorganism Excellent residual effect Effective for up to 6 hours	External use only Can cause permanent eye and internal ear damage Avoid use on mucous membranes
Chlorhexidine gluconate in alcohol base Concentration: 0.5%	Excellent residual effect	External use only Can cause permanent eye and internal ear damage Avoid use on mucous membranes
Ethyl or isopropyl alcohol (70%, 91.3%)	Very rapid acting Denatures protein and breaks down microbial cell wall Effective against gram-positive and gram-negative No residual effect	External use only Do not use in eyes, mouth, or mucous membranes Has a drying effect Flammable
Triclosan 1%	Intermediate acting Interruption of hormonal activity in the microbial cell Effective against gram-positive and gram-negative bacteria, tuberculosis	FDA has banned this antiseptic from all consumer and hand hygiene products Found in urine and breast milk (https://federalregister.gov/d/2017-27317) (Final rule effective 12/20/2018)
Chloroxylenol, parachlorometaxylenol 1%–3.75%	Effective against gram-positive and gram-negative bacteria Bactericidal Disrupts the cell wall	External use only Do not use in eyes Can cause skin irritation

FDA, US Food and Drug Administration.

4. Methicillin-resistant *S. aureus* is a common bacterium resistant to many antibiotics. It is spread by direct contact from contaminated wounds or hands (https://www.cdc.gov).

Transmission by Droplet

Droplet transmission can occur when microorganisms travel by respiratory droplets. Respiratory droplet particles are larger than 5 mm and can travel up to 3 feet. Coughing, sneezing, exhaling, and talking can aerosolize microorganisms into the air, which land on surfaces capable of causing infection.

Droplets spread diseases, including common cold, chicken pox, influenza, bacterial meningitis, strep throat, tuberculosis (TB), whooping cough, measles, mumps, diphtheria, and pertussis.

Some personnel harbor microorganisms such as *Staphylococcus* and *Streptococcus* that do not affect their own bodies. These individuals are referred to as **carriers**. Carriers spread these microorganisms by sneezing, talking, and coughing without showing signs of overt disease. Carriers can be identified through a nasopharyngeal culture. If the culture comes back positive, the individual can be treated with an antimicrobial nasal spray or cream to decolonize the nose. Droplet precautions include:

1. Masks must cover the nose and mouth and be worn within 3 feet of patient care.
2. Masks should be removed by the ties. Masks are never worn around the neck.
3. Keep talking to a minimum.
4. People with respiratory infections should not be permitted in restricted areas.
5. Patients with respiratory infections should also wear a mask.
6. Certain respiratory infections such as TB may require a special mask (N95) for patients and staff.

Transmission by Airborne Particles

Fomites are items that are contaminated by microbiologic particles. Particles floating in the air can enter the surgical site, causing an SSI. Particulates from surfaces such as the floor, desks, tables, lights, surgical equipment, and instruments may be forced into the air, increasing the number of circulating microorganisms. Particles are generated from surgical plume and vaporization, and carried by forced air warmers. Movements of personnel in the OR stir up many particles, leading to SSIs. OR personnel can minimize the dispersal of airborne microbes by performing the following actions:

1. Damp dust all horizontal surfaces before the first procedure of the day.
2. Decrease surgical plume with suction evacuation devices.
3. Isolate the surgical site with barriers such as drape.
4. Keep traffic in and out of the room to a minimum.
5. Keep all OR doors closed to maintain HVAC (heating, ventilation, and air conditioning) positive pressure in the room.

Transmission by Blood and Bodily Fluids

Some common diseases are spread by contact with bodily fluids, mucous membranes, or percutaneous injury with sharps. Proper personal protective equipment (PPE) and Standard Precautions must be strictly followed by OR personnel. Personnel are at risk for needlesticks, glove punctures, splashing of bodily fluids, saliva, secretions, and direct contact with blood (Table 2.2).

| TABLE 2.2 | Common Microorganisms in an Operating Room Environment |

Microorganism	Usual Environment	Mode of Transmission
Staphylococci	Skin, hair	Direct contact
	Upper respiratory tract	Airborne
Escherichia coli	Intestinal tract	Feces, urine
	Urinary tract	Direct contact
Streptococci	Oronasopharynx	Airborne
	Skin, perianal area	Direct contact
Mycobacterium tuberculosis	Respiratory tract	Airborne, droplet
	Urinary tract	Direct contact
Pseudomonas	Urinary tract	Direct contact
	Intestinal tract	Urine, feces
	Water	Water
Serratia marcescens	Urinary tract	Direct contact
	Respiratory tract	Water
Clostridium	Intestinal tract	Direct contact
Fungi	Dust, soil	Airborne
	Inanimate objects	Direct contact
Hepatitis virus	Blood	Bloodborne
	Body fluids	Direct contact

From Phillips, N. (2017). *Berry and Kohn's operating room technique* (13th ed.). St. Louis, MO: Elsevier.

What Can a Perioperative Nurse Do to Reduce the Transmission of Microorganisms?

1. Bathe daily with soap and water; shampoo hair.
2. Personnel who sweat excessively should bathe with an antibacterial soap, focusing on areas that contain sweat and oil glands (head, axillae, and genital area).
3. Wear clean, close-fitting OR scrub attire. Nonsterile team members wear long sleeves. Warm-up jackets should be fully closed at all times. Immediately change soiled scrub suits (including sweat).
4. Remove jewelry: rings, wrists, neck, hanging earrings, and facial piercings.
5. Cover hair (including facial hair) in the restricted areas. Bald heads shed dander.
6. Wash hands before entering the OR. Perform hand hygiene before and after donning gloves.
7. Cover any cuts or wounds on hands. Personnel with nonintact skin on the hands or arms should not scrub.
8. Wear gloves when handling bodily fluids and specimens.
9. Correct contamination errors immediately.
10. Wear mask correctly.

Transmission of Prion Disease

A **prion** (infectious protein particle that lacks nucleic acid) is a nonliving protein-based helical structure. Without DNA or RNA, they can mutate and form clumps of protein in the brain that look like holes in a sponge (spongiform). These nonliving proteins cannot be deactivated by heat, drying, freezing, most chemicals, and radiation.

There are two forms of prion disease, one affects humans and the other animals.

Human Form of Prion Disease

Transmissible spongiform encephalopathy (TSE) is rare family of prion diseases that cause fatal neurologic disorders. The human form is **Creutzfeldt-Jakob disease (CJD)**. It is a rare disease that becomes fatal. Findings include:

1. **Diagnosed** only by brain tissue biopsy.
2. **Sporadic manifestation:** Patient has no known risk factors, but it can be hereditary.
3. **Acquired by transmission:** It is introduced by contaminated blood, instruments, growth hormone, brain tissue, dural grafts, or consumption of infected cattle.
4. CJD usually presents in older people because of prolonged development periods. **New variant type CJD** can present in younger individuals. Symptoms include dementia, muscle spasms, and severe neurologic problems.

Animal Forms of Prion Disease

Animal forms of prion disease include **bovine spongiform encephalopathy (BSE)** in cattle (mad cow disease) and **scrapie** in sheep and goats.

Managing Surgical Procedures With Suspected Prion Contamination

1. Wear recommended PPE.
2. Remove all nonessential equipment from the room. Cover all noncritical work surfaces with disposable drapes (including floors).
3. Disposable patient drapes and instruments are recommended.
4. Clean environmental surfaces with 1:10 bleach solution for 15 minutes.
5. Do not flash instruments for use in other patients.
6. Avoid high-powered instruments such as drills to minimize the risk for aerosolization.
7. Notify surgical processing department and isolate soiled instruments. Keep the instruments moist. See Chapter 10 for more information about caring for prion-contaminated instruments.
8. Soak instruments in sodium hypochlorite 1:10 (NaClO bleach) or sodium hydroxide 40 g (NaOH Lye):1 L H_2O for 1 hour, then rinse well with water. The chemicals must be rinsed well or could create a noxious gas when processed in autoclave.
9. Process unwrapped in gravity displacement sterilizer (60 minutes at 272°F) or prevacuum sterilizer (18 minutes at 274°F). Isolate instrument set and do not use in patient care until biopsy results return as negative per facility policy and procedure (https://www.cjdfoundation.org).

Appropriate Attire and Personal Protective Equipment

Appropriate attire for the surgical suite provides a safe barrier from microorganisms to protect both the surgical team and the patient. OR surgical attire consists of close-fitting scrub suit, mask, head cover, and shoe covers if necessary.

Proper attire worn in specific zones has a purpose to prevent the contamination from outside sources to the patient. PPE (gowns, gloves, masks, eyewear, and shoe covers if necessary) worn by personnel protects them from blood, bodily fluids, and disease. Appropriate attire and PPE worn correctly reduces the risk for patient SSIs.

1. Proper attire worn in **specific zones** has shown a reduction of microorganisms on inanimate objects and the body. All personnel are responsible for the safety of their patients. By following facility dress code policies and procedures the reduction of microorganisms into the patient environment can be minimized. The unrestricted, semirestricted, and restricted areas have guidelines and policies for specific OR attire.
   a. The **unrestricted area** has no specific clothing requirements and includes street clothes. This area is of importance because it includes dressing rooms where street clothes are changed into OR attire. Outside clothing and personal items can harbor microorganisms and pet dander, which can easily be transferred to other surfaces. Considerations for the unrestricted area include:
      1) Personal hygiene should include daily bathing with an antimicrobial soap and application of deodorant (body odor is from the multiplication of microorganisms found in follicles and hair). Fingernails and hair should be clean and groomed (including facial hair and eyebrows). Makeup should be simple and not flake.
      2) Scrub attire should be changed in the designated location adjacent to the semirestricted area. Clean attire provided by the facility should be donned daily (no home-laundered scrubs). When donning scrub attire, avoid contact with contaminated areas such as the floor. Shoes should be clean and for the perioperative area only.
      3) Remove any jewelry that cannot be contained inside the scrub attire (rings, bracelets, and watches increase bacteria counts on skin).
      4) Identification badges should be secured where they are visible and cleaned often. Lanyards should not be worn.
      5) Personal items, such as purses, backpacks, cell phones, and tablets, should remain secure in the unrestricted area and not brought into the OR.
   b. The attire for the **semirestricted area** includes the basic scrub suit and hair (head) cover. The scrub suit and hair cover should be worn in the correct manner. Scrub suit and hair cover are not considered PPE. These items worn in the semirestricted area should follow the dress code for proper attire. Guidelines for the scrub suit include:
      1) All perioperative personnel (professional and nonprofessional) should don clean, hospital-laundered scrub attire daily. Select the correct size from approved scrub attire (loose scrub suits can disperse cells into the air or drag on the floor).
      2) If a two-piece suit is worn, the top should be tucked into the pants or fit closely to the body. Personal underclothing (T-shirts) not fully contained under the scrub suit should not be worn.
      3) Do not place clean scrub suits into personal lockers; they can become contaminated from personal items. Worn scrub suits or jackets placed into lockers can contaminate personal belongings.
      4) Soiled scrub suits should be changed immediately and placed directly into dirty laundry container (shower if necessary). Worn attire (single use or reusable) should remain at the facility and returned to the designated area for laundering.

5) Hair is considered a gross contaminate because it can harbor bacteria such as *S. aureus*. The purpose of covering the hair and head is to contain or minimize the shedding and dispersal of microbes. Bald heads can shed dander. The selection of a head cover, donning it correctly, and how to remove it can keep microorganisms to a minimum (Fig. 2.3).
   a) Don head cover before the scrub suit to prevent contamination from shedding. The head cover or hood should be clean and cover all hair, scalp, nape of the neck, and sideburns (beards should be fully covered).
   b) Do not comb or brush hair when wearing a scrub suit (dander and hair can contaminate the scrub suit).
   c) If a cloth cap is permitted, it should be made of tightly woven, low linting material and washed daily by an accredited laundry facility. For personnel wearing cloth caps, turbans, or head garments, a disposable bouffant style cap should cover the entire garment.
   d) Head cover should not be removed by personnel wearing scrub attire when leaving the perioperative area.
   e) Remove hair cover when changing into street clothes or going outside the building. Single-use head covings should be disposed of and not worn again.
c. Appropriate attire in the restricted area for nonscrubbed personnel includes the basic scrub suit, hair cover, long-sleeved jacket, and mask.
   1) Warm-up jackets
      a) Long-sleeve jackets should be fully closed, snapped, or buttoned. Covering arms with long sleeves helps to contain shedding from the skin.
      b) The jacket should fit close to the body to prevent it from bellowing or touching sterile areas.
      c) Long sleeves worn during the patient skin prep may contain the skin squames from dropping onto the patient.
      d) A clean jacket should be worn each day.
   2) Masks
      a) The mask should be donned correctly and not permitted to hang around the neck. Do not cross the strings when tying. Masks are part of PPE worn to protect the patient and environment (Fig. 2.4).
      b) A fresh mask should be donned for each new patient or procedure. Masks should cover the mouth and nose (prevent venting at the sides). Select a mask that is comfortable and fits the contours of the face. Masks must be worn when scrubbing or entering a room in process and not removed until after cleanup.
      c) Only one mask should be worn. Wearing two masks defeats the filtration of the product and causes side venting.
      d) Masks filter the droplets expelled from the mouth and nose during talking, breathing, coughing, and sneezing (talking should be limited). Masks filter 99% of particles larger than 5 mm.
      e) Change the mask immediately if it becomes wet or soiled. Remove a mask by the ties or strings. After removal of the mask, the wearer should perform hand hygiene.
      f) High-efficiency particulate air filtration masks (HEPA) are individually fitted for cases with smaller particles such as TB, viruses, laser, and electrosurgical unit plume.
      g) Patients with communicable respiratory disease or compromised immune conditions should wear a mask during transport until intubated during general anesthesia.

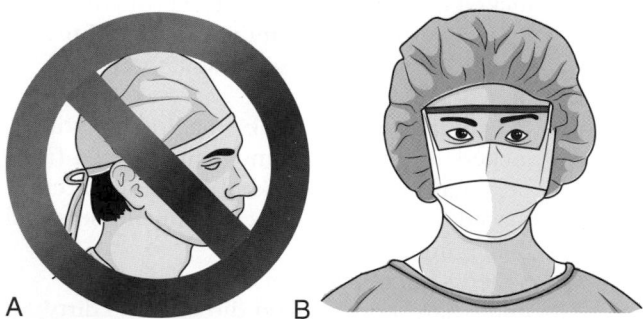

Figure 2.3 (A) Skull cap does not cover all hair and should not be worn. (B) All hair must be covered. (From Phillips, N. [2017]. *Berry and Kohn's operating room technique* [13th ed.]. St. Louis, MO: Elsevier.)

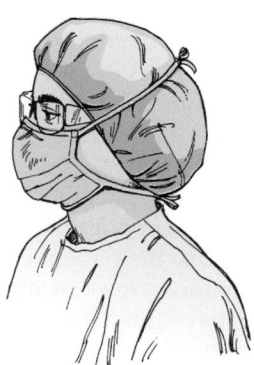

Figure 2.4 Mask covers nose and mouth and conforms to the facial contours. Upper strings are tied at back of head; lower strings are tied behind neck. (From Phillips, N. [2017]. *Berry and Kohn's operating room technique* [13th ed.]. St. Louis, MO: Elsevier.)

3) Eyewear
   a) All team members at the sterile field must wear appropriate protective eyewear. This is an Occupational Safety and Health Administration (OSHA) requirement. Eyewear is part of PPE and should be facility approved (Fig. 2.5).
   b) If personal glasses or spectacles are worn, they should be cleaned and covered by a face shield. Protective eyewear must have side shields.
   c) Eyewear is selected according to the procedure or risk for splashing or splatter. Different styles of eyewear are available from reusable, single-use, antifog, to eyewear attached to masks.
   d) Specific laser eyewear should be worn based on the laser type and optical density.
4) Footwear
   a) Shoes should be specific for the OR and left at the facility (no street shoes). Shoes should be comfortable nonporous material, such as leather or other synthetic material, and easily cleaned.
   b) OSHA requires that all shoes be enclosed with no open backs. They should have a low heel with nonskid bottoms. No sandals or clogs. Orthotic inserts are acceptable.

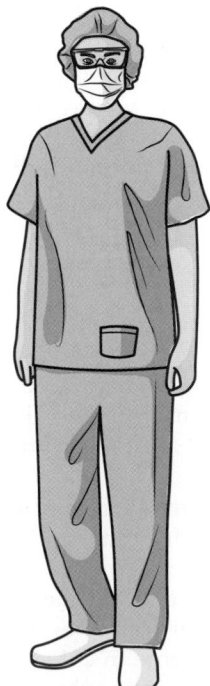

Figure 2.5 Appropriate attire for the restricted area in preparation for scrubbing. (From Phillips, N. [2017]. *Berry and Kohn's operating room technique* [13th ed.]. St. Louis, MO: Elsevier.)

c) Single-use shoe covers or high booties should be available as part of PPE if there is anticipation of contamination. Shoe covers must be removed before leaving the OR.
5) Gloves
   a) Gloves can be nonsterile or sterile. Both types of gloves are worn when handling any contaminated item, blood, or bodily fluid. Sterile and nonsterile single-use gloves are discarded immediately after use. Avoid touching clean items with contaminated gloves.
   b) Nonsterile gloves can be latex, vinyl, or nitrile. Latex is avoided if personnel or patient is sensitive to latex. Most facilities have converted to nonlatex products.
   c) Sterile gloves are worn by perioperative team members during patient prepping, catheterization, and other actions that require sterile handling.
   d) Sterile gloves are packaged individually for use in invasive procedures. Double gloving is recommended.
   e) Special gloves for radiation and chemical handling are available. Some facilities have sterile Kevlar woven gloves for orthopedic procedures where the glove could be easily torn handling heavy instrumentation.
   f) A colored indicator glove may be worn under a second pair of gloves if double gloving. The colored glove (usually green or blue) will show through if the outer glove is perforated during the surgical procedure.
6) Cover apparel
   a) OR attire should not be worn outside the OR suite. Cover apparel is a controversial topic. All perioperative personnel should follow their facility policy regarding attire outside the OR suite.
   b) If a scrub suit must be covered for a short time in an unrestricted area, a jacket, gown, or lab coat may be worn. The warm-up jacket should be changed into a clean one before reentry into the semirestricted or restricted areas. Lab coats should be clean and laundered daily.
   c) Scrub suits and lab coats should not be worn to outside offices and then back into the OR without changing into fresh OR attire.
   d) A clean one-piece jumpsuit, head cover, mask, and shoe covers may be worn in the semirestricted and restricted area for a short time for facility personnel or visitors.
   e) Scrub suits should not be worn outdoors. Street clothes should be worn when going outside.

Patient and Personnel Safety

Patient and personnel safety should be taken into consideration when selecting and laundering attire. Pathogenic organisms, including endospores, carried on attire can put personnel and patients at risk for infections. Personnel can spread these organisms by improper handling of scrub attire. The laundering and storage process of surgical attire should be taken into consideration.

1. Accredited laundry facilities must follow the Centers for Disease Control and Prevention standards and Healthcare Laundry Accreditation Council practices for selection and laundering of scrub attire. Accreditation requires industrial standards for water temperature, cleaning chemicals, mechanical action, textile recommendations, and cycle times.
   a. Facility scrub attire and hospital linen should be made from fabrics that are tightly woven and low linting.
   b. Woven textiles can be stain resistant or made of antimicrobial fabric requiring special laundering.
2. Attire can be processed in the healthcare facility or sent to an accredited location.
   a. Dirty linens and scrub suits are placed in waterproof containers that prevent the transmission of microorganisms while in motion. Soiled laundry is sorted and handled by personnel wearing PPE.
   b. Wash-water temperatures can reach up to 160°F, and monitored drying times can kill most bacteria.
3. Clean linens and attire should be stored in an area free from environmental contamination. All clean items should be covered or enclosed to remain clean.
   a. Storage parameters meet National Fire Protection Association (NFPA) requirements concerning fire safety.
   b. Storage should be 1 to 2 inches from the wall, 6 to 8 inches from the floor, and 12 to 18 inches from the ceiling.
4. **Home-laundered scrub attire**
   a. Scrub suits should never be taken home. Soiled scrub suits brought out of a facility can contaminate the outside environment, such as cars, personal items, and home.
   b. Home laundering is not monitored for temperature or microorganism destruction. The highest temperature of home laundry machines reaches approximately 110°F and is not consistent. Studies have shown that home laundering is not effective in removing microorganisms from attire.
   c. Bacteria and endospores can contaminate the home washing machine and be transferred to the personal clothing of the family.
   d. Microorganisms and pet dander can be brought back into the facility from home.

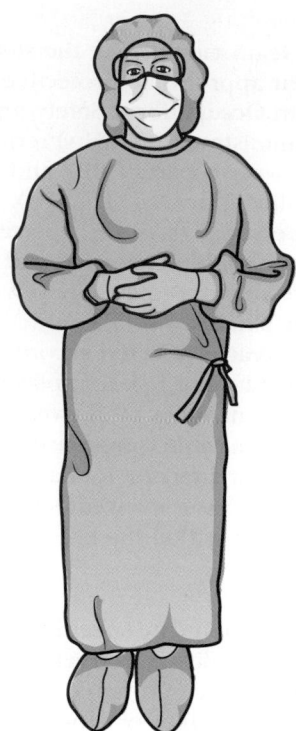

Figure 2.6 Appropriate attire for the sterile scrubbed person in the restricted area. The gown and gloves are worn over the scrub suit. Hair cover, protective eyewear, and mask are worn. (From Phillips, N. [2017]. *Berry and Kohn's operating room technique* [13th ed.]. St. Louis, MO: Elsevier.)

Sterile Attire

Sterile gowns and gloves are donned by the surgical team to permit them to enter the sterile field. The gowns and gloves are donned in a specific manner to maintain sterility. PPE for the scrubbed surgical team consists of mask, eyewear, sterile gowns and gloves, and shoe covers if needed.

The characteristics of gowns and how to don them, and the different types of gloving will be reviewed in this section (Fig. 2.6).

Sterile Gowns

1. The sterile gown is the impervious barrier that protects the wearer from blood, microorganisms, and fluids from the sterile field. The sterile gown also protects the patient from contaminants borne by the members of the team. Sterile gowns can be reusable or disposable.
2. Gowns should be made from a tightly woven material or paper to prevent fluid from soaking through the material. Gowns come in a variety of sizes, such as XS, S, M, L, XL, XXL, etc. Selection should permit full coverage. Sometimes sizes or materials are special ordered. Gowns come in colors that reduce glare. Blue or green are commonly used.
3. Gowns should be fire resistant and meet the standards of NFPA.

Principles of Gowning and Gloving

Self-gowning for a sterile procedure must always be done from a surface separate from the main sterile field. Gloving for a sterile procedure can be done in several ways depending on the circumstance. Methods of gloving include open gloving, closed gloving, open assisted gloving and closed assisted gloving.

1. **Self-gowning**
   a. A gown should be opened on a clean, separate surface away from the sterile field. The Mayo stand may be used. Never gown and glove from the sterile field.
   b. After scrubbing, the hands are dried using one end of the drying towel for each hand. Discard the towel. After drying hands, the gown is ready to be donned.
   c. Lift the gown up by the middle fold without touching the wrapper. The neck line should be facing up (Fig. 2.7).
   d. Grasp the inside of the gown near the armholes and let it unfold (Fig. 2.8).

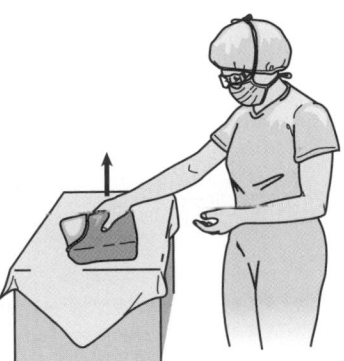

Figure 2.7 Scrub person, picking up gown below neck edge, lifts it directly upward and steps away to avoid touching the edge of the wrapper. Note that inside of wrapper covers the table. Gown is folded inside out. (From Phillips, N. [2017]. *Berry and Kohn's operating room technique* [13th ed.]. St. Louis, MO: Elsevier.)

   e. Extend the arms through the sleeves without letting the hands go through the cuffs. The circulating nurse stands behind the scrubbed person and pulls the gown over the shoulders by reaching inside the gown.
   f. The circulating nurse ties the inner waist tie and secures the neck closure. The rest of the tying-in happens after the scrubbed person dons sterile gloves. Disposable gowns have sterile wraparound ties in the front of the gown attached to a tag (Fig. 2.9).

2. **Closed gloving** is the method used when the hands are not exposed through the sleeves of the gown. This method is recommended when setting up a sterile field. Sterile gloves are opened on a separate surface before scrubbing (Fig. 2.10).
   a. The sterile gloves are applied without extending the hands through the cuffs. The cuffs are not impervious and are not considered sterile once the gloves are applied.
   b. Once the gloves are applied, the sterile wraparound tie tag (still attached to the long end of the tie) is passed to the circulating nurse, who passes behind the scrubbed person. The scrubbed person holds the short tie. The scrubbed person takes the long tie from the tag and turns to the left to close the gown. If the tie drops from the tag, it is considered contaminated. Both ends are secured in the back of the scrubbed person by the circulating nurse (Fig. 2.11).
   c. Never turn the back to the sterile field or tie the gown by placing the tag under something on the sterile field.
   d. If double gloving, the second outer pair of gloves can be applied after tying from the sterile field.

3. **Assisted gowning and gloving** other team members: The sterile scrubbed person assists the surgeon and other team members don their sterile gowns and gloves.
   a. Scrubbed members coming in with wet hands will be handed a clean towel from the scrubbed person

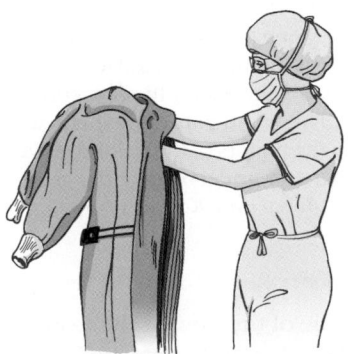

Figure 2.8 Scrub person, putting on gown, gently allows the gown to unfold away from body and then slips arms into sleeves without touching sterile outside of the gown with bare hands. (From Phillips, N. [2017]. *Berry and Kohn's operating room technique* [13th ed.]. St. Louis, MO: Elsevier.)

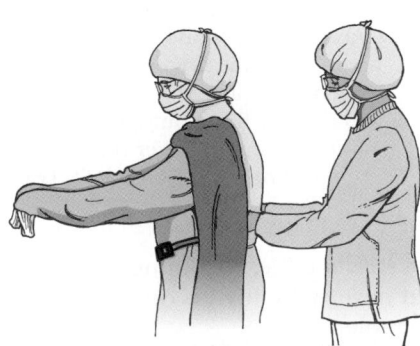

Figure 2.9 Circulating nurse ties the inner waist ties of the sterile gown. (From Phillips, N. [2017]. *Berry and Kohn's operating room technique* [13th ed.]. St. Louis, MO: Elsevier.)

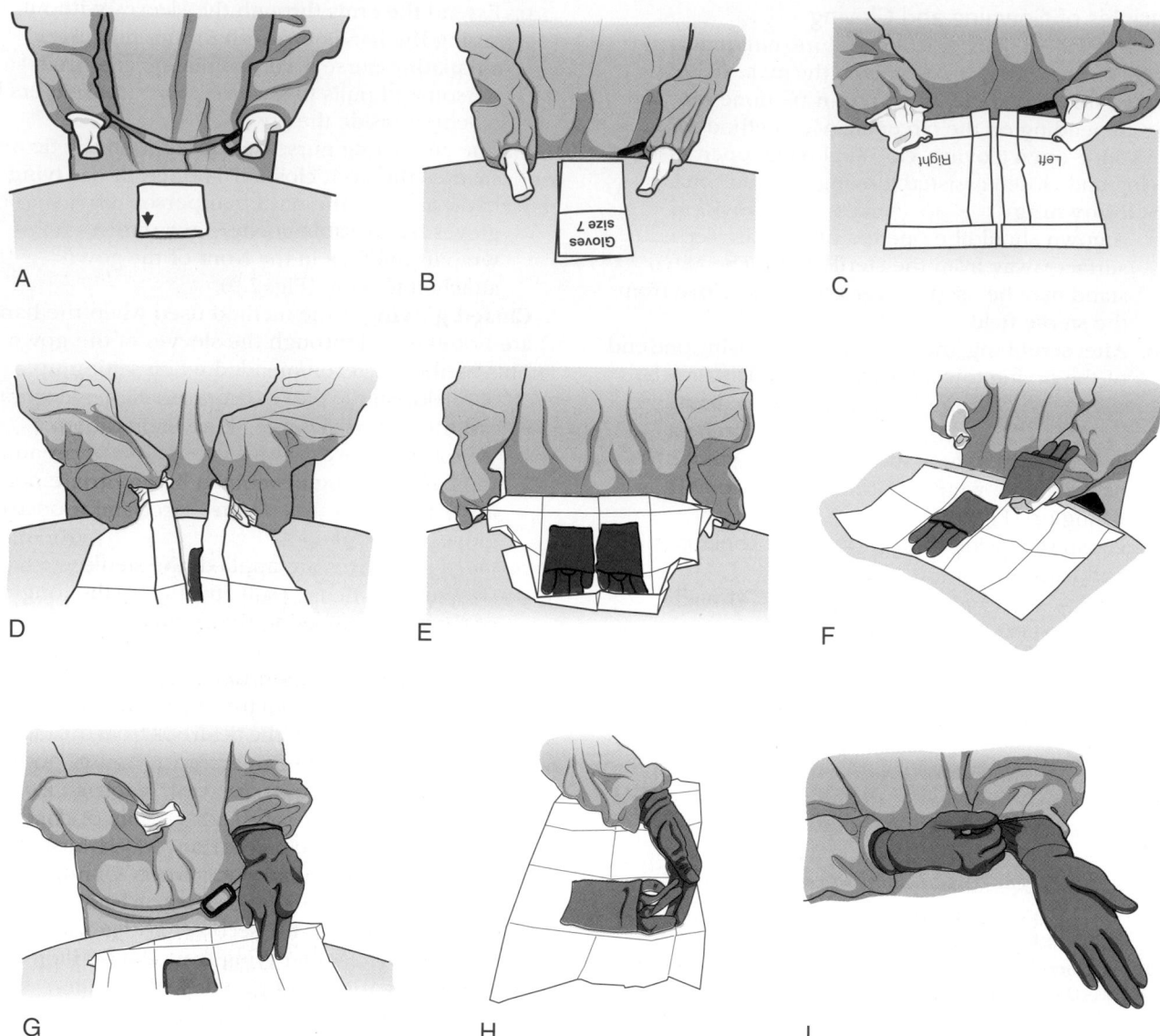

Figure 2.10 Closed gloving. The scrub person opens the glove wrapper on a sterile field with hands contained inside sleeves and cuffs. (A) Primary one-fourth fold. (B) Secondary half fold. (C) Open folded wrapper is labeled "right" and "left." Gently pull lower wrapper flap down. (D) Grasp inner corner of the wrapper and pull open. (E) Fold bottom flap under the glove wrapper to hold the paper open. (F) As the hands remain within the cuffs at all times, grasp the fingers of the first glove with the opposite cuffed hand and flip directly over onto the wrist of the supinated hand. (G) Grasp the upper and undersides of the glove cuff and begin to pull the glove over the first cuffed hand. Work the fingers into the glove until it is fully on the hand. The white part of the first cuff must be completely covered. (H) With the sterile gloved hand grasp the fingers of the second glove and directly flip it onto the second cuffed hand. (I) Grasp the upper and undersides of the glove and pull it up and over the second cuff. (From Phillips, N. [2017]. *Berry and Kohn's operating room technique* [13th ed.]. St. Louis, MO: Elsevier.)

from a sterile table. Incoming team members should never take towels or gowns from a sterile table.

b. The scrubbed person lifts a folded gown and unfolds it, holding it near the shoulders; the hands should be protected by forming a cuff on the sterile side of the gown. The team member should keep his or her arms stretched out and place them into the sleeves (Fig. 2.12).

c. If the hands are pushed all the way through the cuffs, the scrubbed person gloves the team member using the **open-assisted method**. Care is

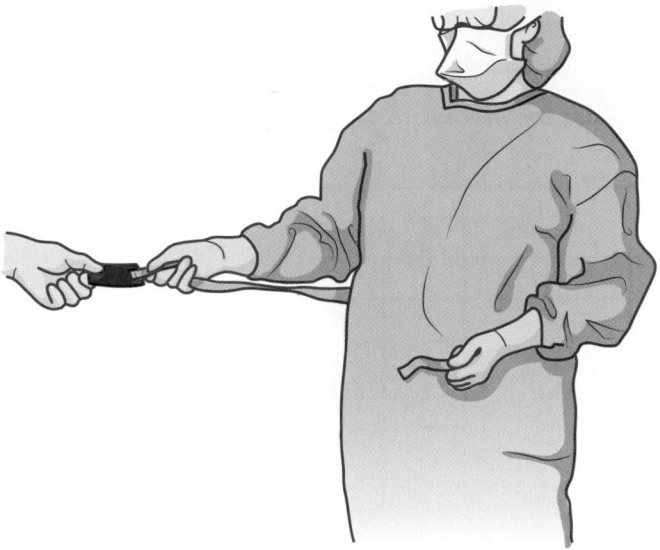

Figure 2.11 The circulating nurse ties in the sterile scrub person. The scrub person hands the paper tag that holds the long right wraparound tie to the circulating nurse while holding the shorter left tie. The nurse walks behind the scrub person and passes the long sterile tie to the scrub person without touching anything but the removable paper tag. (From Phillips, N. [2017]. *Berry and Kohn's operating room technique* [13th ed.]. St. Louis, MO: Elsevier.)

taken by the scrubbed person not to touch the bare hands of the person being gloved. Usually start with the right glove (Fig. 2.13).

   d. If the hands remain inside the cuffs, the gloving is referred to as **closed assisted gloving**. The gloves are applied to the cuff-covered hands. This is the preferred method.

4. **Open gloving** is the method used when the hands are exposed through the cuffs of the sterile gown.

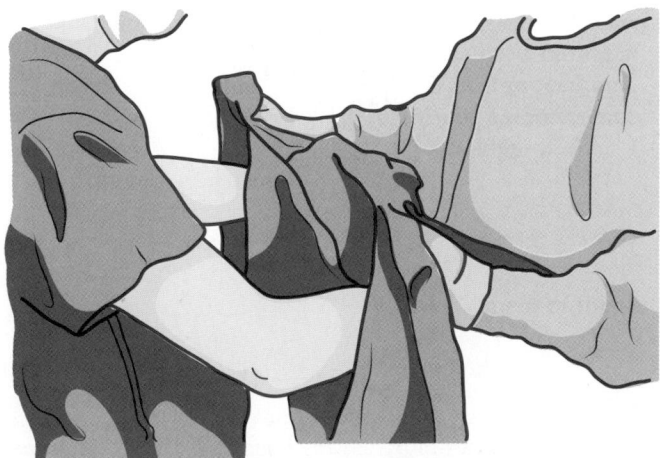

Figure 2.12 Gowning a team member by holding the armholes open and protecting hands inside sterile surface of the gown. (From Phillips, N. [2017]. *Berry and Kohn's operating room technique* [13th ed.]. St. Louis, MO: Elsevier.)

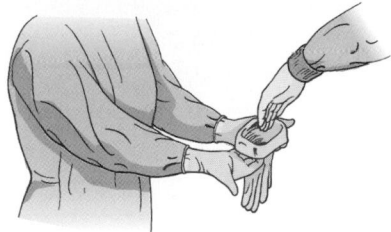

Figure 2.13 Gloving a team member by open-assisted method. (From Phillips, N. [2017]. *Berry and Kohn's operating room technique* [13th ed.]. St. Louis, MO: Elsevier.)

The gloves are open on a separate surface away from the sterile field. Care is taken not to touch the outer surface of the glove when picking up the first glove by the cuff (Fig. 2.14).

   a. Open gloving is recommended when changing a contaminated glove. Closed gloving should never be used to change contaminated gloves when wearing a gown. The cuffs are contaminated and will contaminate the sterile gloves as they are applied.

   b. The circulating nurse may grasp the contaminated glove near the palm wearing protective gloves and pull the glove off, causing it to turn inside out. A sterile team member should use the open-assisted method to reglove the hand.

   c. Open gloving is used by personnel performing the skin prep or placing a urinary catheter. No gown is worn. Hand hygiene is performed before and after wearing any gloves for any reason.

5. Removing or changing the contaminated gown and gloves: If the gown is contaminated during a surgical procedure, both the gown and gloves must be changed. If only the sleeve is contaminated, a sterile sleeve can be applied to cover the area without having to change gloves. When removing the gown and gloves for contamination or at the conclusion of the case, the gown is removed first, followed by the gloves. The following principles apply:

   a. The contaminated person must step away from the sterile field and untie the front tie of the gown. The circulating nurse opens the back of the neck and the back waist ties to decrease the risk of the team member reaching around and touching the scrub suit with bloody gloves.

   b. The contaminated person pulls the gown away from and rolls it away from the body (Fig. 2.15). Dispose of the rolled-up gown in the biohazard trash. Do not just rip the gown off from the body. Contaminants can be aerosolized or be deposited on the scrub suit.

   c. The gloves are removed one by one. (A) The first glove is grasped and removed without touching

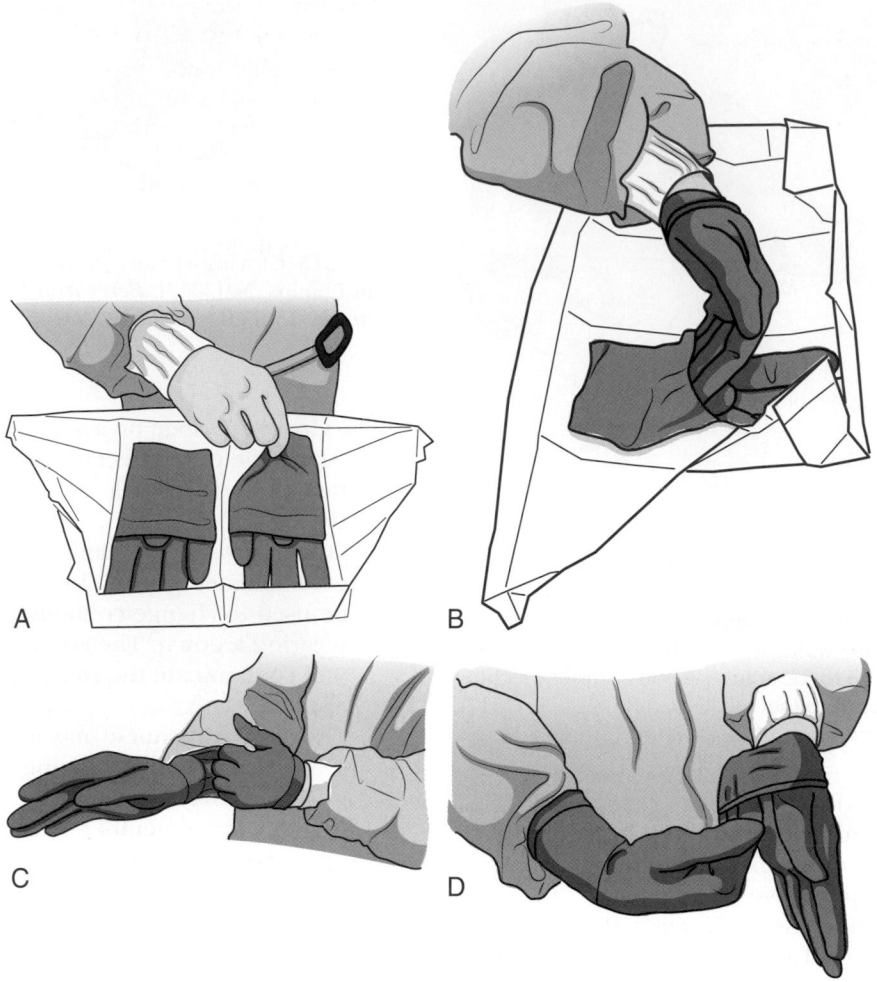

Figure 2.14 Open gloving. (A) The wrapper is opened without touching the inner surface. The first inner glove cuff is grasped without touching the sterile surface and slid over the first hand. The first cuff remains folded. (B) The first gloved hand is slid into the second cuff on the sterile surface. (C) The second glove is applied all the way up and over the knitted cuff. (D) The first cuff is now pulled over the knitted cuff. (From Phillips, N. [2017]. *Berry and Kohn's operating room technique* [13th ed.]. St. Louis, MO: Elsevier.)

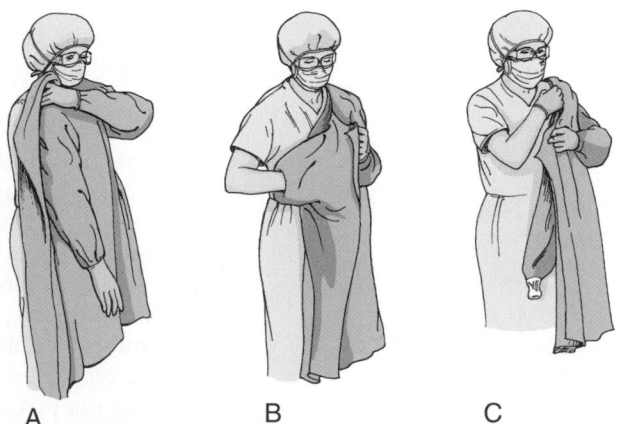

Figure 2.15 Sequence of scrub person removing soiled gown at end of surgical procedure. The gown is removed before the gloves. Clean arms and scrub suit are protected from contamination outside of gown. Do not reach behind the gown to untie the back strings. Have someone untie the back. (A) With gloves on, grasp the front shoulder of gown and pull forward. (B) In pulling gown off arms, make sure that gown sleeve is turned inside out to prevent contamination of scrub attire. (C) The other shoulder is grasped with the other hand, and the gown is removed entirely by pulling it off inside out and rolling it away from body. (From Phillips, N. [2017]. *Berry and Kohn's operating room technique* [13th ed.]. St. Louis, MO: Elsevier.)

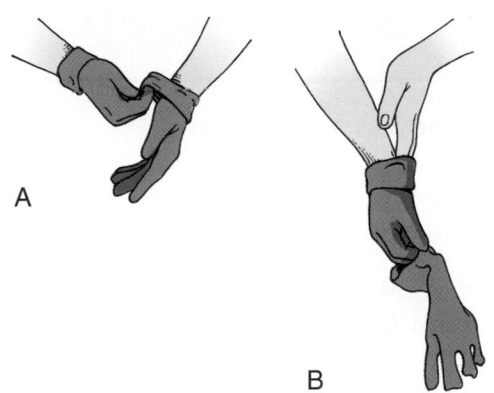

A

B

Figure 2.16 Scrub person removing the contaminated gloves. (From Phillips, N. [2017]. *Berry and Kohn's operating room technique* [13th ed.]. St. Louis, MO: Elsevier.)

the skin (glove to glove). (B) The second glove is removed by sliding the bare finger into the cuff against the skin of the gloved hand and rolling off without touching the bloody external surface (skin to skin) (Fig. 2.16).

d. Rescrubbing is not necessary if the gown and gloves are intact. A fresh sterile gown may be donned. A team member should use the assisted open gloving method to reapply the fresh sterile gloves. The closed method may be used if the hands have not passed through the cuffs during the regowning process.

e. If double-gloved and only the outer glove is contaminated, the circulating nurse can remove the outer glove and the team member can reapply a fresh outer glove.

f. At the conclusion of the case, hand hygiene is performed upon removing the contaminated gown and gloves.

Great importance is placed on hand hygiene and OR attire. The materials and composition are designed to enhance the protective qualities for the patient and perioperative personnel. Sterility and cleanliness cannot be compromised without placing the patient in a vulnerable position for a hospital-acquired infection. An emphasis is also placed on preventing infectious material from the facility entering the home environment. Attire in the OR is not about making a fashion statement, but about preventing the spread of infection.

LEARNING ACTIVITIES

INSTRUCTIONS: Complete the word search puzzle. Use the clues to help identify the words.

```
V W V M U Z D H L E D X H T O A F A N D S V X J H F O B S X
S N H M A X Y E F N G J J P N E P F P D G R Q T Y A Z N T G
O R I E R S K I O N M H C E O R X W E E Q O J N Q L O D A U
K H R G J W K I I A X V L R A O I O U D E P U V A I E D P S
Q R A T W M R V O H I Q O S P B G M G N J T J O T T G G H C
R S Y N W P O T L Z G S S O G I G S I J S D G A C E S G Y R
Z G V Y D L Z N M L F E E N O C A W T Q K C Z I N T C N L U
M I I Q G H E Z V P U Y D T Y Z D Y V V K I R B V D G D O B
N S J N A G Y X Z V W N G O X C Y Q Y I L T T U R K A K C S
Y N E P O W X G D Z H R L P Y Q L Q B O S U V Z B U K U O U
Q P M H Q U E K I N X F O E O Z V W S E B S M H D B S J C I
O U T F S H R I V E H O V R G A H O R Z R L T S H W E H C T
O A Q O U E S G N M N J I S K D R I E Y I E P A A N F D U I
P U I N I B P Q L U N E N O Z E M H V F J S I B T I C W S R
K J E R E F K A E O T F G N A E Y P O J M D Q F Y W H Z C Q
U T R Y W T R S R R V E L G S F D I N C B V O C O H N S O E
O A T X Y N X V J A Z E S I B O B G E B W M N B K D J U U N
C R L S L X T Z A V T A S I H D K H K M O S L N N K L E A N
C T Y T O M G S H P D E X O G E N O U S T E A I V O R L N B
E O V Z U Z Z A U P O O S I L I A R G O W N H M G X Y J I L
```

CLUES

1. Microorganisms that need oxygen to survive
2. Particles stirred up into the air from movement of OR personnel
3. Name of the slime secreted by bacteria that is difficult to remove from instrumentation
4. Which method of scrubbing should be the first of the day?
5. Individual who does not get sick from harboring microorganisms
6. Preferred method of gloving when setting up a sterile field
7. The surgical scrub should be completed 2 inches above this
8. Outside form of contamination
9. These should be worn when handling any contaminated item
10. This impervious barrier protects the wearer from blood and microorganisms at the sterile field
11. First line of defense in preventing the spread of microorganisms
12. This piece of PPE should be worn within 3 feet of patient care as part of droplet precautions
13. Preferred method of gloving when changing a contaminated glove
14. Can cause infection to the host or spread to a patient
15. Main source of transmission of microorganisms
16. Infectious protein particle that lacks nucleic acid; difficult to deactivate
17. Attire not considered PPE
18. This area requires a basic scrub suit and head cover
19. Self-gowning and gloving should be done from a(n) _____ surface
20. Hair is a gross contaminate and can harbor which type of bacteria?
21. These members should wear a warm-up jacket or long sleeves during a case

LEARNING ACTIVITIES ANSWERS

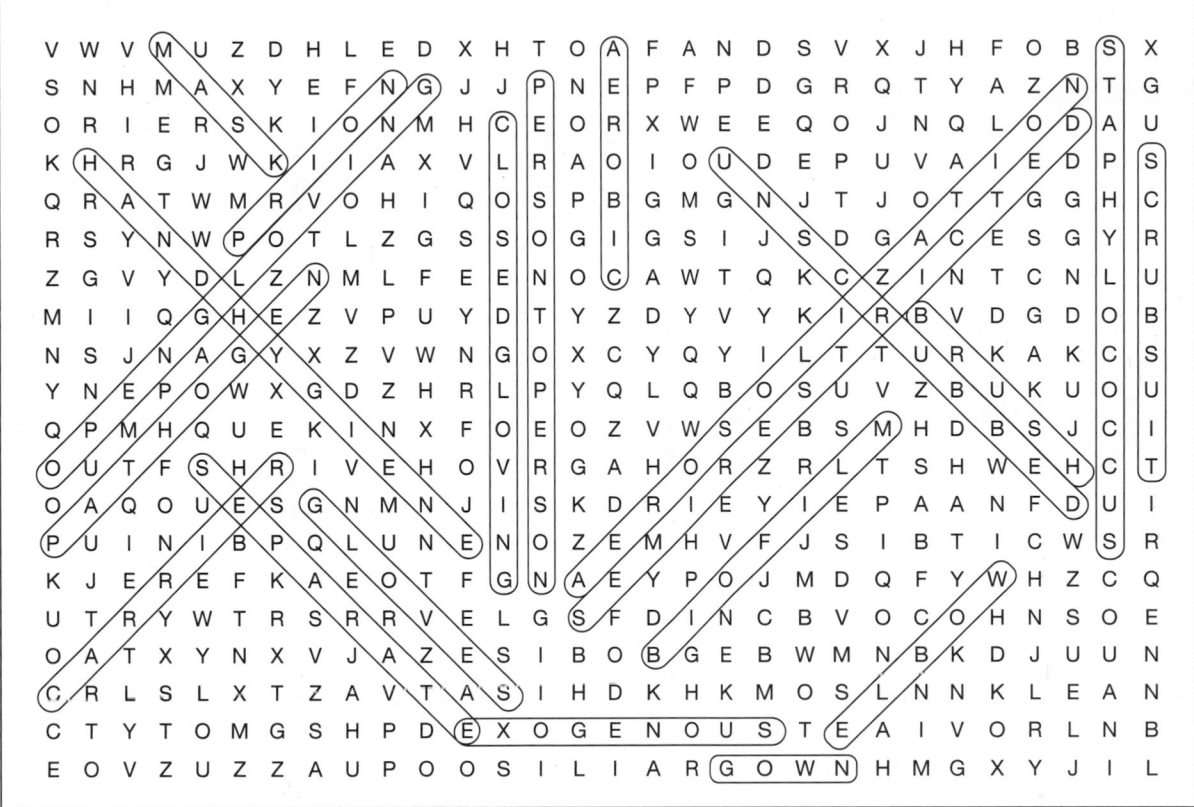

1. Aerobic
2. Aerosolization
3. Biofilm
4. Brush
5. Carrier
6. Closed gloving
7. Elbow
8. Exogenous
9. Gloves
10. Gown
11. Hand hygiene
12. Mask
13. Open gloving
14. Pathogen
15. Person to person
16. Prion
17. Scrub suit
18. Semirestricted
19. Separate
20. *Staphylococcus*
21. Unscrubbed

Aseptic and Sterile Techniques

Aseptic and sterile techniques are two different practices. A nonsterile person practicing aseptic technique may open a sterile package to the sterile field, but may not manipulate the sterile item within the field. Sterile technique means everything must be sterile that comes into contact with a sterile field. Only sterile persons can manipulate sterile items within the sterile field. The perioperative registered nurse demonstrates the knowledge to differentiate the techniques based on scientific principles and recommended practices.

What Is Aseptic Technique?

Aseptic technique means without dirt or contamination. Aseptic technique is the method of practice to reduce the transmission of microorganisms. This technique is applied in many other settings such as clinics, doctors' offices, outpatient surgery centers, hospitals, and any practice to reduce the transmission of microorganisms. This is sometimes referred to as clean technique. Microorganisms are present in air and on every object. No environment is 100% free from microorganisms, including the operating room (OR).

Principles of Aseptic Technique

1. Principles of aseptic technique for unsterile persons include:
   a. Perform recommended hand hygiene.
   b. Patient care items are handled with gloves to protect the caregiver and patients.
   c. Some items start out sterile but can be used in unsterile circumstances.
   d. Items are not considered sterile if processed unwrapped without processing indicators.
   e. Contamination is kept to a minimum and avoid cross contamination.
   f. Cleaned, disinfected, or decontaminated items are safe to handle with bare hands.
   g. Items that are not sterile are used on intact skin and mucous membranes.
   h. Disposable items are not reused.
   i. Unwrapped items should be stored in a clean, dry core area and processed according to the manufacturer's recommendations.
   j. Skin is not sterile; the process of skin prepping is aseptic.

Circulating Nurse

1. The circulating nurse is a nonsterile team member who must have good judgment and use aseptic technique. Aseptic technique is used before, during, and after procedures. Some tasks performed by the circulating nurse using aseptic technique include:
   a. Check all supplies for package integrity, cleanliness, and that they are free from moisture.
   b. Make sure room equipment such as the OR bed, tables, and horizontal surfaces have been cleaned with appropriate facility disinfectant. All surfaces must be dry before room setup.
   c. Open custom packs or back table covers by edges only and open wrapped supplies without touching the inside of the wrapper or container. Do not reach over the sterile field or remove items when not in sterile attire.
   d. Dispense sterile items to the field without tossing or touching sterile areas.
   e. Dispense medications and solutions to the sterile field without splashing or touching the unsterile container to the field.
   f. Keep a safe distance of at least 12 inches from the sterile field. Do not walk between two sterile fields. Reduce activity near the sterile field.
   g. Touch only the ends of cords and tubing of sterile connections after they are tossed off the sterile field.
   h. Dispose of contaminated items in correct biohazardous bags or trash containers.

What Is Sterile Technique?

Sterile technique means free from all living microorganisms including endospores. Sterile technique is a higher controlled process where microorganisms are absent or reduced to as low as possible. Sterile technique is used in any environment where surgery or invasive procedures are performed.

AORN has established guidelines for sterile technique. The guidelines provide recommendations for creating a sterile field, maintaining the field, and safety.

1. **Principles of sterile technique** performed by a sterile team member include:
   a. Sterile team members wear appropriate attire for the OR (clean scrub suit, hair cover, mask, eyewear, shoe covers as appropriate) and perform

a surgical scrub before donning sterile gowns and gloves for entering the sterile field.

b. Only sterile scrubbed personnel may handle items on sterile tables or in the field.

c. Only sterile items are used in a sterile field. Items are considered sterile by cleaning, decontamination, wrapping, or packaging before sterilization according to the manufacturer's recommendations. Outside and inside indicators/integrators show the sterilization process was complete.

d. Sterile items are used on mucous membranes, nonintact skin, and introduction into the vascular system.

e. Sterile items are used on body parts prepped with antiseptic agent.

f. An open sterile field is event related; there is no time limit.

g. Contaminated items are immediately discarded.

2. The scrub person is a sterile team member who performs a surgical scrub and dons appropriate sterile attire to establish the sterile field. Scrubbing, gowning, and gloving were discussed in Chapter 2. The scrub person must have a strong surgical conscience and knowledge to remedy any issue relating to contamination or questionable sterility. Duties of the sterile scrub person include:

a. Performs surgical hand hygiene and dons the sterile gown and gloves from a surface separate from the main sterile field using the closed gloving method.

b. Establishes the sterile field and counts all items with the circulating nurse.

c. Receives any additional sterile instruments or supplies such as staplers, endoscopic equipment, solutions, and medications from the circulating nurse.

d. Assists other sterile team members with gowning and gloving.

e. Creates a sterile field around the patient with sterile drapes.

f. Maintains and monitors the sterile field and sterile team members throughout the surgical procedure.

g. Breaks down the sterile field at the end of the procedure and prepares soiled instruments for processing.

h. Transports the soiled instruments to the decontamination area for processing.

3. The "Eight Ps" of Operating Room and Sterile Field Setup and Management table gives both the circulating nurse and scrub person some basic points on the role they play for setting up the room and sterile field. The Eight Ps are listed as follows with points of consideration in Table 3.1:

a. **Proper placement:** Room equipment and surgical instruments on the field are positioned in a useful manor.

b. **Proper function:** Test equipment and surgical instruments before use.

c. **Place it once:** Place items where they belong and do not keep moving them around for efficient use.

d. **Point of contact:** Point of contact refers to aseptic delivery of items to the sterile field, passing instruments to the surgeon's hand, or use of a neutral zone for sharps.

e. **Position of function:** Position items the way they are to be used both on the field and around the room.

f. **Point of use:** Refers to easy access for immediate-use items in the room and on the sterile field.

g. **Protected parts:** Delicate or potentially harmful items are secured on the field or in the room.

h. **Perfect picture:** Organized room and sterile field are picture-perfect at a glance before the patient enters the room.

Preparing for a Sterile Field Begins With Preparing the Room

1. **Preparing the room for the first procedure of the day.** The room is prepared by both the circulating nurse and the scrub person before opening sterile supplies in the room. All personnel in the room must be wearing appropriate surgical attire (scrub suit, warm-up jacket, and mask).

a. Lights and all horizontal surfaces are damp dusted with approved disinfectant solution and a clean cloth to remove settled particulate matter.

b. The clean OR bed should be in the correct position and appropriate for the procedure. The OR bed must be the correct weight-bearing surface for the weight of the patient.

1) Necessary attachments must be immediately available.

2) Positioning aids must be immediately available.

c. Arrange equipment around the room in position of use. Examples:

1) Electrosurgical unit (ESU)

2) Headlight if planned for use

d. Check the contents of the case cart for completeness. Gather any additional needed supplies from the sterile core.

e. Check all packaged items for cleanliness, expiration date as appropriate, package integrity, and external sterilization indicators.

f. "If in doubt, throw it out"—do not use any item if sterilization is questionable. Return questionable reusable items to processing department with the load number intact in case other items processed in the same load need to be removed from service.

2. Prepare the sterile field as close to the time of use as possible. Once a sterile field is open, it must be in view at all times and never left unattended.

A custom pack or sterile table cover is opened on a clean, dry surface to act as a barrier. Wet surfaces can contaminate the cover if it soaks through the drape.

TABLE **3.1** The "Eight Ps" of Operating Room and Sterile Field Setup and Management

The "Eight Ps" to Consider When Preparing for a Surgical Procedure	Environment Considerations for the Circulating Nurse	Sterile Field Considerations for the Scrub Person
Proper Placement Items should be placed so they will not need to be moved during the procedure.	Suction canisters, tourniquet, and the electrosurgical unit (ESU) need to be stationary. The operating room (OR) lights should be directed toward the field.	The Mayo stand and instrument table should not be moved during the procedure. Drapes may not be moved on the patient's skin.
Proper Function Items should be tested for safety and usefulness before they are needed, to prevent delay in the case.	Test the ESU, tourniquet, laser, and other equipment before the patient enters the room.	Test the efficiency of instruments (e.g., scissors, needle holders, clamps) as they are needed.
Place It Once Items should not be manipulated during the procedure. Energy and attention should not be diverted to resetting the field.	The OR bed should be in the right place for the procedure. The dispersive electrode should not be moved or displaced.	When setting up the field, each item (e.g., a basin) should be placed where it will be used during the procedure with minimal handling.
Point of Contact Items used within the field could cause harm or be rendered useless if they do not reach the intended point of contact.	The circulating nurse should evaluate the delivery of items to the sterile field. Some items (e.g., staplers) should be handed; others can be transferred in other ways.	The scrub person should be aware of the passing of instruments and how they are securely placed in the waiting hand of the surgeon or first assistant.
Position of Function Items should be positioned so they will be usable during the procedure.	The use of a C-arm, laser with articulating arm, or microscope should be preplanned so they may be positioned while the procedure is in progress.	When passing instruments, they should be placed in the surgeon's hand in a usable way. For example, the curve of the instrument should match the curve of the hand.
Point of Use Items should be as close to the area of use as possible.	Pour solutions directly into the basins; open and hand sponges or sutures directly to the scrub person as they are needed.	Basins should be placed close to the edge of the table so the circulating nurse can pour without requiring the basin to be repositioned. The ESU pencil holder should be close to the field for safe containment of the tip.
Protected Parts Items and surfaces should be rendered safe for the patient and the team.	Cords, cables, and tubing should be secured and appropriately directed away from the field. Pad the OR bed and patient as appropriate. Use safety belts.	Apply jaw liners to instruments during setup. Hand instruments with care to avoid causing injury with the tip or sharp surface. Do not lay items on or against the patient's body.
Perfect Picture Items within and around the field should not be at risk for causing harm or becoming damaged. The environment should not be cluttered.	The entire room should appear neat and tidy. The door should be closed, and the temperature and humidity should be appropriate. Forethought to having a clear path for the crash cart or setup emergency equipment is essential.	The sterile field should remain neat and orderly, with instruments and supplies within easy sight and reach. Consistency fosters a sense of comfort and confidence in the scrub role.

The examples used for each *P* will vary according to the type of procedure and equipment, the position of the patient, and the surgeon's preference. The Eight Ps apply to both the scrub person and the circulating nurse.

Guidelines for opening a table cover include (Figs. 3.1 and 3.2):

a. Remove the unsterile plastic outer wrapper and position the sealed custom pack in a position to cover the intended sterile. Place it once, do not move it around. The package will indicate which direction the opened ends will cover.

b. Break the secured paper seal. Some custom packs open envelope style with the first flap opened toward the rear of the table. The side flaps open to the sides. The last flap is unfolded toward the user. Never reach over the exposed sterile surface. Touch only the edges that will overhang the table.

c. Some custom packs open side to side. The first side is opened followed by opening the second side. Move to the end or side of the table and place hands under the edge of the table cover and complete the opening on that side. Move to the opposite side and finish. The entire tabletop will be covered with a sterile surface.

d. Avoid fanning the drape or creating unnecessary bellowing. This can cause movement of microorganisms in the air.

e. The edges and sides of tables are not considered sterile.

3. Opening sterile items onto the sterile field must be done without contaminating the item or sterile field. Opening items in specific manner reduces the chance of contamination (Fig. 3.3).

a. All packaged items must be checked for integrity and external indicators checked for sterilization before opening.

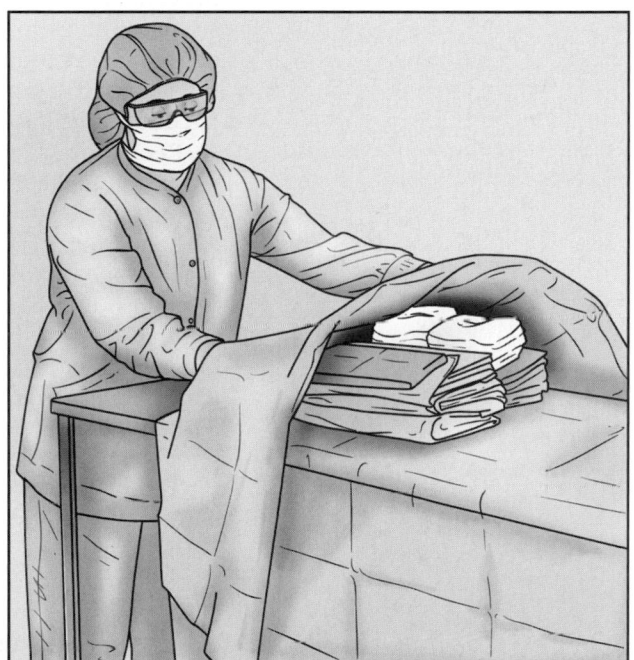

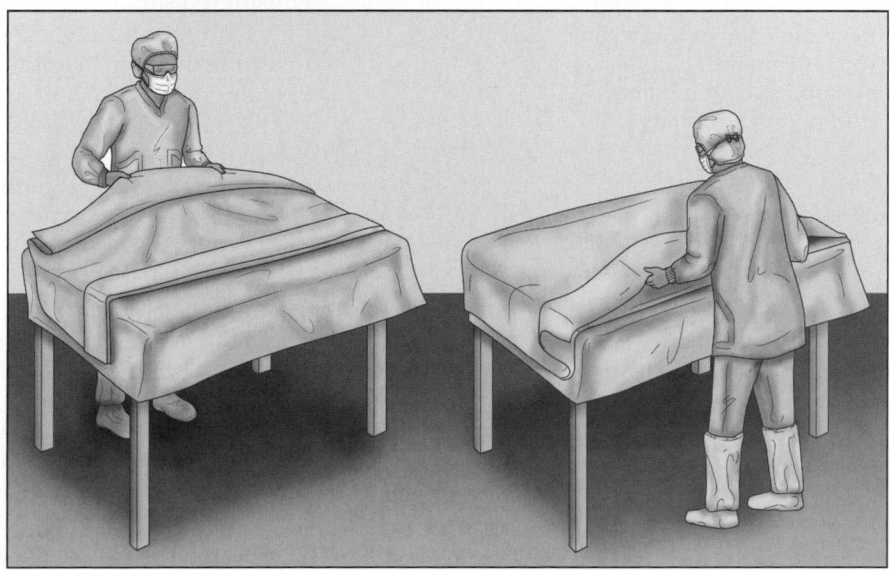

Figure 3.1 Circulating nurse opening table cover. (From Rothrock, J. [2019]. *Alexander's care of the patient in surgery* [16th ed.]. St. Louis, MO: Elsevier.)

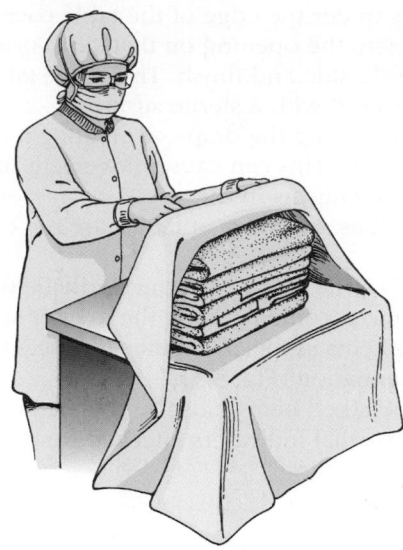

Figure 3.2 Opening square-fold sterile pack. Wrapper is lifted back while keeping hands on the outside. Hands are in folded cuff to avoid contaminating contents of pack. Area touched falls below unsterile table level; sterile inside of wrapper (now table cover) remains sterile. (From Phillips, N. [2017]. *Berry and Kohn's operating room technique* [13th ed.]. St. Louis, MO: Elsevier.)

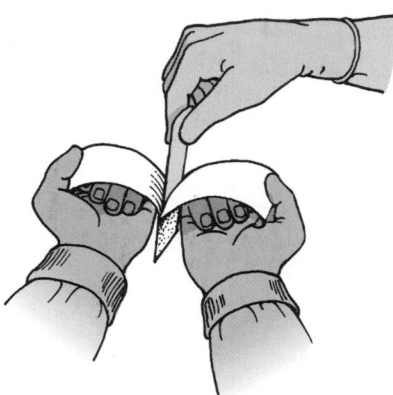

Figure 3.3 Scrub person taking contents from suture packet opened and held by circulating nurse. Scrub person avoids touching unsterile outer wrapper. (From Phillips, N. [2017]. *Berry and Kohn's operating room technique* [13th ed.]. St. Louis, MO: Elsevier.)

b. When opening a small sterile item wrapped envelope style: The sealing tape is broken. The first flap is unfolded away from the body; the sides are turned down and tucked into the hand. The last flap is opened toward the body. Avoid hovering or reaching over sterile contents. Do not let the flaps fall back onto the contents. The item can be delivered to the sterile field. If the item is double wrapped, then both wrappers are opened before dispensing to the sterile field.

1) Instrument sets wrapped envelope style are opened on surfaces such as a ring stand or small table. The first flap is opened away from

the body and the side flaps opened to the side without passing the hands over the exposed sterile tray surface. The final flap is opened toward self.

2) If the set is double wrapped, the second wrapper is opened in the same manner before the scrubbed person retrieves the tray for the sterile field.

c. The inside of a wrapper is considered sterile within 1 inch of the edges as a margin of safety. Edges are considered contaminated.

d. Wrapped items that are dropped to the floor can become contaminated by forcing air in or out of the package. If opened for use, the item's wrapper could shed particulate from the floor onto the sterile field.

e. Peel packs should be stored on their sides to prevent rupture of the pack during processing or storage. Check for holes and that the heat-sealed edge is intact. Some packs that contain sharp items may have tip protectors or may be double-peel packed for safety.

1) Peel packs should have processing indicators on the inside and outside of the pack.

2) Open a peel pack by peeling the edges over the hands to prevent contamination. Do not tear package open or let contents slide over the edges. Edges are not considered sterile.

f. When opening instruments in rigid containers, the outer container is considered unsterile. Check the external processing indicator and the integrity of the seals. To open the container, break the seals and release the locks. The lid is lifted vertically and tilted toward the body to remove. The inner surface of the lid should be dry and the filter intact. Some filters in the lids contain an additional sterilization processing indicator.

1) Never open suture or other sterile items into the rigid container. The edges are not considered sterile.

2) The scrub person will grasp the inner sterile instrument basket without touching the outer container, and lift it out and away toward the sterile field.

3) When the basket is removed, the circulating nurse should check the bottom filter in the container.

Other Considerations

Other considerations regarding the sterile field include remaining items delivered to the scrub person, zones of sterility, and preparing gowns and gloves for the additional surgical team (Fig. 3.4).

1. The scrub person sets up their sterile table by efficiently placing items in position of use. The drapes are arranged in the order of use. During the setup process, the scrub person places sterile basins near the edge of the table. The circulating nurse pours solutions without reaching over the sterile field or splashing.

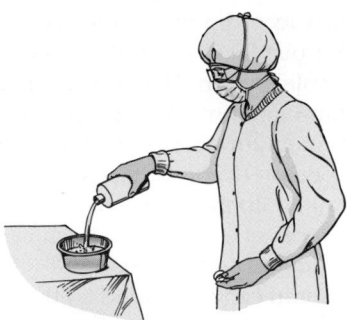

Figure 3.4 Circulating nurse pouring sterile solution into sterile basin. Note that only the lip of bottle is over the basin. The unsterile person avoids reaching over the sterile field. (From Phillips, N. [2017]. *Berry and Kohn's operating room technique* [13th ed.]. St. Louis, MO: Elsevier.)

    a. Solutions are poured in one motion. Once poured, the lip of the bottle is considered contaminated. The bottle may not be recapped for sterile use.

    b. The scrub person immediately labels the basin after the pouring is complete. Do not label the basin ahead of time in case the wrong solution is poured in the wrong basin.

    c. Medication delivery to the field is discussed in Chapter 8.

2. The scrub person must be aware of the **zones of sterility**.

    a. The scrub person always faces sterile areas and never turns the back to the sterile field.

    b. Tables are sterile only on the top and at table level.

    c. The front of a gown is sterile from the chest to the level of the sterile field and from the cuffs to 2 inches above the elbows (Fig. 3.5).

    d. Cuffs of gowns are considered unsterile under gloves because they can retain moisture from perspiration. Cuffs are not impervious.

    e. Hands are kept above the waist, not above the neckline. When in sterile attire, keep hands in sight at all times, elbows close to sides. Avoid folding arms because of risk for contamination. The armpits are not considered sterile (Fig. 3.6).

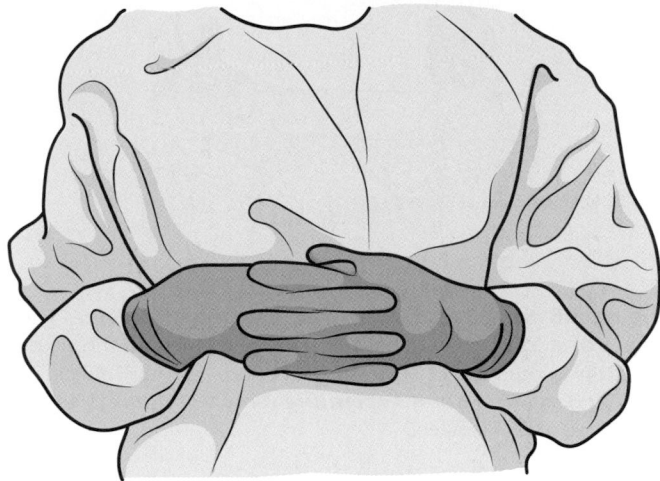

Figure 3.6 Sterile personnel keep hands in sight at or above waist or level of sterile field. Gowns are considered sterile only in front from chest to the level of sterile field, and the sleeves from above elbows to cuffs. (From Phillips, N. [2017]. *Berry and Kohn's operating room technique* [13th ed.]. St. Louis, MO: Elsevier.)

    f. The back of a gown is not sterile because it is not in view.

    g. The patient or surgical site sets the level of sterility for the team. The patient may be positioned in a manner that has more than one level (Fig. 3.7).

    h. If one member of the surgical team sits for the procedure, the whole team must sit. The zones of sterility are altered when seated and the front of the gown is lower (Fig. 3.8).

3. The scrub person prepares gowns and gloves for additional team members. The scrub person can gown and glove other team members from the sterile field or from another separate surface. Gowning and gloving of team members entering the sterile field is discussed in Chapter 2.

    a. Gowns are selected based on the size of the person.

    b. Some surgeons request gowns made of certain materials or with hoods for orthopedic surgery.

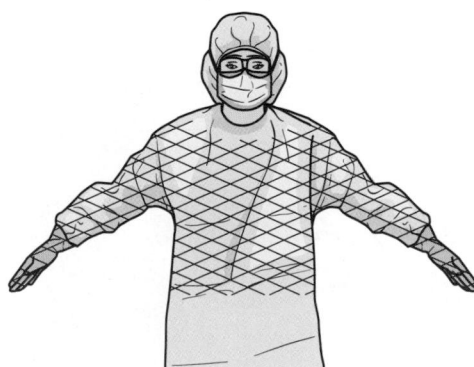

Figure 3.5 Zones of sterility on front of gown. The zones of sterility can change based on position of draped patient and sterile team. (From Phillips, N. [2017]. *Berry and Kohn's operating room technique* [13th ed.]. St. Louis, MO: Elsevier.)

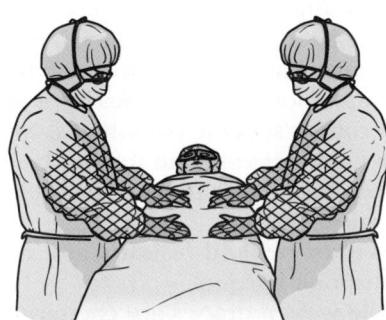

Figure 3.7 Zones of sterility when standing at sterile field with patient as the baseline for the level of the sterile field. (From Phillips, N. [2017]. *Berry and Kohn's operating room technique* [13th ed.]. St. Louis, MO: Elsevier.)

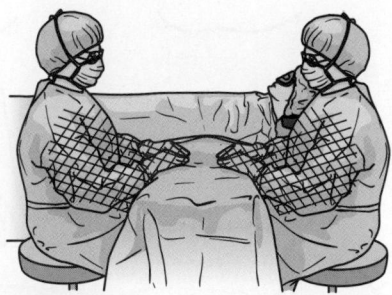

Figure 3.8 Seated team for upper extremity procedure. The zones of sterility change based on the placement of the team in relation to the type of surgical procedure. (From Phillips, N. [2017]. *Berry and Kohn's operating room technique* [13th ed.]. St. Louis, MO: Elsevier.)

c. The scrub person should have the requested glove sizes and type of glove for each team member.

d. Double gloving is recommended. Use a half-size larger pair first covered by actual size glove as the outer pair. This method creates extra space without compression of the hands.

Sterile Drapes, Towels, or Sheets

Sterile drapes, towels, or sheets create a barrier that establishes a sterile field. The barrier reduces the risk for microorganisms passing from an unsterile area to the sterile area. Do not use perforating towel clips to secure drapes; they create holes and increase the risk for contamination. The sterile areas are created on tables, equipment, and patients where a sterile procedure takes place. Drapes come in disposable single-use or reusable material forms. Whichever form of drape is used, it should have certain qualities and be handled with sterile technique.

1. Characteristics of sterile drapes
   a. Drapes should be durable and withstand the process of sterilization at the manufacturer's facility.
   b. All drapes must meet the NPFA requirements for fire safety. Most drapes are flame retardant, but can ignite if exposed to an ignition source. Fire safety is discussed in Chapter 5.
   c. Disposable drapes are commercially packaged for single use and are preferred for surgical use. Some styles are designed for specific-sized instrument tables. Disposable drapes are preferred.
   d. Fenestrated nonwoven drapes have openings that are precut for specific body areas. Nonwoven drapes must never be cut to size, because they shed cellulose fibers that act as foreign bodies in the surgical site.
   e. Drapes must be fluid resistant and create strikethrough barriers.
   f. Reusable woven drapes are chemically treated to provide an adequate barrier. Laundering diminishes the barrier quality over repeated washings.
      1) Reusable woven drapes must be low linting, free of holes, and processed in an accredited

facility according to fabric recommendations. They must be inspected for wear.
      2) Reusable woven drapes and towels that are contaminated must be placed in leakproof containers for transport to the laundry facility.

2. The scrub person drapes items such as tables, Mayo stands, x-ray equipment, microscopes, the patient, and other pieces of equipment. Each item may have a specific drape and technique.
   a. A Mayo stand can be draped so that it can be used as a working space above the patient. Points for draping a Mayo stand are as follows (Figs. 3.9 and 3.10):
      1) Open the drape so it is in position with an opening in the cuff.
      2) Place hands under the large cuff and fold the drape so it does not fall below the waist.
      3) Place a foot on the base of the Mayo stand so it does not move during the draping process.
      4) Slide the drape over the Mayo stand like a pillowcase.

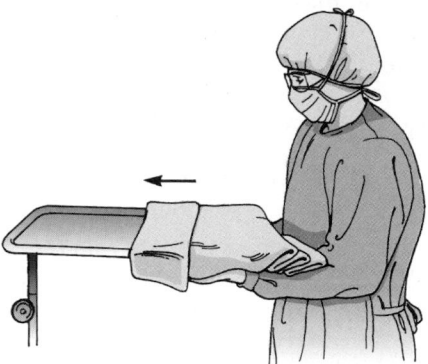

Figure 3.9 Starting to drape Mayo stand. Scrub person's hands are protected in cuff of drape. Folds of drape are supported on arms, in bend of elbows, to prevent their falling below waist level. Foot is placed on base of stand to stabilize it. (From Phillips, N. [2017]. *Berry and Kohn's operating room technique* [13th ed.]. St. Louis, MO: Elsevier.)

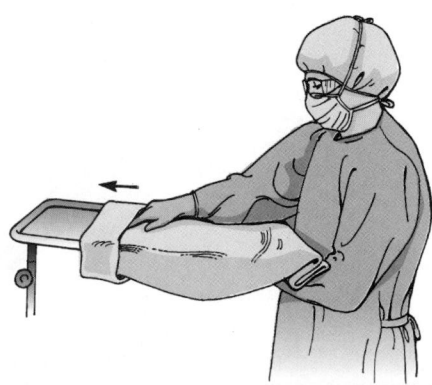

Figure 3.10 Completing draping of Mayo stand. Hands are protected in cuffs. (From Phillips, N. [2017]. *Berry and Kohn's operating room technique* [13th ed.]. St. Louis, MO: Elsevier.)

5) Tuck in extra material along the top surface under the tray.
6) Do not reach to pull the open end of the drape down. The circulating nurse can reach inside the Mayo cover to pull it down over the pedestal.

  b. Draping a small table while in sterile attire (Fig. 3.11)
1) Cuff the drape over the gloved hands for protection.
2) Place the sterile drape edge toward self first.
3) Then finish covering away from self.

  c. Draping a large table while in sterile attire
1) Hold drape toward middle of table; gently let it settle into position for opening (Fig. 3.12).
2) Unfold toward self (Fig. 3.13).
3) Stand back far enough so the gown does not touch the unsterile table.
4) While protecting the gloved hands, unfold away from self (Fig. 3.14).

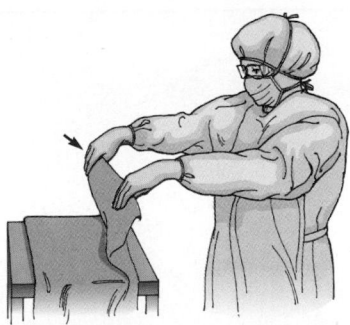

Figure 3.13 Scrub person unfolding sterile table drape. Scrub person stands back from unsterile table and unfolds drape first toward self. Note that hands are inside sterile cover to protect them. (From Phillips, N. [2017]. *Berry and Kohn's operating room technique* [13th ed.]. St. Louis, MO: Elsevier.)

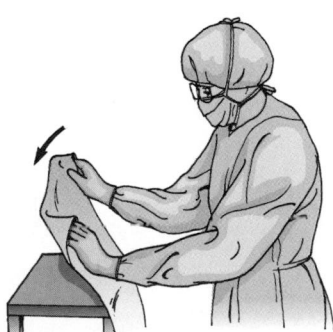

Figure 3.11 Sterile scrub person draping a small table. Sterile personnel avoid reaching over unsterile field. The scrub person therefore drapes the unsterile table first toward self, then away. Gown is protected by distance, and hands are protected by cuffing drape over them. (From Phillips, N. [2017]. *Berry and Kohn's operating room technique* [13th ed.]. St. Louis, MO: Elsevier.)

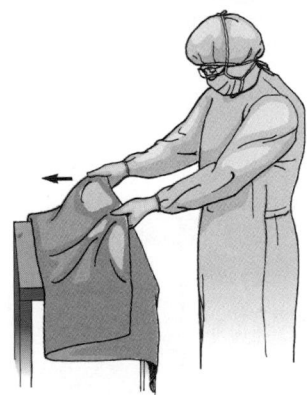

Figure 3.14 Scrub person continuing to unfold sterile table drape. Note that the hands are inside sterile cover for protection. Scrub person may now move closer to table because the first part of unfolded drape now protects gown. (From Phillips, N. [2017]. *Berry and Kohn's operating room technique* [13th ed.]. St. Louis, MO: Elsevier.)

Creating a Sterile Field Using Drapes

Creating a sterile field using drapes can be tricky and can be specialized to a procedure. Principles to remember include:

1. Antiseptic skin preparation solutions must be dry before draping. Pooling of an alcohol-based solution can be a fire hazard. Fumes can accumulate under the drapes and ignite if an ignition source is activated.
2. Have drapes stacked in the order of use. Smaller drapes may be placed before the large main fenestrated drape. An overlay adhesive, clear, plastic drape or a style impregnated with iodine may be used. The incision is made directly through the plastic surface.
  a. If towels are used to square off a surgical site, do not reach over the site to place. Walk around the OR bed to place them. If handing towels or drapes to the surgeon, hand them from the same side as the person receiving them (Fig. 3.15).
  b. Do not let your gown or gloves touch any unsterile area or the patient's skin.

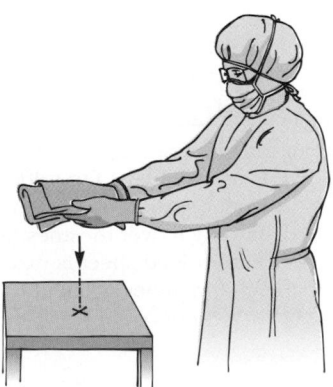

Figure 3.12 Draping large unsterile table. Scrub person holds sterile fan-folded table drape high and drops it on center of table, standing back from table to protect gown. (From Phillips, N. [2017]. *Berry and Kohn's operating room technique* [13th ed.]. St. Louis, MO: Elsevier.)

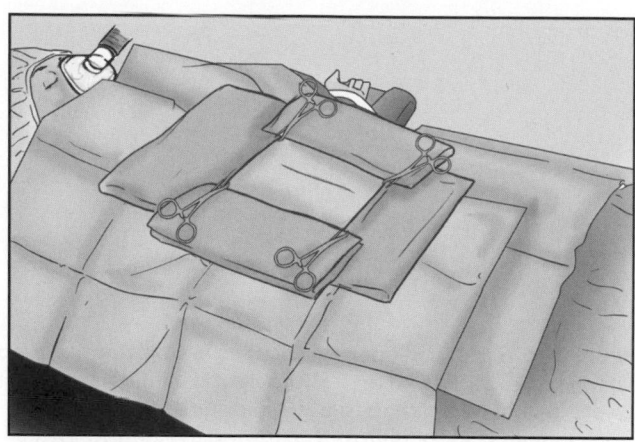

Figure 3.15 Abdomen may be draped with four sterile towels, which are secured with nonperforating towel clamps. Standard method of placement of disposable towels is used. (From Rothrock, J. [2019]. *Alexander's care of the patient in surgery* [16th ed.]. St. Louis, MO: Elsevier.)

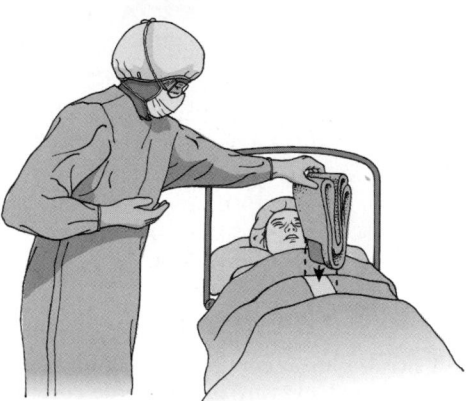

Figure 3.16 Draping with sterile laparotomy sheet. Scrub person carries folded sheet to table. Standing far back from OR bed, with one hand, scrub person places the fenestration of the sheet on patient so that opening in sheet is directly over prepped skin area. A second sterile team member helps complete the opening of the drape over the body from the opposite side of the table. (From Phillips, N. [2017]. *Berry and Kohn's operating room technique* [13th ed.]. St. Louis, MO: Elsevier.)

c. Handle drapes as little as possible and ask for assistance if draping cannot be done without contamination.

d. Hold drapes high enough so they do not touch unsterile areas or fall below the waist.

e. Place the drape over the incision site and unfold toward the bottom of the bed, then unfold toward the top. Nonwoven drapes usually have arrows that provide directions for application (Figs. 3.16 through 3.18).

f. Do not move drapes once they are placed. Place them only once. Moving or repositioning drapes can contaminate the surgical site.

Maintaining the Sterile Field

Maintaining the sterile field is the job of all surgical team members. The scrub person and the circulating nurse

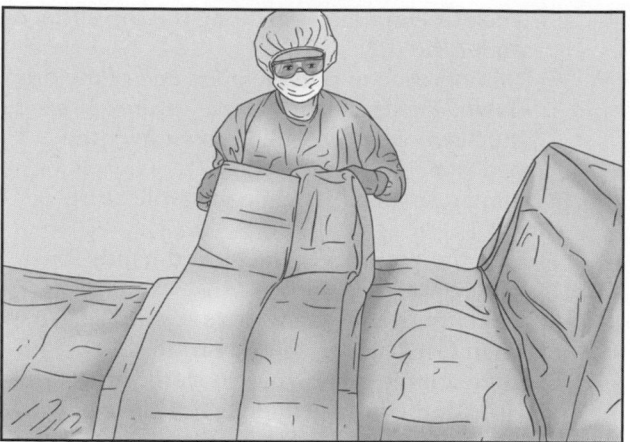

Figure 3.17 Placement of laparotomy sheet. Identification of top portion of the laparotomy sheet helps the scrub person readily determine correct placement of the drape. After placing the folded laparotomy sheet on the patient, with fenestration of sheet directly over site of incision outlined by sterile towels, the scrub person unfolds drape over sides of patient and bed. (From Rothrock, J. [2019]. *Alexander's care of the patient in surgery* [16th ed.]. St. Louis, MO: Elsevier.)

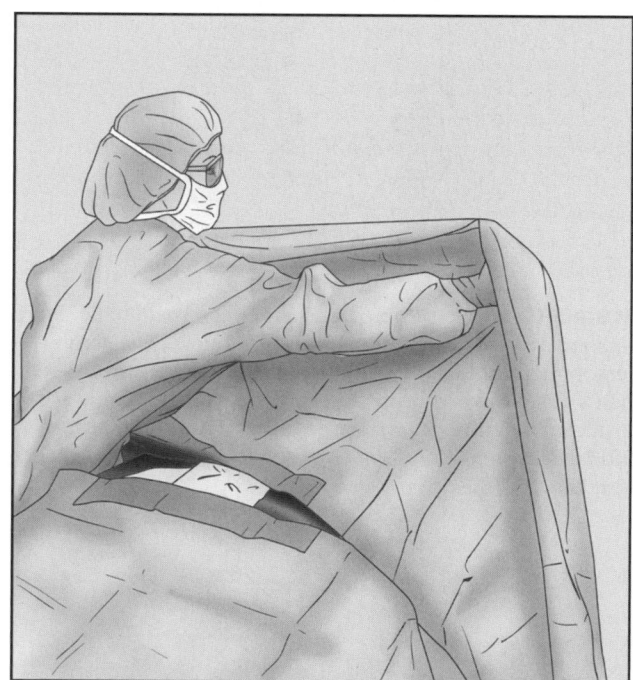

Figure 3.18 Laparotomy draping continued. Scrub person protects gloved hands under cuff of fan-folded laparotomy sheet and draws the upper section above fenestration toward the head of the bed, draping it over the anesthesia screen. The bottom portion of the fan-folded sheet is extended over the foot of the bed in a similar manner. (From Rothrock, J. [2019]. *Alexander's care of the patient in surgery* [16th ed.]. St. Louis, MO: Elsevier.)

monitor the activities within the sterile field. The circulating nurse is the second set of eyes and may observe a breach in technique while the sterile team is working.

1. The sterile team must not lean on instrument tables or against unsterile surfaces (intravenous [IV] poles or

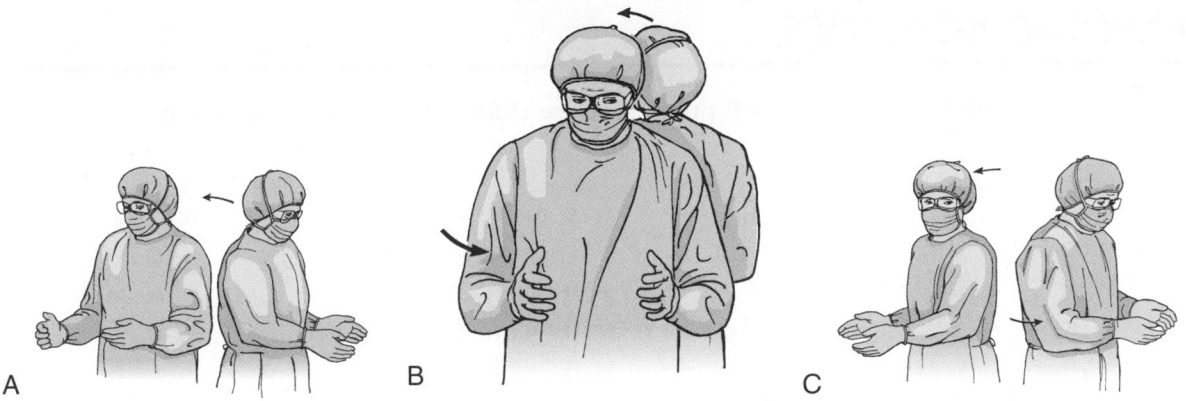

Figure 3.19 Sequence of one sterile person going around another. They pass each other back to back, keeping well within the sterile area and allowing a margin of safety between them. (From Phillips, N. [2017]. *Berry and Kohn's operating room technique* [13th ed.]. St. Louis, MO: Elsevier.)

machinery). Items could be knocked from the table or the person leaning could be injured on a sharp instrument.

2. Never lean on the draped patient's body. This could cause a pressure injury to the patient without realizing what has happened.

3. Do not sit unless the whole team sits for the procedure. There is no excuse for sitting while waiting for the case to begin or for a test result from pathology. If a sterile team member sits, the level of sterility of the gown is compromised and must be changed.

4. Any item that falls over the sterile instrument table edge or draped patient is considered contaminated (i.e., suture tail or sponge).

5. Sterile team members pass each other back to back or face to face (Fig. 3.19).

6. Sterile team members must not go outside the sterile field. To do so risks contamination of the gown or gloves.

Any contamination of the sterile field or sterile team must be corrected immediately. No compromise in sterility or suspicion of compromise is acceptable.

The circulating nurse and scrub person must work together as a team to maintain a high level of sterility. Patients depend on the skills and knowledge of the team to keep them safe and free from SSIs. All team members, sterile or unsterile, must be diligent and provide the highest level of patient care.

LEARNING ACTIVITIES

INSTRUCTIONS: Complete the word search puzzle. Use the clues to help identify the words.

```
N J R H L W E X B R G D U S T E D B P A T I E N T A K T U B
O Y Q A G J J O T J A J B S G F U Q G L R M P N R S O H L K
C H M D P J E X I R H H S J J H D R Y R R B O O D P N M V I
X G K D A Z X C E M O E V Y E N N W C Q A J O N P P U A C N
G E P W C W U T S B U N S T E R I L E D Z E L S V P E G O T
U N E S C M O V E D O Q I I T J C N E E X Z I T Y T H T X E
K D R W S P L A S H I N G E Z E G T D A Q W N E H U E H W G
P O F D K F H Z O N E S M N A V A P H C O M G R W O V E H R
L S O K K G G B J E D G E S K L I D I F K Q D I D A V Z R I
L P R H V R W U K W W D N M E V G T X B A M H L U Q Y E S T
X O A A F T G N D W W G D R T B P G Z Q Y C E E W F S A R Y
L R T U X G O A Y S V U T E N E I K B K J Q E U X O E R Z R
M E I J O M E T C M N N T U S G C O N T A M I N A T E D Q Z
K S N B J W T T F Y E B O A S C P S W W Y D D X V U U P D K
K K G A T W B E R V U V P S I C H E Z W A D F X X W O S F D
B S I C O K V N E U K H W H O L E E N U P I J M E B D Y T X
H A T K M Y H D A V M F U B G Q P J S Y A N S X G T I U N G
Y R R K Y M T E E H G E S H B K R S O T F K O T D B O W T O
U L J M D R R D M B Q H J C O N S C I E N C E I I I M S G H
Y A D C N J E O V S A J Y P Z L G Y J Q C X F D A V E Z F X
```

Clues

1. Without dirt. _____ technique reduces the number of microorganisms.
2. The scrub person never turns his or her _____ to the sterile field.
3. The front of the gown is sterile from the _____ to the level of the sterile field.
4. A scrub person must have a strong surgical _____ to remedy any issue relating to questionable sterility.
5. The lip of a solution bottle is considered _____ after some has been poured.
6. A custom pack or sterile table cover is opened on a clean _____ surface.
7. Lights and horizontal surfaces should be damp _____ before the first procedure of the day.
8. When opening a peel pack, the _____ are not considered sterile.
9. Sterile means free from all living microorganisms including _____.
10. An open sterile field is _____.
11. Sterile team members pass each other back to back or _____ to face.
12. All packaged items should be checked for _____.
13. Drapes should not be _____ once placed.
14. The circulating nurse is a _____ team member.
15. "If in doubt, throw it _____."
16. Never reach _____ a sterile field.
17. The _____ sets the level of sterility for the team.
18. Do not use _____ towel clips to secure drapes. Integrity can be jeopardized.
19. An alcohol-based prep solution can be a fire hazard from _____ under the patient.
20. The circulating nurse should pour solutions without reaching over the table or _____.
21. Masks should be removed by the _____.
22. Tables are sterile only on the _____ and at table level.
23. An open sterile field should never be left _____.
24. The cuffs of the gown are considered _____.
25. While draping, do not let them fall below the _____.
26. If one member of the surgical team sits, the _____ team must sit.
27. The scrub person must be aware of the _____ of sterility.

LEARNING ACTIVITIES ANSWERS

INSTRUCTIONS: Complete the word search puzzle. Use the clues to help identify the words.

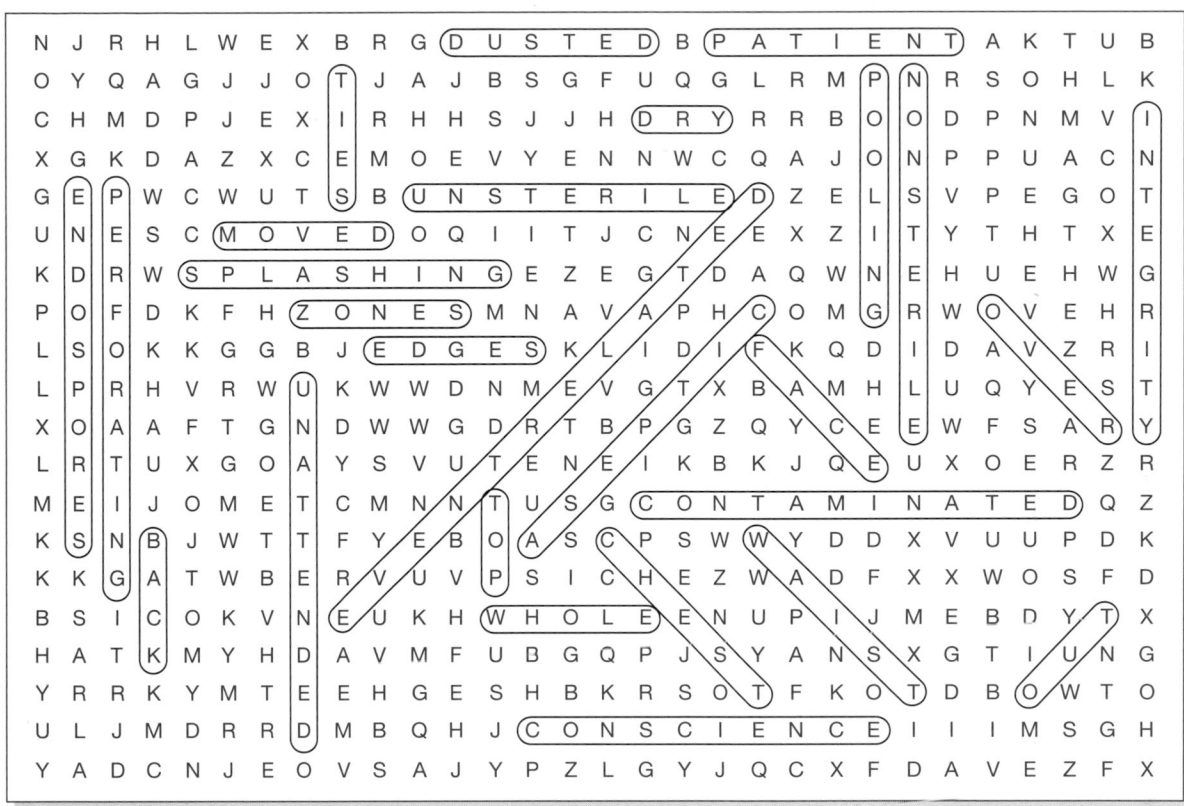

1. Without dirt. **Aseptic** technique reduces the number of microorganisms.
2. The scrub person never turns his or her **back** to the sterile field.
3. The front of the gown is sterile from the **chest** to the level of the sterile field.
4. A scrub person must have a strong surgical **conscience** to remedy any issue relating to questionable sterility.
5. The lip of a solution bottle is considered **contaminated** after some has been poured.
6. A custom pack or sterile table cover is opened on a clean **dry** surface.
7. Lights and horizontal surfaces should be damp **dusted** before the first procedure of the day.
8. When opening a peel pack, the **edges** are not considered sterile.
9. Sterile means free from all living microorganisms including **endospores**.
10. An open sterile field is **event related**.
11. Sterile team members pass each other back to back or **face** to face.
12. All packaged items should be checked for **integrity**.
13. Drapes should not be **moved** once placed.
14. The circulating nurse is a **nonsterile** team member.
15. "If in doubt, throw it **out**."
16. Never reach **over** a sterile field.
17. The **patient** sets the level of sterility for the team.
18. Do not use **perforating** towel clips to secure drapes. Integrity can be jeopardized.

19. An alcohol-based prep solution can be a fire hazard from **pooling** under the patient.
20. The circulating nurse should pour solutions without reaching over the table or **splashing**.
21. Masks should be removed by the **ties**.
22. Tables are sterile only on the **top** and at table level.
23. An open sterile field should never be left **unattended**.
24. The cuffs of the gown are considered **unsterile**.
25. While draping, do not let them fall below the **waist**.
26. If one member of the surgical team sits, the **whole** team must sit.
27. The scrub person must be aware of the **zones** of sterility.

CHAPTER 4

The Perioperative Environment

The surgical suite is designed with specific areas to promote efficiency and confine contamination. Each area is referred to as a **zone**. Each zone has specific functional requirements for activity, attire, and traffic patterns. The zone design incorporates patient and staff safety, infection control and prevention, security, efficient traffic patterns for entrance and exit, backup systems in case of power failure, and noise control.

Architects create the surgical suite blueprint to include corridors, air handlers, temperature and humidity control, electricity, anesthetic gas delivery, and evacuation systems. Each zone has specific HVAC (heating, ventilation, and air-conditioning) requirements.

The Three Zones Within the Perioperative Department

Unrestricted Area, Semirestricted Area, and Restricted Area

1. Unrestricted area
   a. There are no special requirements for attire. Street clothes are permitted in this area.
   b. Activities in the unrestricted area include patient arrival and admission departments, personnel locker rooms, staff lounges, offices, waiting rooms, phase I and II postanesthesia care unit (PACU), and procedural room entrances.
   c. Public access is limited to appropriate personnel and patients.
2. Semirestricted area
   a. Attire for personnel includes scrub suits and hair/head covering
   b. Areas located in the semirestricted area include storage for clean and sterile supplies, instrument processing areas, scrub sinks, and hallways leading from the unrestricted areas (locker rooms, preoperative admissions, and control desk) to the restricted areas (operating rooms [ORs] and sterile cores).
   c. Access to the semirestricted area is limited to persons accompanied by authorized personnel.
3. Restricted area
   a. Attire for personnel in the restricted area includes scrub suit, hair/head cover, and mask. When performing surgical procedures, the personnel wear sterile gowns and gloves, masks, and additional personal protective equipment (PPE) such as appropriate eyewear (i.e., splash protection or laser).

b. The doors remain closed to facilitate special airflow to minimize microbial transfer.
   c. Access is restricted to authorized personnel.

HVAC is an important part of the perioperative environment for maintaining the lowest microbial count possible for infection prevention using air handlers. Each zone has special requirements for air handling according to the level of risk associated with the activities performed in the area. The fresh air flows through two sets of filters (Table 4.1).

1. **In unrestricted areas**, the HVAC air handlers operate at a level of comfort for patients and personnel, because the risk for microbial transfer is not greater than the risks outside of the perioperative environment. Attire is common with clothing worn at home or outdoors. Sterile supplies are not in use.
   a. The air handlers have the same or similar requirements as the general patient care divisions. In PACU and procedural areas where patient care is performed, air exchanges per hour (ACH) can vary. These are not sterile environments, but external contamination is contained.
      1) PACU ACH: six total exchanges with two outdoor air changes
      2) Procedure room ACH: 15 total exchanges with three outdoor air changes
      3) Endoscopy room ACH: six total exchanges with two outdoor changes
   b. The temperature can range from 68°F to 75°F for comfort.
   c. The humidity can range from 30% to 60%.
      1) PACU humidity can range from 20% to 60%.
      2) Procedure room humidity can range from 20% to 60%.
      3) Endoscopy room humidity can range from 20% to 60%.
   d. No specific pressure gradient is required.
2. **In semirestricted areas**, the HVAC air handlers operate in specific directions at specific rates according to the risk for microbial movement through the area and the potential for patient vulnerability. The HVAC is designed to meet the needs of the specific room.
   a. The air pressure in areas where soiled materials are handled is negative. This minimizes the transference of microbial contamination from soiled instruments and supplies. Instrument

TABLE 4.1 Environmental Controls in Perioperative Areas

Environmental Controls	Class A OR	Class B and C OR	Cesarean Delivery Room	Storage Room	PACU
Pressure	Positive	Positive	Positive	N/A	N/A
ACH	15	20	20	4	6
OA	3	4	4	N/A	2
Humidity[a]	30%–60%	30%–60%	30%–60%	30%–60%	30%–60%
Temperature	68%–73%	68%–73%	68%–73%	68%–73%	70%–75%

ACH, Air exchanges per hour; *N/A*, not applicable; *OA*, outdoor air; *OR*, operating room; *PACU*, postanesthesia care unit.
[a]Humidity is expected to decrease as low as 20% by the 2012 edition of the AIA (American Institute of Architects) Guidelines. The rationale is that the old 30% to 60% is based on the use of flammable anesthetics and the risk of fire by static spark, which is not a consideration in modern times. ©ASHRAE, http://www.ashrac.org. 2017 ASHRAE Standard-170.

cleaning/decontamination areas and housekeeping closets where trash accumulates is a source of aerosolization.
   1) Decontamination room ACH: six total exchanges with two outdoor changes under negative pressure
   2) Sterile storage ACH: four total exchanges with two outdoor changes with positive pressure
   b. The temperature can range between 60°F and 73°F.
   1) Sterile storage should not exceed 75°F.
   2) Decontamination room temperature should be at a comfortable range between 60°F and 75°F.
   c. Humidity may vary in decontamination areas because hot water generates steam from cleaning instruments that is not necessarily controllable. No specific humidity setting is recommended.
   1) Sterile storage humidity should not exceed 60%. Higher humidity can cause sterile packages to absorb moisture, causing capillary pass-through and contamination.
   2) Decontamination areas have no specific humidity recommendations.
   d. Environmental control is supported by closed doors and positive pressure in adjacent cleaner areas (OR) with negative pressure in less clean areas, such as the decontamination room.
3. **In restricted areas**, the HVAC air handlers play a larger role in minimizing microbial transfer and airborne contamination by observing stringent controls.
   a. The ACH in the OR is 20 total exchanges with four changes of outdoor air. The incoming outdoor air is filtered through a series of two filters before passing into the OR.
   b. The temperature range is between 68°F and 75°F. Patients in the OR are directly affected by the temperature in the room. Avoiding extremes of temperature (either too cold or hot) is critical for patient metabolism, infection control, as well as sterile team comfort.
      If the room temperature is excessively warm, the patient can experience fluid loss by

perspiration. Very young, elderly, and critical patients, such as burn patients, require a warmer room temperature to maintain homeostasis. Research has shown that prewarming the room to 78°F can benefit patients at risk for hypothermia.
   c. The humidity should be between 20% and 60%. Excessive humidity can cause condensation in sterile packages, leading to contamination entering through the external surface of the wrapper by capillary action.
   d. The air pressure is a positive flow to decrease the risk for airborne contamination from adjacent, less clean areas. The positive airflow moves out of the room when the doors open and lowers the chance for pulling contaminants into the OR, sterile storage, and clean workroom areas. The doors must remain closed to maintain the positive pressure gradient. Leaving the door open can cause a strain on the HVAC system, causing equalization of airflow with the hallway.

Additional Environmental Considerations
Substerile Room
1. **Warming cabinets** usually have two chambers, one for blankets/patient gowns and another for irrigation solutions. Other materials should not be stored in this cabinet.
   a. **Blanket/patient gown section** should not be set above 130°F. The rate of heat dissipation against the patient's skin at 130°F is comfortable and least likely to cause hyperthermic areas on the patient's skin. The temperature of the heated blanket decreases significantly within 5 minutes of removal from the warmer. The temperature of the warming unit should be checked and documented daily.
   b. **Irrigation solution section.** Each manufacturer designates maximum solution storage temperatures and expiration dates for their warmed products determined by evidence-based

studies. These instructions are referred to as IFU (instructions for use).

In 2018, one supplier, Baxter (https://www.baxter.com/ or 1-800-933-0303), posted specific warming temperatures, expiration dates for warmed solutions, and disposal instructions for prewarmed products. The expiration date printed on the packaging or container applies to room-temperature (not more than 77°F) solutions that have not been warmed. Association of peri-Operative Registered Nurses (AORN) guidelines recommend measuring the temperature of the solution before irrigation. The irrigation is safe for use at 104°F.

1) Irrigation solutions in unopened plastic pour bottles may be warmed to 122°F for up to 60 days. Stocking personnel should clearly mark each pour bottle to indicate the removal date. If the solution is warmed longer than the manufacturer's recommendation, the concentration and pH changes and renders the product unstable for patient use.

2) If an unopened pour bottle of irrigation solution is removed from the warming cabinet and allowed to reach room temperature, it may not be returned to the warmer. The solutions in plastic pour bottles may not be warmed more than once.

   If the warming expiration date has been reached and the unopened bottle has been removed from the warmer, the bottled solution may be allowed to remain available for patient use at room temperature until the manufacturer's printed expiration date.

   Once a bottle of solution is uncapped and opened, it may be poured only once and not recapped. The outer lip of the bottle is considered contaminated and may not be poured into a sterile basin.

3) Intravenous (IV) solution bags more than 150 mL inside their outer plastic wrapper/pouch may be warmed at 113°F for 14 days. If warmed at 150°F, the warming duration may not exceed 72 hours. If the IV solution (still in its pouch) has passed its warming expiration date, it may be used at room temperature until the manufacturer's printed expiration date, but not rewarmed.

4) Prevention of patient hypothermia is supported by the use of prewarmed sterile IV and irrigation solutions. ECRI recommends that solutions can be warmed to 110°F. Before use, the temperature decreases when poured into a nonheated basin or pitcher.

   The AORN *Guidelines for Perioperative Practice* indicates that preheated solutions are safely used at 104°F. The temperature should be measured at the point of use before administration.

2. Just in time or immediate-use instrument sterilization.
   a. Sterilization of instruments in the substerile room autoclave or other sterilizer is not recommended for routine use. This method, referred to as "flashing," is used only in an emergency or other urgent situation when no other alternative is available. Facilities should have adequate supplies of backup instrumentation to avoid "flash" sterilization.
   b. If an instrument must be "flash" sterilized, it first must be cleaned and processed according to the manufacturer's recommendations. Each instance of "flash" sterilization should be documented for quality control. Documentation provides information concerning the need for additional instrumentation.
   c. Specific processing and sterilization is discussed in Chapter 10.

Laminar Airflow

Laminar airflow is a high-pressure air movement system designed to flow from a cleaner area to a less clean area. Actual air exchanges are close to 60 per hour. A series of air returns are located at a lower level to minimize contamination by air circulation. Opening and closing the door disrupts the flow of air. Not every room is equipped with laminar airflow. Laminar flow is sometimes installed and used in orthopedic ORs in some facilities.

1. Horizontal flow travels from one wall to a grill in an opposite wall. Potential particulate transfer from items in the flow path is a possibility. Care is taken not to walk through the air stream to prevent contamination.

2. Vertical flow begins in the ceiling and terminates in vents located in the lower portions of the wall. The air flows past fixtures and lights. Unclean lights and suspended monitors can shed dust and particulates as the air passes over the surface. Personnel leaning over the field can deposit skin and hair cells in the surgical site borne by the air current (Fig. 4.1).

Ultraviolet Light

1. Ultraviolet (UV) light used in combination with low ACH is beneficial because of longer light exposure to the microorganisms. UV lights can be used after appropriate use of detergent and disinfection to clean surfaces. When used as a decontamination device, personnel in the vicinity must wear protective eyewear and clothing to prevent eye and skin injury.

2. UV is used in an unoccupied room where no patient is receiving care, and ACH can be lowered for the duration of the low-level disinfection process. It does not sterilize, but it does kill some bacteria, fungi, and viruses. UV acts by denaturing protein and DNA.

3. Higher ACH causes the movement of microorganisms and decreases UV exposure time to microbial surfaces.

4. Prolonged skin and eye exposure to UV can be harmful.

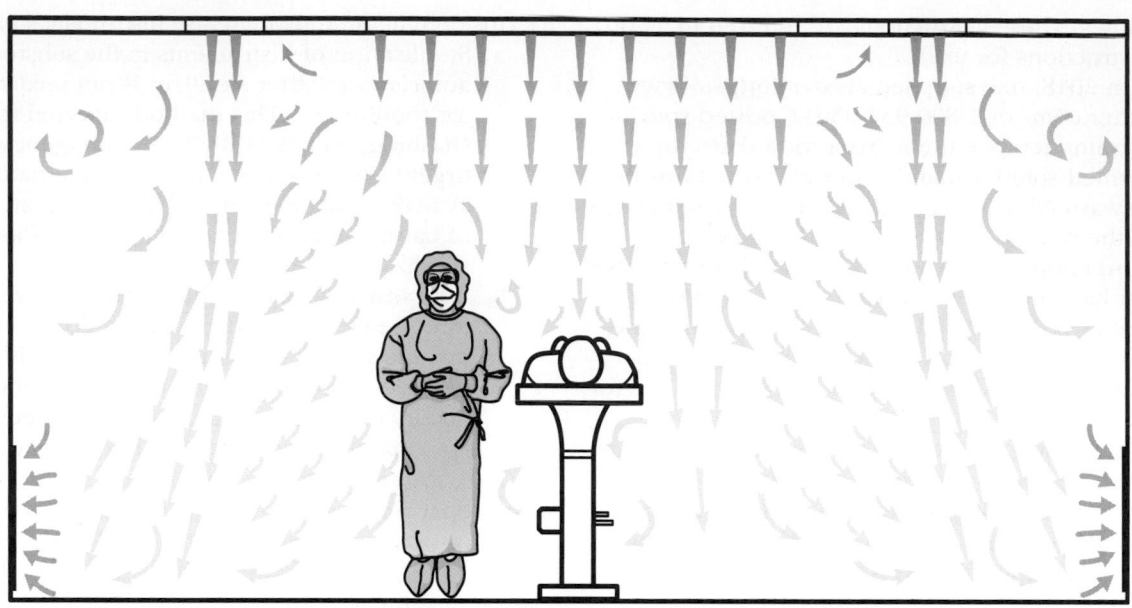

Figure. 4.1 Vertical airflow pattern with downdraft air curtain. (From Phillips, N. [2017]. *Berry and Kohn's operating room technique* [13th ed.]. St. Louis, MO: Elsevier.)

Sanitation in the Operating Room is a Multipart Process

An orderly room minimizes confusion and chaos for the planned cases for the day. Excess equipment and supplies interfere with traffic patterns and present possibilities for contamination and error.

1. **Preparing the room before a patient is brought for surgery.** Check for the necessary equipment: OR bed (appropriate for procedure and patient body weight), electrosurgical unit as appropriate, instrument table(s), Mayo stand, kick buckets, linen and impervious trash hampers (clean and biohazard), sharps disposal container, prep stand, suction apparatus, headlamp (as necessary), endoscopic equipment and machinery, and any other items needed for the specific case.
   a. All surfaces should be damp dusted (and dry) before bringing sterile supplies into the room.
   b. Because surfaces are not saturated as in terminal cleaning, no particular dwell time is necessary.
   c. Dry dusting causes skin cells, microorganisms, fibers, and other contaminates to become airborne.
   d. Begin dusting with the highest horizontal surfaces, especially the spotlights and ceiling-suspended articulating arms (booms and monitors). These are exposed to vertical laminar airflow and could direct particles into the sterile field. All horizontal surfaces should be wiped before setting out sterile packages.
   e. When the room is ready, bring in the case cart and begin opening the sterile packs. Ensure there is a safe pathway for traffic as the patient is brought into the room. Think ahead to leave a path for emergency equipment should the need arise.

2. **Turnover between cases** does not begin until the current patient leaves the room. It is not appropriate to begin cleaning before that time.
   a. The scrub person, still wearing gown, gloves, and PPE (i.e., eyewear, mask), begins to break down the instrument table.
   b. The drapes and other biological trash are discarded in the biohazard trash. The entire instrument set is disassembled and placed open in the bottom of the instrument tray. Some facilities use enzymatic foam or solution to coat the instruments in preparation for decontamination and processing.
   c. Remaining solutions should be evacuated into the suction system or carefully disposed of into the appropriate sink while wearing the appropriate PPE.
   d. All instruments and reusable equipment from the sterile field are placed in the covered case cart. The instrument table drape is discarded in the biohazard trash with all the used disposable sponges and towels. Sharps are disposed of in the sharps disposal container. The scrub person removes the contaminated gown and gloves and places them in the biohazard trash.
   e. The scrub person, still wearing PPE, dons nonsterile examination gloves to take the case cart to the decontamination department. Hands should be washed after removing the gloves used for transport.
   f. The environmental services personnel, wearing PPE, remove trash and linen from the room.
   g. The OR bed and attachments, any control panels, door handles, phones, plastic keyboard and foot pedal covers, and horizontal surfaces are cleaned

with an Environmental Protection Agency/ hospital–approved disinfectant for the manufacturer's recommended dwell time.

h. Any other visible soil is cleaned. The floor is damp mopped 3 to 4 feet around the OR bed and any area where soil may be present, including step stools. Studies have shown that a microfiber mop head may be more effective than string mop.

i. The cleaning process should flow from cleanest to dirtiest areas using a fresh mop for each room cleaning.

j. Care is taken not to aerosolize cleaning solutions because they may be harmful to the skin and respiratory system. The force of the spray can disperse microorganisms.

k. For larger spills containing blood, a mixture of 1:10 sodium hypochlorite (bleach) and water solution is used for cleaning.

l. Fresh bed linen and impervious trash can/linen hamper liners are used.

3. **Terminal cleaning at the end of the day.** Disinfectant solutions are used to saturate surfaces except equipment and machinery vulnerable to damage from moisture.

a. All surfaces should be wiped with hospital-approved disinfectant solution. The cleaning should start at the highest surfaces (lights, booms, and ceiling tracks) and work down to lowest tables and under table shelves and kick buckets.

b. Wheels and casters should be rolled through the disinfectant solution.

c. Standard room equipment and machinery, such as electrosurgical unit and anesthesia machine, sitting stools, step stools, and cabinet handles are wiped with disinfectant cloths.

d. Air intake grills are wiped with disinfectant.

e. The entire floor is mopped with a clean mop and disinfectant from the cleanest periphery to the most soiled areas, including under the OR bed.

f. Some facilities use UV-C light (mercury or pulsed xenon) to denature DNA, or hydrogen peroxide misting (on nonporous surfaces) to kill some endospores (*Clostridial* species: *C. difficile*, tetanus, and gangrene) and bacteria (*Staphylococcus* and *Streptococcus*) as a supplement to terminal disinfection of the room. These processes take 30 to 50 minutes to complete. Personnel should not be in the room during this adjunct disinfection process to prevent potential injury to skin or eyes.

Some UV-C light disinfection machines are designed to deliver rapid pulses and can be used between cases. They also measure and record usage for compliance documentation. UV-C units can be contained within the HVAC vents to kill airborne microorganisms.

4. **Noise and distractions in the OR** environment are significant causes for human error and potential injury to patients. Some noise in the OR is unavoidable. However, excessive nonessential talking and activities should stop during critical periods of patient care. Complex activities should not be interrupted. The creation of a *no interruption zone* (NIZ) should be established. NIZ is recommended by AORN and The Joint Commission to support patient safety.

a. Examples of **critical periods of patient care** in the NIZ include, but are not limited to, the following activities:
   1) Surgical briefings that discuss patient condition or care
   2) Surgical counts and medication distribution to the sterile field
   3) Anesthetic induction and emergence of the patient
   4) Specimen management

b. Distractions to consider include the following:
   1) *Cell phones:* Texting and social media notification tones cause an interruption of thought patterns. These should be silenced or turned off completely.
   2) *Tablets and other personal computers:* Personal electronics should not be permitted in OR unless necessary for patient care. They are also a source of contamination when taken from room to room. If used in patient care information or photography, the concern for encryption and security is important. Approved devices should be password protected.
   3) *Alarms:* Audible alarms should be set to a level where they are heard, but not so loud other necessary communication is not discernable.
   4) *Music:* Sources should not be loud enough to block necessary communication and divert the attention of the team.
   5) *Intercoms or telephones:* They should be used as needed to convey information to areas outside of the room to minimize the need to leave the surgery in process. Cautious use of the intercom is necessary if the patient is awake or under local anesthesia.
   6) *Unnecessary conversations:* These can create confusion in auditory processing of valuable information between the surgical personnel, causing a disruption in the flow of the procedure.
   7) *Metallic and powered instrumentation:* Management of metallic and powered instrumentation should be as quiet as possible. Machinery not in use should be on standby or turned off to minimize noise.
   8) *Traffic:* Maintain limited traffic flow in and out of the room, not only for infection control, but to avoid the distraction to the surgical team.

The perioperative nurse should understand the geographic zones of the perioperative environment. Traffic patterns, attire, and activities that take place in each zone of the perioperative environment must be strictly monitored. Understanding and observing the proper attire, traffic patterns, and activities for each area of the perioperative environment are important for patient safety and the prevention of infection. The perioperative nurse demonstrates the knowledge by following the recommended guidelines for the environment of the OR.

LEARNING ACTIVITIES

MULTIPLE CHOICE

INSTRUCTIONS: Identify the choice that best completes the statement or answers the question.

1. How many total air exchanges and outside air changes are required for an endoscopy room?
   a. 4 total and 2 outdoor
   b. 6 total and 6 outdoor
   c. 6 total and 2 outdoor
   d. 2 total and 6 outdoor

2. Attire for the semirestricted area includes:
   a. Scrub suit, mask, and hair cover
   b. Scrub suit and hair cover
   c. Scrub suit, hair cover, and eye protection
   d. Scrub suit

3. What attire is required for the restricted area?
   a. Scrub suit, hair cover, mask, and sterile gown
   b. Scrub suit, hair cover, and mask
   c. Scrub suit, hair cover, sterile gown, and gloves
   d. Scrub suit, hair cover, mask, sterile gown, gloves, and eyewear

4. What is considered personal protective equipment (PPE)?
   a. Scrub suit, sterile gown, and gloves
   b. Scrub suit, hair cover, and mask
   c. Sterile gown, gloves, and mask
   d. Scrub suit, sterile gown, mask, and eyewear

5. Which area does not require special attire and street clothes are permitted?
   a. Restricted area
   b. Instrument processing area
   c. Semirestricted
   d. Unrestricted

6. The decontamination room should have how many total air exchanges and how many outdoor exchanges under negative pressure?
   a. 4 total and 4 outdoor
   b. 3 total and 2 outdoor
   c. 6 total and 2 outdoor
   d. 2 total and 2 outdoor

7. Sterile storage areas should be under positive pressure with how many total air exchanges and outdoor exchanges?
   a. 4 total and 2 outdoor
   b. 2 total and 6 outdoor
   c. 4 total and 6 outdoor
   d. 6 total and 6 outdoor

8. How many air exchanges are required for the restricted areas and OR?
   a. Positive pressure
   b. 15 total and 2 outdoor
   c. Negative pressure
   d. 20 total and 4 outdoor

9. Humidity in the OR should not exceed which percentage or condensation can form?
   a. 20%
   b. 60%
   c. 50%
   d. 75%

10. The warming unit for blankets and patient gowns should not exceed what temperature?
    a. 100°F
    b. 104°F
    c. 120°F
    d. 130°F

11. Unopened irrigation solutions may be kept in a warmer for how many days?
    a. 14 days
    b. 60 days
    c. 7 days
    d. 30 days

12. At what temperature is warmed irrigation solution safe to use?
    a. 110°F
    b. 122°F
    c. 104°F
    d. 130°F

13. All of the following are true about an uncapped and opened solution bottle except:
    a. Recap and use if it is still warm
    b. Outer lip is considered contaminated
    c. Can be poured only once
    d. Cannot be recapped

14. To be efficient, when should turnover between cases begin?
    a. During the case
    b. While the patient is waking up
    c. When the patient leaves the room
    d. During the first count

15. Before the first procedure of the day, what activity should take place to prepare the room?
    a. Damp dust
    b. Bring in case cart
    c. Dry dust
    d. Position equipment

16. To prevent patient injury or error, distractions should be avoided by establishing which type of zone?
    a. No interruption zone (NIZ)
    b. Quiet zone only during time out
    c. Reduction of noise
    d. No talking zone

LEARNING ACTIVITIES ANSWERS

1. c
2. b
3. b
4. c
5. d
6. c

7. a
8. d
9. b
10. d
11. b

12. c
13. a
14. c
15. a
16. a

CHAPTER 5

Maintaining a Safe Perioperative Environment

Professional organizations make recommendations supported by evidence, but stricter controls are formally enforced by professional agencies. Some of these agencies are governmental, bound by law to monitor specific aspects of operating room (OR) activity in the interest of safety for patients and personnel. Failure of a facility to comply with regulations can cause penalties and fines. Regulatory organizations and agencies are described in Chapter 1.

Nongovernmental agencies may have reporting responsibilities to the governmental agencies for safety infractions but may not have the same authority to impose penalties. Other sanctions can ensue, such as loss of accreditation that can translate into financial loss for the facility in the form of lost reimbursement.

Regulation of Safety in the Operating Room

Professional organizations are described in detail in Chapter 1.
1. **Governmental agencies:** Examples of how they interface with the OR are as follows:
   a. OSHA (Occupational Safety and Health Administration): workplace safety
   b. FDA (US Food and Drug Administration): drug and pharmaceutical control
   c. EPA (Environmental Protection Agency): environmental impact
   d. CDC (Centers for Disease Control and Prevention): infection and disease control
   e. NIOSH (National Institute for Occupational Safety and Health): occupational safety
2. **Nongovernmental agencies:** Examples of how they interface with the OR are as follows:
   a. NFPA (National Fire Protection Association): fire safety
   b. AAMI (Association for the Advancement of Medical Instrumentation): safety of surgical instruments and equipment
   c. ANSI (American National Standards Institute): safe use of equipment and toxic materials
   d. APIC (Association for Professionals in Infection Control and Epidemiology): promote best practices in infection control
   e. ACGIH (American Conference of Governmental Industrial Hygienists): occupational safety
   f. IHI/NPSF (Institute for Healthcare Improvement/ National Patient Safety Foundation): patient and personnel safety

   g. TJC (The Joint Commission): certifies the adherence to standards and guidelines

What Are the Potential Safety Hazards in the Operating Room?

Perioperative nurses must be acutely aware of the risks associated with the perioperative environment. Safe practices protect OR personnel and patients. The dangers of the OR can cause immediate or delayed injury.

Physical Hazards
1. Physical hazards in the OR are any risks to physical safety.
   a. Ergonomic risks
      1) Body mechanics
         a) Push, roll, or slide heavy objects rather than lift.
         b) If lifting must be done, use large muscle groups in legs rather than the back. Use a wide base of support. Coordinated lifting to the count of three with adequate numbers of personnel. Use lifting or other moving devices to move patients.
         c) Tables should be at the appropriate working height. Avoid reaching. Use step stools as necessary.
         d) Wear appropriate shoes that are enclosed (no clogs) to maintain balance in the work area.
         e) Proper use of instrument design helps avoid repetitive stress injury (holding retractors, etc.).
      2) Preventing physical injury
         a) Keep floor free from spills and splashes from sterile field, and scrub sink to avoid slipping.
         b) Avoid having cords and tubing strung across walking areas to prevent tripping.
         c) Correctly remove electrical cords from the electric outlet or connection port. To avoid electrical shock, do not cut electrosurgical unit (ESU) cords.
         d) Remove pressurized cords from power equipment after the flow of gas is expelled.
         e) Carefully remove spring-loaded connectors that could cause impact injury (wall-mounted suction or oxygen delivery regulators, etc.).

b. **Radiation (ionizing and nonionizing) risk exposure:** Proximity to any radiation exposure risk is described as the **Nominal Hazard Zone** (NHZ).

1) **X-ray is ionizing** and can cause radiation effects within 24 to 48 hours or up to many years postexposure. Some of the effects include cataracts, hair loss, skin lesions, infertility, and circulatory problems. Long-term effects can include cancer and genetic changes. The duration of exposure is directly related to the severity of the physical effects.

   a) Three main considerations for radiation exposure and effects include: **Time:** What is the duration of exposure? **Distance:** How close is the ionizing force to the exposed person (NHZ)? **Shielding:** What type of barrier is between the person and the ionizing force?

   b) Personnel protection during x-ray use in patient care requires lead shields for the thyroid, eyes, and body for the team. If the wearer may have posterior x-ray exposure, the lead apron must wrap around the entire body. Radioprotective gloves may be necessary if in close proximity to the x-ray beam.

   c) Protection of the patient includes gonad and glandular shielding for body areas not directly under x-ray study.

   d) When using a C-arm, the gonad and other body shielding is placed under the patient, because the ionizing beam comes from beneath the patient. If the direction of the beam is lateral, the placement of the shielding must be between the patient and the x-ray tube (Fig. 5.1).

   e) Dosimeters are worn on the outside of the lead protection by all personnel in the presence of x-ray. A second dosimeter should be worn under the lead apron for comparison with the external monitor. The same spot should be used each time (Fig. 5.2).

      The dosimeter measures cumulative exposure over a period of time. X-ray does not dissipate, it accumulates. Dosimeters are read each month by qualified radiology personnel, and a yearly report is required by OSHA for yearly accumulation measurement.

   f) Pregnant patients and personnel must have lead shielding of the abdomen and uterus. Pregnant personnel may wear a second dosimeter monitor under the lead apron at the waist area to confirm the integrity of the lead apron.

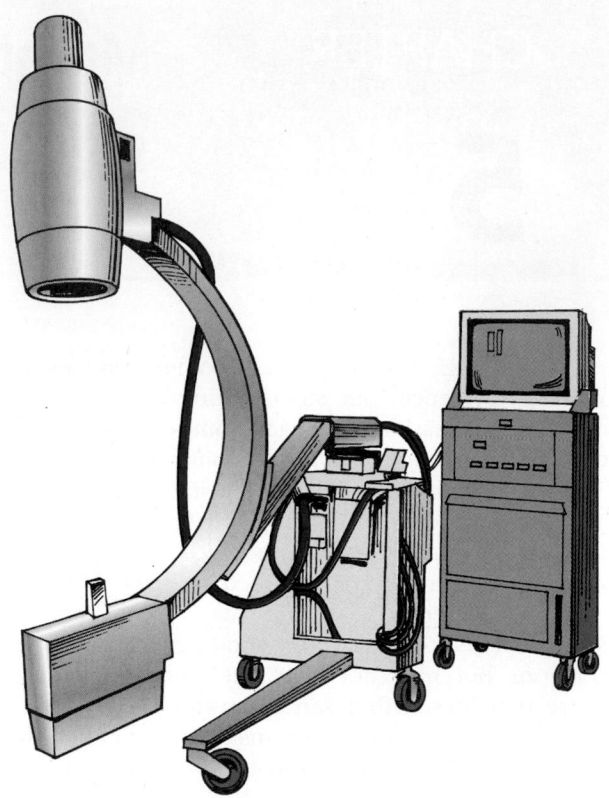

Figure 5.1 C-arm unit. (From Phillips, N. [2017]. *Berry and Kohn's operating room technique* [13th ed.]. St. Louis, MO: Elsevier.)

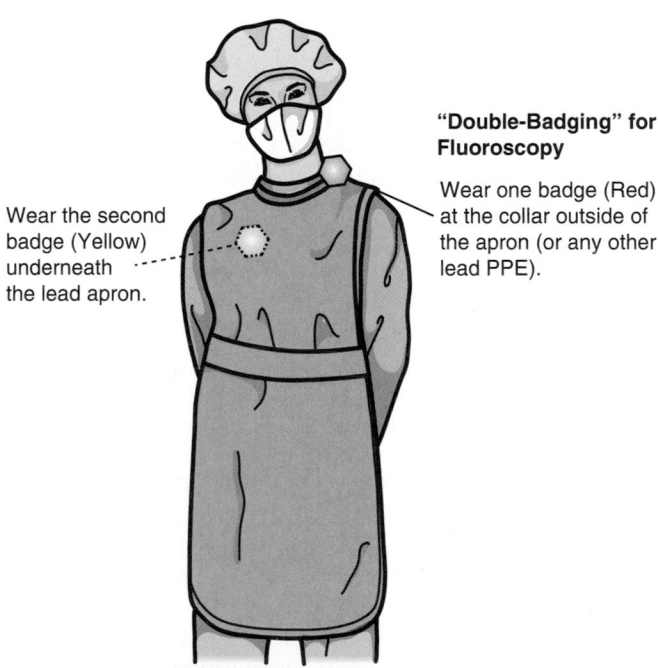

"Double-Badging" for Fluoroscopy

Wear one badge (Red) at the collar outside of the apron (or any other lead PPE).

Wear the second badge (Yellow) underneath the lead apron.

Figure 5.2 Dosimeter monitoring placement. (From Phillips, N. [2017]. *Berry and Kohn's operating room technique* [13th ed.]. St. Louis, MO: Elsevier.)

g) Lead aprons must not be folded but hung or laid flat to prevent cracks in the protective lead surface. A new lead apron should be tested for cracks before first use. Periodic checks for lead integrity should be performed by the radiology department. All lead apron testing should be documented.

h) Lead aprons are cleaned after use with a manufacturer's approved disinfectant.

2) **Nonionizing radiation is emitted by lasers.** It does not accumulate in the body. Lasers operate by transmitting light to different depths in tissue.

The main risks for laser use are burns/fires and eye damage. Lasers must be tested before each use in surgical procedures. Safety for patients and personnel include the following:

a) Doors are closed, and windows covered. Signage on the exterior door indicates type of laser in use (Fig. 5.3). Appropriate optical density protective eyewear is available outside the door in accordance with ANSI standards.

b) Lasers can reflect off shiny surfaces and transmit to an untoward area. Ebonized, anodized, or dull surfaces on instruments protect personnel in the environment. Shiny surfaces in the room must be covered.

c) Lasers can cause a fire. Place saline-moistened radiopaque sterile towels around the surgical site. Sterile saline-moistened radiopaque sponges are used to pack the throat around the endotracheal tube if a laser is used above the xyphoid process, and especially around the head and neck of the patient. Saline-moistened sponges are used in the rectum to prevent methane ignition from

bowel gas in perineal surgery. Vapors from flammable alcohol prep can be ignited if not dry before draping.

d) The cuff/balloon of the endotracheal tube is filled with saline tinted with methylene blue as an indicator of perforation by the laser. Endotracheal tubes are flammable. Laser-specific endotracheal tubes are preferred.

e) Eyes are particularly vulnerable in the presence of a laser. Each laser type has a different wavelength and requires the use of protective eyewear of an appropriate optical density for the type of laser in use. Patient's eyes are protected with saline-moistened eye pads, goggles, and/or sterile corneal shields. Personnel who continually work with lasers should have a baseline retinal scan and periodic scans to ensure eye health.

f) Lasers should be controlled by a laser safety officer who has the authority to place the device on standby or shutdown if the safety of persons in the vicinity is in question. The laser operator should not be circulating or have other distractions during the case.

g) The surgeon must be credentialed by the facility for laser use. The lowest power setting possible is used in the surgical procedure.

h) Smoke from laser use, referred to as plume, is considered a biohazard and is removed via a filtered smoke evacuator.

i) Documentation includes the name of user, laser identification number, and safety precautions employed.

c. **Preventing surgical fires.** AORN has developed a fire safety tool kit to guide perioperative nurses in prevention of surgical fires. All OR personnel must know the location and operation of the emergency gas shut-off valves and fire extinguishers. The fire triangle represents the components necessary for a fire (Fig. 5.4).

1) **Fuel:** drapes, alcohol-based prep solution

2) **Ignition:** ESU, laser, argon beam coagulator, powered equipment, defibrillator, or fiber optic light

3) **Oxidizer:** oxygen, nitrous oxide, or medical air

d. **Fire risk assessment** should be done as part of the time out before a surgical procedure begins. All team members must participate. The fire risk assessment should be documented in the patient's records. This is particularly important if the potential ignition source will be used on a surgical site above the xyphoid process.

e. How can the perioperative nurse control fuel sources in the OR?

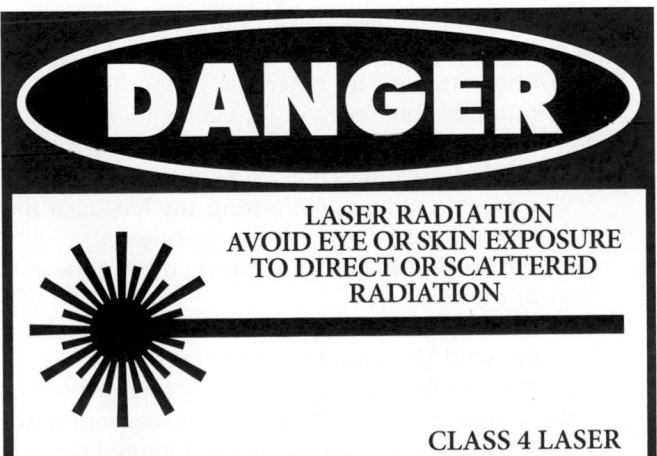

DANGER

LASER RADIATION
AVOID EYE OR SKIN EXPOSURE
TO DIRECT OR SCATTERED
RADIATION

CLASS 4 LASER

Figure 5.3 Laser warning sign. (From Phillips, N. [2017]. *Berry and Kohn's operating room technique* [13th ed.]. St. Louis, MO: Elsevier.)

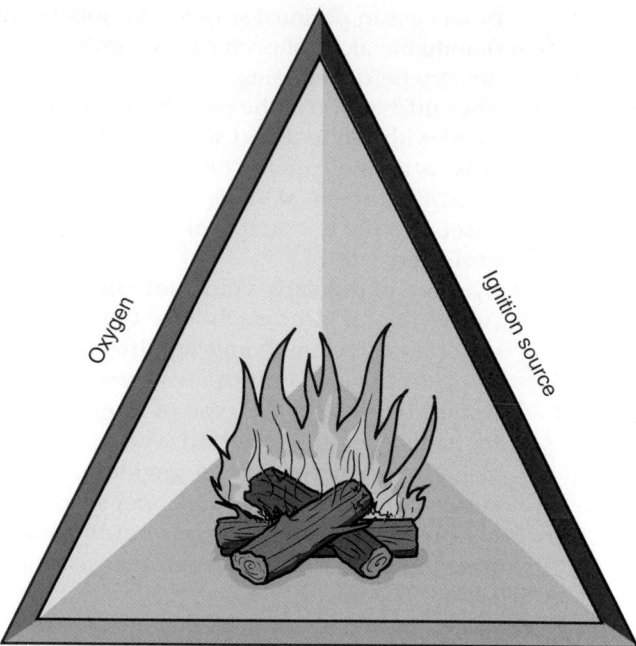

Figure 5.4 Fire triangle. (From Phillips, N. [2017]. *Berry and Kohn's operating room technique* [13th ed.]. St. Louis, MO: Elsevier.)

1) Make sure that alcohol-based antiseptic prep solution is dry before draping to prevent fumes from accumulating under the drapes. Prevent pooling under the patient.
2) Use saline-moistened drapes around the surgical site when a laser is used. Use saline-moistened throat packs around the endotracheal tube.
3) Take extreme care with combustibles on the sterile field, for example, collodion, wound glue, alcohol, liquid from gut suture packs, and tinctures.
4) Coat patient hair with water-soluble gel or lubricant instead of oil-based product.

f. How can the perioperative nurse control ignition sources in the OR?
1) ESU tip must be cleaned and contained in a holder when not in use. ESU must be on the lowest cut-blend setting possible instead of coagulation. ESU is not used near the airway (nitrous, oxygen), open chest/lungs, or distended bowel. The active electrode is controlled and used only by the person activating the handpiece. Check reusable cords for integrity.
2) Laser, ESU, and argon beam coagulator are on standby when not in use and the handpiece is holstered. Only the surgeon can activate the laser or ESU pedal.
3) Check the insulation on ESU instrumentation before use.

4) Use only moist sponges near the active ESU. The rectum must be packed with moist radiopaque sponges when working in the perineal area.
5) Sterile water and/or saline should be on the field for quick use in case of fire on the field. Appropriate fire extinguisher should be immediately available.
   a) Using a fire extinguisher follows this mnemonic: **PASS**
      (i) **P**ull the ring from the handle.
      (ii) **A**im the nozzle at the base of the fire.
      (iii) **S**queeze the handle.
      (iv) **S**weep the spray over the base of the fire.
   b) In the event of a fire, follow this mnemonic: **RACE**
      (i) **R**escue anyone in immediate danger.
      (ii) **A**ctivate the fire alarm.
      (iii) **C**ontain the fire if possible (close the door).
      (iv) **E**xtinguish the fire (some facilities use Evacuate).
6) Fiber-optic cables should not be activated and placed on drapes. Inspect light cables for integrity before use.
7) Use only appropriate-size defibrillator paddles with correct gel.
8) Prevent fluids from spilling into electrical equipment.

g. How can the perioperative nurse control for oxidizers in the OR?
1) The endotracheal tube cuff should be expanded with methylene blue–tinted saline when working in the airway.
2) Suction the airway to clear any oxygen or nitrous oxide when working near the face, mouth, or throat with an ESU or laser.
3) Use saline-moistened packs around the endotracheal tube to prevent oxidizer leaks when working in the mouth or throat.
4) Use a smoke evacuator in small spaces like the mouth for clear vision within the field.
5) Use extreme care when the patient is not intubated but receiving oxygen under a draped head. Supplemental oxygen should be turned off during cautery use. Prevent oxygen buildup under the drape when using any ESU near the face. Inform surgeon of oxygen use.
6) Ensure that the oxygen is turned off at the end of the case.
7) All supplies must be 18 inches from the ceiling to avoid blocking fire sprinklers.

h. **Protection from puncture injury** is addressed in the federal Needlestick Safety and Prevention Act of 2000. Puncture injuries are not limited to needles and blades. Other instruments, such as scissors, trocars, skin hooks, and perforating devices can puncture the skin through a glove.

Employers are required to provide safe work practice policies/procedures and safety-engineered products for use in patient care.

1) Work practice policies and procedures
   a) Use a neutral zone for passing sharps one at a time in the sterile field. Announce when a sharp is placed in the neutral zone. Orient the sharp for surgeon's safe use.
   b) Double gloving. Use indicator gloves as the inner glove. If a puncture happens, the area reveals a color (usually green or blue).
   c) Do not draw medication from a bottle or vial when someone else is holding the container.
   d) Avoid manipulating suture needles by hand when arming or positioning it in the needle holder.
   e) Remove the needle from the suture before tying a stitch.
   f) Use an instrument to retract tissue when suturing.
   g) Never recap needles by hand. Use only a one-handed scoop technique to sheath a needle.
   h) Use an instrument to remove scalpel blades, saw blades, or drill bits.
   i) Cut and cap K-wires or pins after they are passed through the patient's tissue.
   j) Use an instrument to retrieve a needle or blade that has fallen from the sterile field.
   k) Use gauze to open a glass ampule.
   l) Dispose of used sharps in a puncture-resistant biohazard container.

2) Safety-engineered products
   a) Blunt suture needles
   b) Self-capping hypodermic needles or needleless systems
   c) Scalpels: disposable, self-retracting, scalpel blade removal devices

3) Treating an accidental puncture injury during a surgical procedure
   a) Step back from the field and remove glove.
   b) Squeeze blood from the puncture site.
   c) Clean the site with soap and water, alcohol, or iodophor solution.
   d) Apply bandage and report the incident according to facility policy.
   e) Blood will be drawn from the injured person and the patient for baseline examination for infectious disease. The patient will be informed. Follow the facility's policy and procedure.

Chemical Hazards

Each chemical used in the perioperative environment has a material safety data sheet (SDS) available to provide information concerning hazardous potential, precautions, protective measures, exposure limits, first aid measures if exposed, and clean up/disposal instructions.

An emergency spill cleanup kit should be immediately available. The kit should contain appropriate personal protective equipment (PPE) and disposal equipment.

OSHA, NIOSH, and ACGIH set the standards for use of the chemicals in the perioperative environment. OSHA has the legal authority to levy fines for offenses.

1. **Anesthetic gases** can cause DNA mutation and organ damage.
   a. Waste gases are removed by a negative pressure scavenger system attached to the anesthesia machine. Check to ensure that the scavenger circuit is intact.
      Although the anesthesia equipment is maintained by the anesthesia department, when the gas machine is moved, the scavenger hose on the back of the machine can be dislodged.
   b. Overexposure to waste gases can cause birth defects. Pregnant personnel must avoid exposure.
   c. For pediatric cases where rapid sequence induction is used, gases can escape around the facemask used to deliver inhalant anesthesia. Personnel should avoid exposure.
   d. Postanesthesia care unit (PACU) patients expel anesthesia gases in their breath. Air quality in the PACU should be monitored.

2. **Sterilizing agents** used to sterilize heat-sensitive instruments and equipment can be harmful to the airway and eyes even at low-level exposure. The manufacturer's instructions for use (IFU) must be followed.
   a. **Ethylene oxide** is used in a gaseous form. It is a mutagenic and carcinogenic chemical. The sterilized item must be aerated to prevent exposure to the gas.
      1) When the chemical is in contact with water, it forms ethylene glycol, which is toxic.
      2) Inhaled ethylene oxide gas is toxic.
   b. **Glutaraldehyde** emits vapors that irritate the eyes and respiratory tract. Contact dermatitis and hives have been reported. PPE must be worn.
      1) Glutaraldehyde is used only in a container with a secure lid.
      2) It must be mixed according to the manufacturer's instructions and dated for expiration per facility policy.
   c. **Formaldehyde** (formalin) emits fumes that cause respiratory injury, and it is a carcinogen.

3. **Disinfectants** are used to clean and decontaminate the OR after every case. PPE should be worn with each use. The chemical can cause skin and eye irritation. Phenolics and hydrogen peroxide can cause skin burns.
   a. Dilution must be done according to IFU to assure effectiveness. Refer to the SDSs for information concerning the details for the chemical; this is required by OSHA.
   b. Some disinfectants can cause gloves to degrade if concentration is incorrect. Gloves of nitrile or 100% butyl rubber are preferred.

c. Do not use spray bottles because they can cause aerosolization of the disinfectant.

4. **Bone cement is poly methyl methacrylate (PMMA)** composed of a liquid and powdered polymer that is mixed on the sterile field at the point of use. Some forms contain antibiotic compounds. Double-check the patient's allergies before use.
   a. Fumes are flammable. Gloves should be changed immediately after handling the product. Some gloves degrade and break down when exposed to the chemical.
   b. The patient may become hypotensive during use.
   c. Mixing device with a suction port should be used to minimize fume distribution. The mixture has an exothermic effect.
   d. It is an eye irritant and may combine with gas-permeable contact lenses. PMMA irritates the respiratory tract and may cause drowsiness.

5. **Drugs on the sterile field** must not be aerosolized during use. Sensitive personnel could be exposed and have an allergic reaction. Some drugs can be absorbed through mucous membranes of the eyes and ears.
   a. Drugs are dispensed to the field into an appropriate container, then labeled with drug name and strength. Do not prelabel the medicine receptacle.
   b. Antineoplastic drugs may be used in the OR as a controlled irrigation.
      1) Great care is taken to avoid any contact with skin.
      2) Gloves should be changed after handling the drug.
      3) The administering surgeon should be wearing double gloves and remove the outer glove after use of the cytotoxic chemical.

Biologic Hazards

1. **Infectious waste**, blood, and bodily fluids may contain multiple drug-resistant microorganisms, endospores (clostridia and bacillus), HIV, any type of hepatitis, human papillomavirus, fungi, or prions. Biohazards can cause disease through contact with skin, needlesticks, splashes to eyes or mucous membranes, aerosolization, or accidental ingestion.
   a. All infectious and biologic waste must be disposed of in biohazard containers according to facility policies and local laws. Personnel must wear gloves when handling potentially infectious material.
   b. Handwashing must be done after removing gloves.

c. Do not eat or apply lip balm in the semirestricted or restricted areas.
   d. Patients with infectious respiratory conditions must wear a HEPA (high-efficiency particulate air) mask during transport to and from the OR.

2. **Surgical plume** can distribute pathogens, mutated microorganisms and viruses, carcinogens, and other toxic substances that can be absorbed via the respiratory tract and mucous membranes of the eye and ear canal.
   a. High-filtration HEPA masks must be worn by all personnel. Patients not intubated must wear a HEPA mask to prevent respiratory absorption of plume from other parts of the body.
   b. Plume (smoke) is removed with a smoke evacuator. Some ESU plume can be evacuated with conventional suction using an in-line filter.
   c. The smoke evacuator filter must be changed while wearing full PPE.

3. Reproductive implications of exposure to physical and chemical hazards include the following:
   a. *Male:* decreased spermatogenesis and DNA mutations
   b. *Female:* spontaneous abortion and fetal anomalies

4. Allergy and sensitivity can cause anaphylaxis.
   a. Latex particles are carried by glove powder.
      1) Plastic and silicone are safe for use.
      2) NIOSH indicates patients with multiple food allergies such as bananas, potatoes, tomatoes, avocado, papaya, chestnuts, and kiwi are likely to have latex sensitivity or allergy.
      3) Patient history may show skin irritation or respiratory symptoms when handling balloons or rubber gloves.
      4) Care is taken to use nonlatex items if the patient has suspected sensitivity or known allergy (Table 5.1).
   b. Formaldehyde used for specimens can cause allergic or sensitivity reactions.
      1) Carcinogenic
      2) Fumes can be toxic
   c. Disinfectant cleaning agents are respiratory irritants.
   d. Aerosolized medications can be absorbed via mucous membranes of the eyes and ear canals.

The OR can be a dangerous place to work because of fire risks, chemicals, microorganisms, and other hazards. The perioperative nurse should be aware of the risks and take recommended precautions to keep the environment safe.

TABLE 5.1   Care of the Latex-Sensitive Patient

Commonly Used Latex Products	Latex-Free Alternatives	Patient Teaching	Considerations
Anesthesia breathing circuit, endotracheal tube, Ambu breathing bag	Disposable plastic breathing circuits and endotracheal tubes	NA (not applicable)	Dispose of used equipment
Bite blocks for oral surgery	Dental rolls, rolled gauze squares, silicone blocks	NA	Avoid using counted radiopaque sponges
Catheters, enema tips, and drains	Silicone catheters and drains	Instruct patient to report irritation or discomfort in area of drain or catheter	Patients rarely have silicone sensitivity; check product for content in manufacturer's enclosed literature
Electrocardiogram (ECG) leads, dispersive electrodes, pulse oximeter leads	Nonlatex gel pads	Instruct patient to report irritation at application site	Patient may have sensitivity to conductive gel; may need to use water-soluble lubricant
Elastic bandages, antiembolism stockings	White cotton bandages	Instruct patient to report any sensory changes in bandaged part, such as tingling, pain, or loss of sensation	Nonelastic bandages or stockings may restrict movement and have less expansion properties; circulation may become impaired if applied too tightly
Elastic and adhesive tape	Plastic, paper, or silk tape	Instruct patient to report irritation around or under area of tape	Some patients have sensitivity to adhesive rather than tape backing
Elastic bands on surgical caps, shoe covers, urinary catheter leg bags, plastic pants, disposable diapers	Cloth towel or paper caps with ties to cover hair; cloth hook and loop leg bands, cloth diapers	Instruct patient to report irritation around hairline or leg(s)	Cloth diapers will not be impervious to leaks; cloth hook and loop bands may impair circulation to leg
Embolectomy catheters	Silicone catheters	NA	Check composition of entire catheter and balloon
Hypothermia/hyperthermia blanket, hot water bottle, heating pad, mattress cover	Disposable plastic warming blankets and pads	Instruct patient to report irritation or discomfort	Observe for temperature control of device to avoid skin injury
Latex gloves, finger cots	Plastic or other nonlatex gloves	Instruct patient that utility gloves used at home may contain latex	Use nonlatex sterile gloves; vinyl utility gloves for nonsterile activities
Positioning devices, such as egg crate–type, donuts, wedges, rolls	Gel rolls	NA	Roll gel sheets around water bags for added height
Rubber shods	Silicone catheter or plastic tubes	NA	Should be radiopaque; plastic shods are not as pliable
Syringe plungers in plastic syringes	Glass syringes	Instruct patient that plungers in plastic syringes used for self-administered injectable medications contain latex	Air-powered autoinjector device or implantable medication dispensing mechanism is an option at home
Tubing as on blood pressure cuffs and endoscopic insufflators	Disposable plastic tubing and cuff covers	NA	Wrap limb with cotton sheet wadding to avoid contact

LEARNING ACTIVITIES

TRUE/FALSE

INSTRUCTIONS: Indicate whether the statement is true or false.

_____1. It is okay to draw up medication from someone holding a bottle or vial if the needle is clean.

_____2. Double gloving with a colored inner glove is a good idea to reveal a puncture.

_____3. An instrument should be used to remove scalpel blades and saw blades.

_____4. The one-handed scoop technique is acceptable to recap needles.

_____5. If a needlestick occurs, wash the area and report it only if the patient has a disease.

MULTIPLE CHOICE

INSTRUCTIONS: Identify the choice that best completes the statement or answers the question.

6. Which governmental agency is responsible for workplace safety?
   a. FDA
   b. OSHA
   c. CDC
   d. AORN

7. Which nongovernmental agency is responsible for the safety of surgical equipment and instruments?
   a. NFPA
   b. CDC
   c. AAMI
   d. APIC

8. Which organization certifies facilities through adherence of standards and guidelines?
   a. TJC
   b. NIOSH
   c. ANSI
   d. APIC

9. What type of ergonomic injury is common due to poor body mechanics?
   a. Puncture wound
   b. Slipping
   c. Back injury
   d. Tripping

10. Which three factors determine x-ray exposure?
    a. Time, temperature, distance
    b. Time, distance, setting
    c. Time, date, shielding
    d. Time, distance, shielding

11. Where should a dosimeter badge be worn to get an accurate reading of x-ray exposure?
    a. In the pocket of the scrub suit
    b. Outside the lead protection
    c. Don't need to wear one if not having children
    d. Inside the sterile gown

12. Lasers operate by which method?
    a. Transmission of light
    b. Optical density
    c. Reflection
    d. X-ray

13. What type of risk is associated with the use of lasers?
    a. Ear damage
    b. Sunburn
    c. Eye damage, fires, and burns
    d. Puncture wound

14. To reduce reflection of a laser beam, what precautions can be taken?
    a. Wear a lead apron.
    b. Keep door closed.
    c. Use ebonized instruments.
    d. Use shiny instruments.

15. When preparing for a laser procedure, what safety precautions should the perioperative nurse have in place?
    a. Laser-specific eyewear
    b. Laser sign on exterior of door
    c. Smoke evacuator
    d. All of the above
16. Who is responsible for controlling the laser and has the authority to place it on standby or shut it down?
    a. Circulating nurse
    b. Laser safety officer
    c. Surgeon
    d. Laser representative
17. Which patient safety measure for laser use can the anesthesia provider take in the case of fire?
    a. Use a cuffed endotracheal tube filled with tinted saline.
    b. Use an LMA.
    c. Avoid using oxygen.
    d. Cover the patient's eyes with a dry towel.
18. What documentation is required for laser use?
    a. The name of the procedure
    b. The name of the laser
    c. User name, laser identification number, and safety precautions used
    d. Laser name, user name, and representative name
19. Which mnemonic is followed for fire extinguisher use?
    a. RACE
    b. ACGIH
    c. NFPA
    d. PASS
20. In the event of a fire, what is the second step of the fire mnemonic?
    a. Activate alarm.
    b. Run.
    c. Contain the fire.
    d. Extinguish the fire.
21. Anesthetic gases are hazardous. How should they be removed?
    a. Breathing circuit
    b. Blue hose
    c. Suction
    d. Purple scavenger system
22. Which substance can cause eye and respiratory irritation for staff in the OR?
    a. Glutaraldehyde
    b. Ethylene oxide
    c. BONE cement (PMMA)
    d. Formalin

MATCHING
INSTRUCTIONS: Place the treatment of a needlestick in order.
    a. Follow facility policy for baseline blood draws.
    b. Clean site.
    c. Move away from the sterile field and remove the glove.
    d. Squeeze blood from the puncture.
    e. Apply bandage and report incident.
_____23. Step 1
_____24. Step 2
_____25. Step 3
_____26. Step 4
_____27. Step 5

LEARNING ACTIVITIES ANSWERS

TRUE/FALSE

1. F
2. T
3. T
4. T
5. F

MULTIPLE CHOICE

6. b
7. c
8. a
9. c
10. d
11. b
12. a
13. c
14. c
15. d
16. b
17. a
18. c
19. d
20. b
21. d
22. c

MATCHING

23. c
24. d
25. b
26. e
27. a

CHAPTER 6

Preoperative Patient Care

The patient planning to have a surgical procedure relies on the perioperative team for safe and efficient care. Provision of preoperative care is based on knowledge of physical and psychosocial assessment of the patient. The first phase of care establishes a baseline by which to measure the patient's condition throughout the stay in the facility.

The process begins with the surgeon's assessment, and the patient is determined to need a surgical procedure. The collaboration between the preoperative nurses and the surgeon builds the foundation for the patient's perioperative plan of care. The preoperative nurses use data gleaned from the surgeon's assessment and laboratory reports as the beginning of the nursing process.

The nursing process generates the plan of perioperative care. A comprehensive surgical checklist as part of **Universal Protocol** is initiated, and this is used throughout the patient's course in the perioperative environment. See The AORN Surgical Checklist Figure 1-2 in Chapter one.

Nursing Process

Assessment

Identify the patient with at least two methods (name and birth date). Apply wrist or ankle band as appropriate. Parents or guardians can identify a child or adult who is incapable of completing the identification process. Confirm the presence of the signed consent to treat, and that informed consent has been obtained. Are DNR (do not resuscitate) or AND (allow natural death), orders, living will, advance directive, or durable power of attorney present in the medical record? See Chapter 1 for an expanded outline of the nursing process.

Two aspects of patient assessment by the preoperative nurse include a brief review of systems and a brief head-to-toe observation (Box 6.1).

1. **Brief review of systems** includes the data retrieved from laboratory reports and other medical professionals reviewed by the preoperative nurse.
   a. **Laboratory results.** Ensure that all ordered preoperative tests have been performed and the results are available for review. Inform the surgeon and the anesthesia provider of any abnormal or critical results (Tables 6.1 and 6.2).

1) Laboratory results are reported electronically in most instances. The reference range accompanies each entry. Any abnormality is indicated by a capital H or L in the same line. Critical-level results may be augmented by a series of asterisks (***).
2) Reference ranges (also known as expected values) are measured by units of scale. Each facility uses a particular scale for reference that may differ according to whether conventional, metric, or SI units are used. Not every facility in the United States uses the same unit of measurement, so it may vary between institutions.
3) Drugs, comorbidities, pathology, meals, or time of day can cause interference with some of the results. Some results will differ according to sex. Females and menstrual cycles are examples. Extremes of age have an influence on some results.

   b. **Scans, x-rays, and other diagnostics.** Reports of preoperative magnetic resonance imaging (MRI), computed tomography (CT), or other radiologic examinations are available. A report from the radiologist reading the test should be available. Are the reports of ordered preoperative diagnostic tests available in the medical records?
   c. **History and physical (H&P) examination.** The H&P must be completed and available. The preoperative diagnosis and the planned surgical procedure are included. The H&P should include any comorbid conditions and routine medication regimen. Previous surgical procedures and associated medical diagnosis are described. The H&P should be current within the policies and procedures of the facility.
   d. **Physical examination by preoperative nurse**
      1) Compare baseline vital signs (temperature, pulse, blood pressure, pulse oximetry) with the vital signs in the medical record. Any abnormal vital signs are documented and reported to the surgeon and anesthesia provider.
      2) Record allergies and sensitivities. Ask about reaction when exposed to the substance.
      3) Discuss NPO status and last meal.
      4) When were any herbals and/or medications last taken? Any use of over-the-counter medications?

COMPREHENSIVE SURGICAL CHECKLIST

Blue = World Health Organization (WHO)   Green = The Joint Commission - Universal Protocol (JC) 2013 National Patient Safety Goals   Orange = JC and WHO

PREPROCEDURE CHECK-IN	SIGN-IN	TIME-OUT	SIGN-OUT
In Holding Area	Before Induction of Anesthesia	Before Skin Incision	Before the Patient Leaves the OR
Patient/patient representative actively confirms with Registered Nurse (RN):	RN and anesthesia care provider confirm:	Initiated by designated team member All other activities to be suspended (unless a life-threatening emergency)	RN confirms:
Identity □ Yes Procedure and procedure site □ Yes Consent(s) □Yes Site marked □ Yes □ N/A by person performing the procedure **RN confirms presence of:** History and physical□ Yes Preanesthesia assessment □ Yes Diagnostic and radiologic test results □ Yes □ N/A Blood products □ Yes □ N/A Any special equipment, devices, implants □ Yes □ N/A	Confirmation of: identity, procedure, procedure site and consent(s) □Yes Site marked □ Yes □ N/A by person performing the procedure Patient allergies Yes N/A Difficult airway or aspiration risk? □ No □ Yes (preparation confirmed) Risk of blood loss (greater than 500 mL) □ Yes □ N/A # of units available _____ Anesthesia safety check completed □ Yes **Briefing:** All members of the team have discussed care plan and addressed concerns □ Yes	Introduction of team members □ Yes **All:** Confirmation of the following: identity, procedure, incision site, consent(s) □ Yes Site is marked and visible □ Yes □N/A Relevant images properly labeled and displayed □ Yes □ N/A Any equipment concerns? **Anticipated Critical Events Surgeon:** States the following: □ Critical or Nonroutine steps □ Case duration □ Anticipated blood loss **Anesthesia provider:** □ Antibiotic prophylaxis within 1 hour before incision □ Yes □ N/A □ Additional concerns? **Scrub and circulating nurse:** □ Sterilization indicators have been confirmed □ Additional concerns?	Name of operative procedure Completion of sponge, sharp, and instrument counts □ Yes □ N/A Specimens identified and labeled □ Yes □ N/A Any equipment problems to be addressed? □ Yes □ N/A **To all team members:** What are the key concerns for recovery and management of this patient? _____ _____ _____ _____ _____ _____ June 2013 **⟁ AORN**
Include in Preprocedure check-in as per institutional custom: Beta blocker medication given (SCIP) □Yes □N/A Venous thromboembolism prophylaxis ordered (SCIP) □Yes □N/A Normothermia measures (SCIP) □Yes □N/A			

The Joint Commission does not stipulate which team member initiates any section of the checklist except for site marking. The Joint Commission also does not stipulate where these activities occur. See the Universal Protocol for details on the Joint Commission requirements.

5) Any prosthetics, contact lenses, or dentures? Any surgical procedures involving implants? Any pacemaker or internal defibrillator?

6) Any history of self or family complications during surgery or anesthesia?

7) Any systemic (musculoskeletal or neurologic) mobility problems?

8) Will the patient's size or body weight affect the type of instrumentation or operating room (OR) bed weight limit?

9) Are any of the preoperative nurse's assessment findings different from the data in the H&P? Any differences must be brought to the attention of the surgeon and anesthesia provider.

BOX 6.1   Assessment by the Preoperative Nurse Using Brief Review of Systems and Brief Head-to-Toe Observation

Review of Body Systems (Brief History)

- Is the patient a reliable historian, or is a family member translating or communicating on his or her behalf?
- Is the patient taking any medication on a regular basis (e.g., heart or blood pressure medications)? This should include vitamins, hormones, or herbal preparations.
- Does the patient have any allergies? What are the patient's reactions when exposed to the offending substance? Is the reaction localized or systemic?
- When was the patient's last meal and oral intake? If this is an emergency, what were the foods in this meal? Red foods may falsely imply gastrointestinal bleeding if the patient vomits.
- Has the patient ever had any surgery before? This may reveal a condition that requires special positioning or other modification to the standard plan of care.
- Has the patient experienced any complications during previous surgeries?
- Does the patient wear contact lenses or prosthetic parts?
- Does the patient have any trouble moving limbs?
- Is the patient extremely large or small? This may indicate the need for additional instruments or a weight-appropriate operating room (OR) bed.
- Is the patient aware of the procedure being performed?
- Are laboratory studies and blood work reports included with the chart? Are they current?

Head-to-Toe Assessment (Brief Physical)

- Is the patient here for a scheduled procedure, urgent or emergent care, or possibly a redo from an earlier surgery? This may alter the needed supplies for the case.
- Is the patient a child or adult? Is a parent present?
- Observe the color of the patient's skin and body tissues.
- Listen to the sound of the patient's voice as he or she speaks. Is it raspy or breathless? Is the patient coughing? Note any odors on breath or body.
- Touch the patient's skin as the dialogue progresses. Is it cool, hot, damp, dry, or in any other condition? This assessment can be performed as part of shaking hands. Does the patient have a weak or strong handshake or grasp? Is the patient shaky?
- Is there eye contact, and do the eyes move appropriately?
- Is one or the other eyelid drooping? Is the patient crying?
- Does the patient have enough physical coordination to point to the surgical site? Has the correct site been marked per facility policy and procedure?
- Does the patient appear to understand what is being said? Can the patient speak and respond appropriately?
- Does the patient have a Foley catheter or an ostomy? Is the patient continent?
- Are intravenous (IV) fluids running? Is the line infusing? Are additives in the container?
- Is the correct surgical site marked with the surgeon's initials?

Most of these assessment activities can be performed simultaneously in just a few minutes and may lead to additional nursing diagnoses that require a modification of the plan of care.

From Phillips, N. (2017). *Berry and Kohn's operating room technique* (13th ed.). St. Louis, MO: Elsevier.

---

2. **Brief head-to-toe assessment** and reaffirmation of identification
   a. Objective observations by the preoperative nurse
      1) Observe behavioral mannerisms and psychosocial affect. Does the patient make eye contact? Is the patient crying or emotionally distracted? Is the patient relatively calm? Does the patient interact with family or significant other? Does the patient confirm understanding of the surgical procedure and what to expect postoperatively? Is a language barrier present? Is a translator needed? Confirm that the patient has an adult to provide a ride home.
      2) Confirm the surgical site and planned procedure. Ask the patient to point to and describe the surgical site. The surgeon, postgraduate medical student, advanced practice nurse, or physician assistant, if attending the surgical procedure, should **mark the surgical site** with initials or a mark designated by the facility. Areas that cannot be marked are confirmed in a manner approved by the facility. The nurse should document the marking process in the patient's record.
      3) Observe the patient's skin color and characteristics. Is the patient cold or diaphoretic? Are any reddened areas or injuries present? Does the patient have tattoos on or near the surgical site?
      4) As the patient breathes and speaks, is the vocal quality clear without congestion or cough? Is the speech slurred or understandable? Is there any particular odor to the breath or body?
      5) Is the patient able to move all extremities? Any complaints of pain? Any neurologic deficits?
      6) Any catheters, intravenous (IV) lines, drains, or ostomies?
      7) Body piercings, jewelry, hair pins, and prosthetic appliances are removed. Disposition of personal effects is documented in the patient's medical record. The items are secured. Nail polish is removed to facilitate the use of pulse oximetry and observe the color of the nailbeds.

TABLE 6.1   2018 Normal Blood Chemistry Laboratory Values and the Influences on Results

Blood Component	Normal Values for Adult 2018	Examples of What Can Influence the Result
ALP (alkaline phosphatase)	32–117 unit/L	Elevated: recent meal, antibiotics, metastatic cancer, healing fracture Decreased: pernicious anemia, malnutrition, celiac disease, hypothyroidism
ALT (alanine aminotransferase)	7–38 unit/L	Elevated: smoking, heart failure, hemolytic disease Decreased: essential hypertension
AST (aspartate aminotransferase)	13–35 unit/L	Elevated: myocardial infarction, hepatitis, mononucleosis, muscle trauma, burns Decreased: pregnancy, renal dialysis, ketoacidosis
Ammonia	15–50 μmol/L	Elevated: liver disease, gastrointestinal bleeding, heart failure, hemolysis, alcoholism Decreased: essential hypertension, malignant hypertension
Albumin	3.9–4.9 g/dL	Elevated: acute infection, burns Decreased: malnutrition, liver disease
Amylase	56–190 international unit/L	Elevated: mumps, pancreatitis, necrotic bowel, peptic ulcer, cholecystitis, ketoacidosis, ectopic pregnancy Decreased: intravenous (IV) glucose = false negative, oxalates
Anion gap	9–18 mmol/L	Elevated: acidosis, renal disease Decreased: multiple myeloma
Bilirubin (total)	0.2–1.3 mg/dL	Elevated: jaundice, anabolic steroids, antibiotics, antimalarials, dextran, codeine, diuretics, epinephrine Decreased: barbiturates, high-dose aspirin, caffeine
BUN (blood urea nitrogen)	7–21 mg/dL	Elevated: hypovolemia, burns, dehydration, myocardial infarction, sepsis, renal disease Decreased: liver failure, fluid overload, malnutrition, pregnancy
Calcium (Ca)	8.5–10.2 mg/dL	Elevated: hyperparathyroidism, bone metastasis, lymphoma, excess vitamin D, tuberculosis Decreased: low pH value, prolonged tourniquet time, fat embolism, pancreatitis, anticonvulsants, heparin, diuretics, estrogen, malnutrition
Chloride (Cl)	97–105 mmol/L	Elevated: androgens, saline infusion, cortisone, eclampsia, metabolic acidosis, respiratory alkalosis, estrogen, nonsteroidal antiinflammatory drugs (NSAIDs) Decreased: corticosteroids, diuretics, bicarbonates
CPK (creatine phosphokinase)		Elevated: skeletal muscle injury, myocardial infarction, alcoholism Decreased: connective tissue disease
Creatinine	0.58–0.96 mg/dL	Elevated: kidney disease, diabetic nephropathy, rhabdomyolysis, acromegaly, aminoglycosides, chemotherapy, cephalosporins Decreased: muscular disease
CO_2 (carbon dioxide)	22–30 mmol/L	Elevated: metabolic alkalosis, vomiting, starvation, emphysema Decreased: renal failure, aspirin toxicity, metabolic acidosis, ketoacidosis
Glucose	74–99 mg/dL	Elevated: diabetes, stress, myocardial infarction, antidepressants, corticosteroids, diuretics, lithium, aspirin toxicity, pancreatitis Decreased: alcohol, anabolic steroids, insulin, propranolol, insulinoma, hypothyroidism, Addison's disease, liver disease, starvation
Magnesium (Mg)	1.5–2.2 mEq/L	Elevated: renal insufficiency, hypothyroidism, Addison's disease, uncontrolled diabetes, antacids, laxatives, lithium Decreased: malnutrition, malabsorption, diuretics, antibiotics, alcoholism, diabetic acidosis
Phosphate (P)	0.8–1.5 mmol/L	Elevated: renal failure, acromegaly, rhabdomyolysis, hypoparathyroidism, bone metastasis, laxatives, IV glucose, advanced lymphoma or myeloma, hemolytic anemia, acidosis Decreased: chronic antacid use, hypoparathyroidism, sepsis, alkalosis, hyperinsulinism, vitamin D deficiency, osteomalacia, malnutrition

(Continued)

TABLE 6.1   2018 Normal Blood Chemistry Laboratory Values and the Influences on Results—cont'd

Blood Component	Normal Values for Adult 2018	Examples of What Can Influence the Result
Potassium (K)	3.7–5.1 mmol/L	Elevated: renal failure, hypoaldosteronism, hemolysis, infection, acidosis, dehydration Decreased: burns, gastrointestinal distress, diuretics, ascites, licorice, insulin, cystic fibrosis, trauma
Protein, total	6.3–8.0 g/dL	Elevated: multiple myeloma, lupus, androgens, anabolic steroids, corticosteroids, growth hormones Decreased: malnutrition, pregnancy, burns, enteropathy, uropathy, increased IV crystalloids, oral contraceptives
Sodium (Na)	136–144 mmol/L	Elevated: anabolic steroids, antibiotics, clonidine, corticosteroids, laxatives, oral contraceptives, diabetes insipidus Decreased: diuretics, heparin, haloperidol, NSAIDs, antidepressants, vasopressin, ACE (angiotensin-converting enzyme) inhibitors, gastrointestinal distress, third spacing, peripheral edema, congestive heart failure

TABLE 6.2   Complete Blood Cell Count and Clotting Profile

Blood Cell	Male	Female
Red blood cells	4.4–5.9×10^6/mL	3.8–5.2×10^6/mL
Hematocrit	40%–52%	35%–47%
Hemoglobin	13–18 g/dL	12–16 g/dL
White blood cells	3500–11,000 mm^3	Same
Differential		
Neutrophils	40%–80%	Same
Eosinophils	0.5%	Same
Basophils	0.2%	Same
Monocytes	3%–8%	Same
Lymphocytes	10%–40%	Same
Clotting profile		
Platelets	150,000–400,000/mm	Same
Prothrombin time (PT)	12–15 seconds	Same
Partial thromboplastin time (PTT)	60–70 seconds	Same
International normalized ratio (INR)	<2.0–3.0	Same

b. Is an IV present and running? What medications are infusing? Have any other medications been administered?

1) Are any preoperative medications ordered before transfer to the OR. Is IV access needed (e.g., antibiotic to be given 1 hour before incision time per SCIP (Surgical Care Improvement Project) protocol?

2) Has the patient had any other ordered preoperative preparation such as antiseptic bath/shower with chlorhexidine or a bowel cleansing?

Nursing Diagnosis

Formulate the nursing diagnosis as defined by NANDA-I (North American Nursing Diagnosis Association International, Inc.; see Box 6.2 and see also Chapter 1 for a description of NANDA-I).

BOX 6.2   Examples of Nursing Diagnoses in the Perioperative Setting That are Actual or Potential Risks

Needs Identified by Nursing Diagnosis
- Knowledge deficit
- Ineffective decision making
- Alteration in spirituality

Problems Identified by Nursing Diagnosis
- Acute pain
- Alteration in body temperature
- Ineffective airway clearance

Health Status Considerations Identified by Nursing Diagnosis
- Exposure to cigarette smoke
- Occupational hazard exposure
- Substance abuse

1. Analysis of the nursing assessment provides the data used in formulation of the nursing diagnosis. The nursing diagnosis corresponds to a specific actual or potential need, problem, or health status consideration. Examples include:
   a. *Need:* knowledge deficit, anxiety relief
   b. *Problem:* health condition such as altered breathing or impaired circulation
   c. *Health status consideration:* occupational risks, smoking, recreational drug use
2. **Nursing diagnosis meshes with the domains of the Perioperative Nursing Data Set (PNDS)**
   a. *Safety:* risks and protection
   b. *Physiologic responses* to treatment
   c. *Behavioral responses*: knowledge and ethical/legal
   d. *Health system effects*

Outcomes
Identify the desired outcomes. The PNDS has identified 39 desired perioperative outcomes specific to patients in surgery. The outcomes are attainable through the nursing interventions. The patient should collaborate as much as possible. Outcomes are measurable and clear. Examples include:
1. **Psychosocial examples**
   a. Patient or support person participates in planning care.
   b. Patient's value system, ethnicity, and lifestyle are incorporated in planning care.
2. **Physiologic examples**
   a. Patient is free from harm caused by thermal sources.
   b. Patient is free from harm caused by positioning for the surgical procedure.

Planning
Through assessment, establishing the nursing diagnoses, and identification of the desired outcomes, a perioperative plan of care is developed. A combination of nursing knowledge of the patient and the planned surgical procedure is the foundation for planning care. The preoperative nurse begins the patient care planning and communicates with the intraoperative team to implement the plan.
1. **Psychosocial examples**
   a. The patient's expressed needs are incorporated into the plan of care.
   b. The patient's religious beliefs are incorporated into the plan of care.
2. **Physiologic examples**
   a. The appropriate positioning devices are prepared for the patient and the planned surgical procedure.
   b. The appropriate warming devices are prepared for the patient and the planned surgical procedure.

Implementation
Perioperative nursing **interventions** are derived from the development of assessment data identified through the nursing process. There are 151 identified perioperative nursing interventions recognized by NANDA-I and the PNDS.
1. **Psychosocial examples**
   a. The patient has signed a blood refusal form for religious reasons.
   b. The child is permitted a stuffed animal in the OR for psychologic comfort.
2. **Physiologic examples**
   a. The patient was safely positioned and secured for the surgical procedure.
   b. The surgical site is prepped with the appropriate antiseptic agent without introducing contamination.

Evaluation
The goal of evaluation is to measure how well the desired outcomes were met through nursing intervention.
1. **Psychosocial examples**
   a. The patient experienced the surgical procedure without demonstrating anxiety.
   b. The patient (and/or family) verbalizes understanding of postoperative instructions.
2. **Physiologic examples**
   a. The patient's skin shows no injury caused by positioning.
   b. The patient is at or returning to normothermia at the end of the surgical procedure.

Hand-Over (i.e., Hand-Off) to the Intraoperative Nurse
Successful communication for safe patient care is evidenced by the studies reported in "Guideline for Team Communication" in AORN's (Association of periOperative Registered Nurses's) 2018 *Guidelines for Perioperative Nursing*.
1. **Professional communication** is critical for the safety of the patient and the team. Communication between perioperative team members is a combination of the spoken word and documented information. Contemporary documentation of patient care is computerized. Formats commonly use a directed form (paper format or computerized) with specific fields to complete in a specific order.

   Universal Protocol (perioperative checklist initially developed by WHO the World Health Organization) can be computerized or a paper format and started in the preoperative care area as part of the "hand-over" protocol. Using the same comprehensive document throughout the perioperative care period establishes a continuity of care for the patient. Each subsequent caregiver adds to the document.

The preoperative nurse communicates verbally in addition to a standardized documented form. Verbal communication during the hand over from the preoperative nurse to the intraoperative nurse should use a standardized format.

Some key elements of a successful patient-oriented exchange include avoiding distractions and meaningless dialogue, and read back of information. Studies have shown that verbally repeating the key points promotes recall and fewer miscommunications. At the conclusion of the exchange, ask if there are any other questions. Communication must always be two-way transmissions. Several mnemonics provide the framework for a standardized verbal communication between caregivers (Box 6.3).

a. Standardized verbal communication techniques: Mnemonic examples include the following:
  1) **SBAR:** situation, background, assessment, recommendations
  2) **I PASS The BATON:** introduction, patient, assessment, situation, safety concerns, background actions, timing, ownership
b. **Barriers to communication** that can lead to errors and potential harm to a patient
  1) **Human factors:** inattentiveness, multitasking, use of nonstandard language, lack of respect for the process, poor communication skills, transmitting inaccurate information, misunderstanding the information
  2) **Environmental factors:** ringing phones, excessive traffic flow, or questionable privacy during exchange
2. **Communication between the preoperative nurse and the intraoperative nurse during the hand-over process**
  a. Identification of patient, procedure, and surgical site/side with patient (or significant other) involvement
  b. Report of nursing assessment: highlight baselines and any abnormal findings
  c. Discussion of any abnormal findings reported to surgeon or anesthesia provider
  d. Location of waiting family or significant other

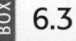

BOX 6.3 | Preoperative Hand-Over Exchange Between the Preoperative Nurse and the Intraoperative Nurse

Patient's Name and Birth Date (Identification Band, Allergy Band, or Other)
• Confirmation with parent or guardian of minor child

Planned Surgical Procedure and Correct Side/Site (Marked)
• Verification of consents and the surgeon's name
• Advance directives

Medical and Surgical History (Baseline Vital Signs, Height, and Weight [in Kilograms])
• Physical mobility issues, include skin condition and NPO status
• Any pain or other discomfort
• Allergies or sensitivities
• Any prosthetics or appliances
• Any communication barriers with patient
• Presence of intravenous (IV) lines or catheters
• Any antiembolic measures ordered
• Any special precautions (i.e., tuberculosis or infectious respiratory condition)

Current Routine Medications and All Preoperative Medication Administration
• Any blood or specialty pharmaceuticals on hold as ordered

Laboratory Reports
• Significant laboratory findings
• Results of scans or x-rays

Location of Family or Significant Other During the Surgical Procedure
• Any psychosocial or spiritual concerns

The surgical process starts with the surgeon's assessment of the patient and determination of the need for surgery. The nursing process begins with assessment and establishing the plan for perioperative patient care. The preoperative assessment and universal surgical checklist guide the perioperative nurse throughout the surgical procedure for continuity of care.

LEARNING ACTIVITIES

INSTRUCTIONS: Complete the word search puzzle. Use the clues to help identify the words.

```
J U P P C Z J B U Y W P R R J N E F B D K T I S Y B H L B M
H L P H A G N G Y B W V K Z B M U P P E I S L F X V Y M B N
U A S X Y A K B A R R I E R S N Y R S E H A D B P B E M E W
O N N P O S P S R R P T H N O J E D S Y C A G E R J N P S N
F V I D P F I N U D G T H I U Z F A S I C W V N N Q Y D O N
J Q Y V O M P C D R Z C T L I R X O S Z N H U I O Z E G J H
A A M C E V Z D A S G A R U R P S Y B J R G O W O S I Y J E
K J L H E R E I J L C I U I Q E H I L B O O P S D R T E G A
W B P D A I S R O I E M C E T P T P N M E C M R O D A I A L
S P V U C W K A F A E X V A D I Y F E G I E N R O C A L C T
S O V Q B Z C I L L S I A N L T C B X G D A I J D C I Z G H
A N J L H F T N B P T S A M E S I A O G L I J K M F E A Z S
T E N G B N A O K C R Y E F I H I L L P I Q A A P J O S L Y
A U Q P E I R R E C R O A S C N O T C E V P G G O N Y H S S
D S N D D P I J X O V S T G S I A K E F Z U O W N V P H D T
T K I R D F B N T A Q K P O S M J T E F Q D N N L O G Y C E
Q I A S Q O O S L F O E J Y C F E P I I R N W W M H S B O M
P U I V D U I D M Z F O H H G O D N O O U S N W C U V I B L
G O J E C H E J A H C P A P N T L Z T W N A R H Y I P S S D
M K M P S Q H M Q U J T J O C A O U T C O M E S S B A R C O
```

1. Brief review of systems or head-to-toe _____.
2. _____ to communication can lead to errors and patient harm.
3. _____ response is part of PNDS that includes knowledge and ethics/legality.
4. Laboratory reference ranges are measured by units of scale. _____ levels may be indicated by "H" or "L" or a series of asterisks (***).
5. Any reports, such as MRI, x-ray, or CT, are _____ reports that should be in the medical record.
6. A parent or _____ can identify a child or adult who is incapable.
7. Verbal communication during the _____ from the preoperative nurse to the intraoperative nurse should use a standardized format.
8. _____ effects is part of PNDS.
9. The _____ should be completed with diagnosis, planned procedure, comorbid conditions, current medications, and previous surgical procedures.
10. _____ requires at least two methods, such as name and birth date.
11. Analysis of the nursing assessment provides the data used in formulation of the _____.
12. _____ generates the plan of care.
13. The perioperative nurse uses _____ observations.
14. _____ are measurable through nursing interventions.
15. Hands-on examination or _____.
16. _____ response to treatment is a domain of PNDS.
17. Through assessment, nursing diagnosis, and desired outcomes, a perioperative _____ of care can be developed.
18. There are four domains of the _____.
19. A nursing diagnosis correlates with a need, _____, or health consideration.

20. The patient's needs and beliefs are expressed through _____ values.
21. _____ is a domain of PNDS that includes risk and protection.
22. _____ is a standardized form of communication: Situation, Background, Assessment, Recommendations.
23. The _____ should be marked with initials and indelible ink by the surgeon or designated person attending the procedure.
24. The comprehensive surgical checklist is part of _____.

LEARNING ACTIVITIES ANSWERS

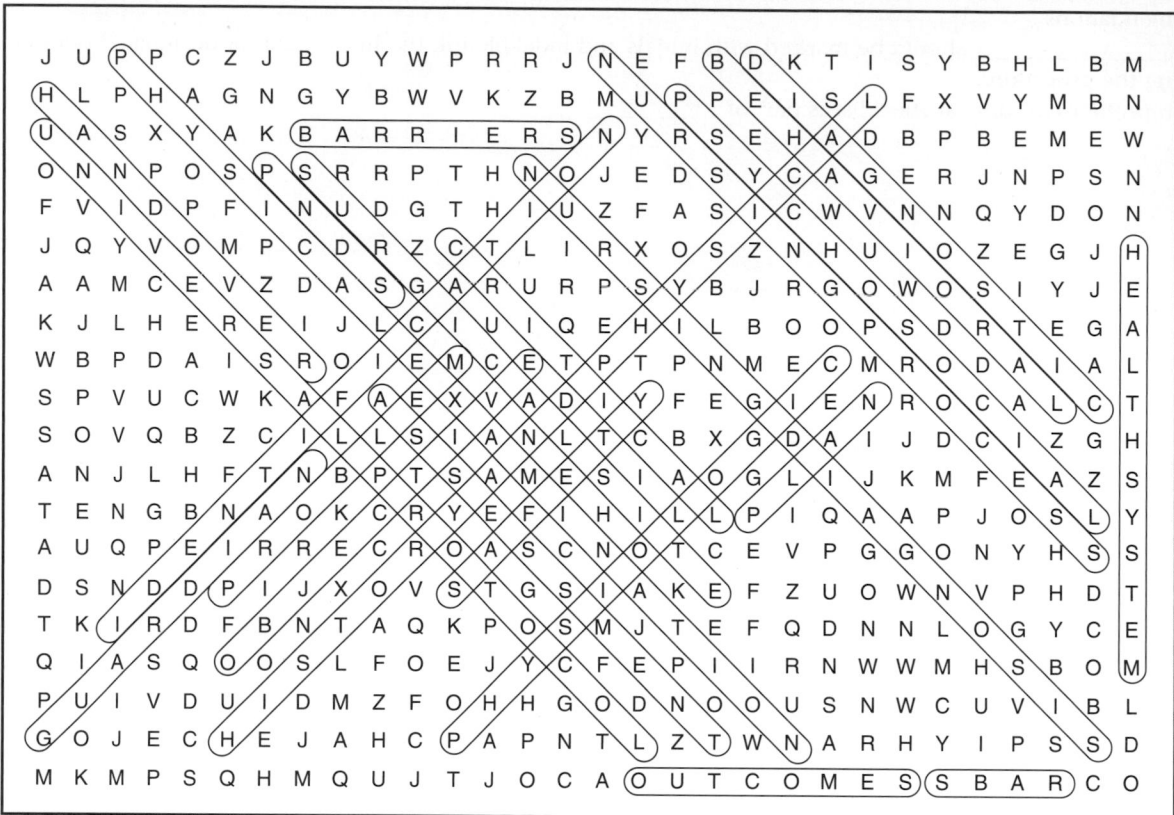

1. Brief review of systems or head-to-toe **assessment**.
2. **Barriers** to communication can lead to errors and patient harm.
3. **Behavioral** response is part of PNDS that includes knowledge and ethics/legality.
4. Laboratory reference ranges are measured by units of scale. **Critical** levels may be indicated by "H" or "L" or a series of asterisks (***).
5. Any reports, such as MRI, x-ray, or CT, are **diagnostic** reports that should be in the medical record.
6. A parent or **guardian** can identify a child or adult who is incapable.
7. Verbal communication during the **hand over** from the preoperative nurse to the intraoperative nurse should use a standardized format.
8. **Health system** effects is part of PNDS.
9. The **history and physical** should be completed with diagnosis, planned procedure, comorbid conditions, current medications, and previous surgical procedures.
10. **Identification** requires at least two methods, such as name and birth date.
11. Analysis of the nursing assessment provides the data used in formulation of the **nursing diagnosis**.
12. **Nursing process** generates the plan of care.
13. The perioperative nurse uses **objective** observations.
14. **Outcomes** are measurable through nursing interventions.
15. Hands-on examination or **physical examination**.
16. **Physiologic** response to treatment is a domain of PNDS.
17. Through assessment, nursing diagnosis, and desired outcomes, a perioperative **plan** of care can be developed.
18. There are four domains of the **PNDS**.
19. A nursing diagnosis correlates with a need, **problem**, or health consideration.

20. The patient's needs and beliefs are expressed through **psychosocial** values.
21. **Safety** is a domain of PNDS that includes risk and protection.
22. **SBAR** is a standardized form of communication: Situation, Background, Assessment, Recommendations.
23. The **surgical site** should be marked with initials and indelible ink by the surgeon or designated person attending the procedure.
24. The comprehensive surgical checklist is part of **Universal Protocol**.

Intraoperative Patient Care

The perioperative nurse circulator receives the patient from the preoperative nurse. Care is taken to relay all pertinent information during the hand over. In most instances the Universal Protocol (comprehensive surgical checklist) initiated by World Health Organization (WHO) is started in the preoperative area, and the baseline data are documented. In some facilities the preoperative nurse is not the person transporting the patient and may call the circulating nurse on the telephone and deliver a verbal report in addition to the comprehensive surgical checklist. The utilization of a universal checklist continues in the operating room (OR) to guide and document each step of the patient care safety and process in the intraoperative phase of the surgical procedure.

Receiving the Patient in the Operating Room

A discussion of times to document can be found in Chapter 1.

Universal Protocol

Universal Protocol is designed to assure that the right patient is having the right surgical procedure on the correct location on the body.

1. A **comprehensive surgical checklist** should contain information concerning the patient's planned procedure, the surgeon, and informed consent. The current history and physical must be available in the patient's medical record. The intraoperative nurse must assess the patient (Box 7.1). Refer to Chapter 6 for details concerning patient assessment.

   Pertinent information is documented, such as baseline vital signs, height/weight, current laboratory and radiology results, medical condition and/or comorbidities, allergies and sensitivities, and any special needs.
   a. **SCIP** is the Surgical Care Improvement Project. The purpose of SCIP is to prevent surgical site infection (SSI). Centers for Medicare and Medicaid Services (CMS) has mandated that preventable SSI will not be reimbursed (Box 7.2).

   Activities associated with increased risk for SSI are closely monitored during intraoperative patient care including appropriate antibiotic prophylaxis, maintaining normothermia, hair removal only as necessary, limited use of urinary catheters, and serum glucose monitoring during the surgical procedure. Documentation of the SCIP protocol is incorporated into the patient's medical record.
   b. **NPSG** are the National Patient Safety Goals established and updated yearly by The Joint Commission. The 2018 NPSGs include correct identification of the patient, improved staff communication, use of appropriate medical alarms, prevent infection, identify safety risks, and prevent mistakes in surgery. The NPSGs are updated each year to reflect current statistics and trends in patient care technology.

2. **Time out** requires all personnel on the surgical team to concur about the following details concerning the patient (identification [ID], health conditions, special circumstances), the surgical procedure, the correct site, the supplies and equipment, and potential risks (e.g., fire) (Box 7.3). The patient should participate as much as possible. Key elements to assure patient safety in addition to the time out include the following:
   a. Each member of the team should be identified and demonstrate respect for each other.
   b. Physical conditions of the OR should be compliant with appropriate heat, humidity, and lighting needs.
   c. Supplies, equipment, implants should be immediately available and appropriate for the intended surgical procedure.
   d. Complete attention by the entire team to the surgical procedure and sterile/aseptic techniques is required.

3. Capsule summary of documentation by the circulating nurse (Box 7.4).
   a. Identification and assessment of the patient (before and after the surgical procedure)
   b. Time entering the OR
   c. Time and type of anesthesia, as well as anesthesia provider(s)
   d. Patient position and positioning devices used
   e. Surgical procedure performed and surgeon
   f. Names and titles of all personnel on the surgical team
   g. All equipment and devices used in the procedure
   h. Skin prep and placement of return electrode; skin condition before and after each activity (i.e., positioning, prepping, and placement of return electrode)

BOX 7.1   Overview of Patient Assessment

Review of Body Systems (Brief History)

- Is the patient a reliable historian, or is a family member translating or communicating on his or her behalf?
- Is the patient taking any medication on a regular basis (e.g., heart or blood pressure medications)? This should include vitamins, hormones, or herbal preparations.
- Does the patient have any allergies? What are the patient's reactions when exposed to the offending substance? Is the reaction localized or systemic?
- When was the patient's last meal and oral intake? If this is an emergency, what were the foods in this meal? Red foods may falsely imply gastrointestinal bleeding if the patient vomits.
- Has the patient ever had any surgery before? This may reveal a condition that requires special positioning or other modification to the standard plan of care.
- Has the patient experienced any complications during previous surgeries?
- Does the patient wear contact lenses or prosthetic parts?
- Does the patient have any trouble moving limbs?
- Is the patient extremely large or small? This may indicate the need for additional instruments or a weight-appropriate operating room (OR) bed.
- Is the patient aware of the procedure being performed?
- Are laboratory studies and blood work reports included with the chart? Are they current?

Head-to-Toe Assessment (Brief Physical)

- Is the patient here for a scheduled procedure, urgent or emergent care, or possibly a redo from an earlier

surgery? This may alter the needed supplies for the case.
- Is the patient a child or adult? Is a parent present?
- Observe the color of the patient's skin and body tissues.
- Listen to the sound of the patient's voice as he or she speaks. Is it raspy or breathless? Is the patient coughing? Note any odors on breath or body.
- Touch the patient's skin as the dialogue progresses. Is it cool, hot, damp, dry, or in any other condition? This assessment can be performed as part of shaking hands. Does the patient have a weak or strong handshake or grasp? Is the patient shaky?
- Is there eye contact, and do the eyes move appropriately?
- Is one or the other eyelid drooping? Is the patient crying?
- Does the patient have enough physical coordination to point to the surgical site? Has the correct site been marked per facility policy and procedure?
- Does the patient appear to understand what is being said? Can the patient speak and respond appropriately?
- Does the patient have a Foley catheter or an ostomy? Is the patient continent?
- Are intravenous (IV) fluids running? Is the line infusing? Are additives in the container?
- Is the correct surgical site marked with the surgeon's initials?

Most of these assessment activities can be performed simultaneously in just a few minutes and may lead to additional nursing diagnoses that require a modification of the plan of care.

From Phillips N: *Berry and Kohn's operating room technique*, ed 13, St. Louis, 2017, Elsevier.

BOX 7.2   Overview of Surgical Care Improvement Project

One hour before incision—fluoroquinolone (ciprofloxacin)
Two hours before incision—vancomycin (Vanocin) (if indicated)
Antibiotic discontinued within 24 hours postoperatively (48 hours for cardiac patients)

Normothermia
Immediate postoperative body temperature 36°C–38°C within 1 hour of the surgical procedure

Appropriate Hair Removal
Hair is removed only as necessary with clippers away from the operating room (OR)

Urinary Catheters
Urinary catheters are removed within 1–2 days of the surgical procedure

Serum Glucose
Maintain serum glucose between 80 and 110 mg/dL for cardiac patients and <200 mg/dL for other patients. Serum A1C should be <7%.

Adapted from Phillips, N. (2017). *Berry and Kohn's operating room technique* (13th ed.). St. Louis, MO: Elsevier.

i. All specimens and implants
j. Count reconciliation; resolution of any incomplete counts
k. Wound class, dressings, and drains
l. All solutions, medications, and doses
m. Time of end of surgical procedure and time of patient exit from OR

Considerations for Accountability

1. **Counts** are a shared responsibility between the circulating nurse and the scrub person. The counts are a verbal process between the circulator and the scrub person and must never be interrupted once started. The process of counting can be manual or automated with computerized machinery with radiofrequency

BOX 7.3	Using Time Out to Prevent Wrong-Site Surgery

- Correct patient?
- Correct position?
- Correct site?
- Correct procedure?
- Correct equipment?
- Correct images? (scans or x-rays in proper orientation)
- Correct implants? (as appropriate)

From Phillips, N. (2017). *Berry and Kohn's operating room technique* (13th ed.). St. Louis, MO: Elsevier.

chips (RFID). Only radiopaque or RFID chipped items should be used as sponges. The facility must have a written policy and procedure for the method of counting and documenting count results.

The entire team has accountability for responsible use of counted items in the sterile field. The surgeon and first assistant may help facilitate counts. No counted item is to be taken from the room during the surgical procedure in process. Everything used in the surgical procedure must be accounted for to prevent retained surgical items (RSI). CMS considers RSI a "never event" and is not reimbursable. RSI must be reported to The Joint Commission (TJC).

Other reasons for accountability in counting include inventory control and prevention of injury if an item is inadvertently left in the linens or trash. The result of counting is reported in the medical record as correct or incorrect. It is not necessary to document item totals in the medical record. All efforts to resolve incorrect counts are documented per the facility's policy and procedure.

a. Packaged sterile items arrive to the OR having been initially counted at the point of origin. This includes instrument trays, sponges, blades, suture/needles, and draping materials. Documentation nomenclature of packaged contents includes enumeration of everything inside. Accountability for confirming the accuracy of the packaged contents is supported by the counting process when opened for use. This count forms the baseline.

Prepackaged items should be counted in the same increments wherein they were packed. When a counted packed item is defective or packed in an incorrect increment, all the items in the package are removed from the sterile field, isolated, and labeled. This product is kept separate from other items used in the surgical procedure in process.

If the patient has not yet been brought to the room, the isolated package may be removed from the room. Any packaging materials should be included in the isolated package in case there is a problem with an entire lot of product.

BOX 7.4	Documentation by the Circulating Nurse in the Operating Room

- Initial assessment of the patient on arrival to the operating room (OR): The identity of the patient and verification of the procedure should be validated. Document the timeout. Correct surgical site should be marked by surgeon's initials.
- Significant times, such as arrival, time out, start, completion, and room exit times
- Disposition of sensory aids or prosthetic devices accompanying the patient on arrival in the OR
- Position, surgical safety devices, and/or restraints used during the surgical procedure
- Placement of monitoring and electrosurgical unit (ESU) electrodes, tourniquets, and other special equipment, and identification of units or machines used, as applicable: The settings and duration of use should be recorded.
- The names and times of all personnel in the room for the procedure
- The type of anesthetic administered and by whom
- The surgical site preparation, the antiseptic agent administered, and by whom
- Medications, solutions, and doses administered, and by whom
- Time-out validation of site, patient, and procedure for the surgical checklist
- A description of the actual surgical procedure performed
- Contact with the patient's family or significant others
- Type, size, and manufacturer's identifying information (lot numbers) of prosthetic implants, or the type, source, and location of tissue transplants or inserted radioactive materials
- Use of x-rays or imaging
- Disposition of tissue specimens and cultures
- Correctness or incorrectness of surgical counts (if incorrect, the remedial measures to locate the lost item)
- Placement of drains, catheters, dressings, and packing: output is recorded if receptacle is emptied in the OR
- Wound classification is designated at the end of the procedure
- Charges to patient for supplies, according to hospital routine
- Piece of equipment sent from OR with patient to unit (e.g., tracheotomy set that accompanies patient after thyroidectomy, wire scissors if patient has had teeth wired together): These items are to be returned.
- Disposition of the patient after leaving the OR
- Any unusual event or complication

Adapted from Phillips, N. (2017). *Berry and Kohn's operating room technique* (13th ed.). St. Louis, MO: Elsevier.

b. During the surgical procedure, anything added for use in the sterile field is counted and added to the tally of counted items.

c. At the closure of a hollow body part, the items in use must be accounted for as counted items. Every item used in a body orifice or cavity must be accounted for to prevent RSI. Examples include throat, vaginal, and rectal packs.

d. As the surgical procedure is ending and the first layers are being closed, the counted items are accounted for to minimize the risk for RSI.

e. When the final layers of tissue are closed, a second reconciliation of counts is performed to affirm that all items have been accounted for and no item has been retained by the patient. Non-radiopaque gauze dressing material should not be dispensed to the sterile filed until the incision is closed and all counts are complete. Never use a counted sponge as a dressing.

f. Some facilities permit aborting surgical counts for reasons related to patient condition or the use of x-ray during the surgical procedure. X-ray should not be used as a substitute for counting and accountability because the patient is exposed to ionizing radiation. During organ procurement a count should be performed as if the donor were a living patient. The facility should have a written policy and procedure for counts involving special circumstances.

g. Items that break or become disassembled during the surgical procedure must be accounted for in their entirety.

h. Great care is taken with items such as clip cartridges, electrosurgical unit (ESU) tip cleaners, syringe caps, suture reels, and other items not always enumerated in the initial counting process. Not all of these items are radiopaque.

i. A count should be done at each change of personnel during a surgical procedure in process. This count should be documented, and the names of the personnel involved are recorded.

j. The process of final counting should begin at the sterile field (patient), next to the Mayo stand, followed by counting on the instrument table. The circulating nurse adds to the final count any item (sponges, needles, or instruments) removed from the field for a total count.

k. The surgeon is notified of all count results and is first to be notified if a count is incorrect and of all efforts employed to find a missing item. All trash, drapes, and linen are searched. An x-ray may be ordered. Results of the count are documented in the patient's record.

l. On rare occasions a patient in extremis is unable to have the surgical procedure completed because of inability to close the site. This patient may be packed with lap tapes and taken to intensive care. The scrub person and circulating nurse count the number of retained items, and the number is documented in the medical record.

When the patient returns for additional surgery the intentionally retained items are removed, counted, and documented. They should be set aside and not mixed with any items involved with the second surgical procedure.

m. All soiled counted items should be disposed of in the appropriate biohazard receptacles at the end of the case when the patient leaves the OR. Sharps boxes must be closed.

2. **Medications** are managed by the circulating nurse and scrub person in the OR. Sterile and aseptic techniques apply to handling medications and drugs in addition to safe practices. Refer to Chapter 8 for information concerning specific medications and pharmaceuticals.

a. The circulating nurse uses aseptic technique when transferring drugs and solutions to the sterile field. The scrub person uses sterile technique when handling drugs and solutions in the sterile field.

   1) Bottled solutions are opened and dispensed to the sterile field in one motion by the circulating nurse. The bottle may not be recapped and the contents used again in the sterile field. Splashing is to be avoided.

   2) The scrub person and circulating nurse check the bottle for integrity, content name, and expiration date before use. They verbalize the name of the product before it is dispensed to the sterile field.

   3) Containers of medication (bags, vials, and ampules) are dispensed to the field by the circulating nurse.

      a) Intravenous (IV) bags are decanted with a pour spout.

      b) Vials can be decanted with a device or drawn into a syringe. The needle should be removed from the syringe and the medication expressed gently into a medicine cup without spraying. It is unsafe for the scrub person to spear a vial the circulating nurse is holding to draw up a drug. Some vials are designed to be opened and poured aseptically. Never pry off a sealed stopper and pour to the field. The edge is not considered sterile.

      c) Ampules are sealed glass containers that can shed glass shards into the drug when opened. These drugs should be drawn up using a filter needle. The filter needle is removed, and the drug is dispensed by the circulating nurse using the syringe.

b. Medications in tubes (lubrication, antiseptics, ointments, and other creams) should be in unit dose packaging. Multidose tubes can cross-contaminate patients.

   1) Small foil packages may not be opened and expressed onto the sterile field. The exterior of

the package is not sterile and could contaminate the patient during the transfer. Some foil packaged products may be included in the custom pack during manufacturer's processing. This packaging is considered sterile and can be used within the sterile field.

2) The medicine cup or basin should be labeled after the drug is dispensed. Do not prelabel containers before the drug is poured to the field. Human error can happen if the wrong drug is accidentally poured into the wrong prelabeled cup or basin. The scrub person and circulating nurse should read the label on the medicine cup aloud.

3) The label should list the drug, dose, and strength. Some facilities require user initials, time, and expiration date on every labeled item. If the solution or drug has a sterile patient delivery device, such as a syringe or Asepto, it must have a matching label. Avoid using abbreviations. Some facilities have sterile preprinted labels. Drugs in unlabeled containers on the sterile field must be discarded.

c. Communication during medication or solution use in the sterile field should use the readback method of repeating the name, strength, and dose as the surgeon asks for and receives the delivery device. Changeover of personnel includes reporting any medications and delivery devices on the sterile field.

d. Policies and procedures should be in place for the use of standing orders and verbal orders for medications.

e. Care is taken to assure that the patient has no sensitivity or allergy to any substance, medication, or pharmaceutical used during the surgical procedure.

f. Delivery to the sterile field should be done in a manner to prevent aerosolization that could expose other sensitive personnel in the OR to an allergen.

g. All drugs or medication administered must be documented in the patient's medical record. Some drug-dispensing machines in the OR automatically charge the patient and may list it as a given medication. If the drug is not administered, it must be charged back into the system. If not charged back into the system, other caregivers may believe that it was given and a medication error could take place.

Intraoperative Nursing Care
Nursing Interventions
1. Patient care during anesthesia administration
   a. **Local anesthesia.** During local anesthesia administration the patient should be monitored for changes in his or her vital signs and generalized condition. All monitoring methods and results should be documented in the patient's medical record.

Local anesthetic systemic toxicity (LAST) is a series of signs and symptoms reported by the patient and also noted by the perioperative nurse during patient monitoring. The first actions in a LAST event are to summon help, maintain the patient's airway with 100% O_2, ACLS (Advanced Cardiac Life Support) or BLS (Basic Life Support) protocol, and establish IV access as necessary. For details concerning local anesthetic medication and reactions, see Chapter 8.

1) The circulating nurse dispenses local anesthesia medication to the sterile field. The scrub person labels the medicine cup after the medication is received. If the drug is drawn from the vial and immediately administered by the surgeon at the same time, the syringe does not need to be labeled.

2) **Monitoring the patient.** A perioperative nurse should be assigned to monitor the patient during the use of local anesthesia when an anesthesia provider is not present. Baseline vital signs are compared with vital signs taken during the surgical procedure. The circulating nurse should not simultaneously circulate and monitor the patient, because full attention is not given to the patient's condition.

3) **Moderate sedation.** The patient will have an IV for the administration of sedation. A qualified perioperative nurse, ACLS preferred, must monitor the patient's vital signs and level of consciousness, and have the knowledge of local anesthetic and sedative drugs.

b. **Spinal or epidural.** The perioperative nurse assists the anesthesia provider with patient positioning for **regional anesthesia.** An important aspect of positioning for this method of anesthesia is to keep the patient's shoulders and hips aligned and the spine straight until flexion is needed by the anesthesia provider for needle placement.

The perioperative nurse is positioned in front of the patient at all times to prevent the risk for falling during lateral or seated spinal/epidural administration. After the injection of anesthesia, the patient is positioned on the OR bed. The patient will need help to straighten the legs on the bed as the drugs take effect. The level of the drug's effect is produced by maintaining the patient's position. Once in position, the anesthesia provider may rotate the OR bed into a slight reverse Trendelenburg's position to keep the drug from traveling too high in the spinal column and causing respiratory distress. The patient's dignity is protected during the positioning process.

1) **Lateral positioning for spinal or epidural.** The patient is positioned on his or her side. The spine is straight, the shoulders and hips are perpendicular to the OR bed, the head and chin are flexed to the chest, and the knees are

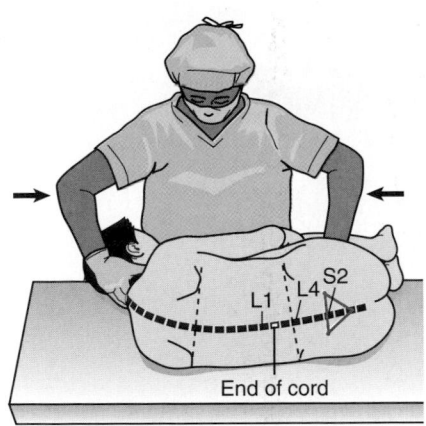

Figure 7.1 Spinal block—lateral position. (From Phillips, N. [2017]. *Berry and Kohn's operating room technique* [13th ed.]. St. Louis, MO: Elsevier.)

flexed and drawn up to the abdomen. The positioning of the head/chin and knees causes the back to be arched without twisting for the placement of the spinal needle or epidural catheter by the anesthesia provider (Fig. 7.1).

2) **Seated positioning for spinal or epidural.** The patient is seated on the side of the OR bed with his or her legs and feet resting on a stool. The spine is kept straight until the head and chin are flexed to the chest. The arms are crossed on a pillow over the abdomen. The back is arched for the placement of the spinal needle or epidural catheter by the anesthesia provider (Fig. 7.2).

c. **General anesthesia** provided through inhaled gases and IV medications. The anesthesia provider assesses the patient for potential complications with the airway, cervical spine mobility, dentition, and any comorbidity that could cause physiologic problems associated with anesthetic drugs.

The perioperative nurse should remain at the patient's side throughout the general anesthetic delivery process to assist the anesthesia provider as needed. See Chapter 8 for the anesthesia provider's role.

1) General anesthesia progresses through four stages. During the first two stages, the patient is easily startled and could overstimulate reflexes. The airway could be compromised. Traffic and noise in the room must be kept at a minimum.

2) Stage 3 is the safe time to begin the surgical procedure. The patient's vital signs are in a safe range, and the airway is patent and controlled.

3) If the anesthetic level reaches stage 4, the patient is in danger. The vital signs are unstable. Respiratory and cardiac arrest are possible. Resuscitation equipment and supplies should be immediately available.

4) **Emergence** from general anesthesia can be a critical time for the patient's safety. Avoid extraneous noise and stimulation. The anesthesia provider regulates the inhalant gases and IV drugs to slowly bring the patient's consciousness and physiologic control back to normal. The patient must be able to breathe without assistance and maintain normal blood pressure and pulse. The patient is at risk for vomiting and aspiration until pharyngeal reflexes are recovered. Suction must be immediately available.

2. **What is the perioperative nurse's role during intubation?** The patient will be supine and may need special positioning to facilitate airway access and maintenance. The patient's physiology can make intubation difficult if the neck is short and the airway is obscured. Additional pillows may be needed to elevate the head 25 degrees (Fig. 7.3).

a. **Sellick's maneuver** (cricoid pressure). The perioperative nurse is sometimes asked to assist with intubation if the patient has a full stomach and might regurgitate during the placement of the endotracheal tube. The cricoid cartilage is compressed to occlude the esophagus until the cuff on the endotracheal tube is inflated. The

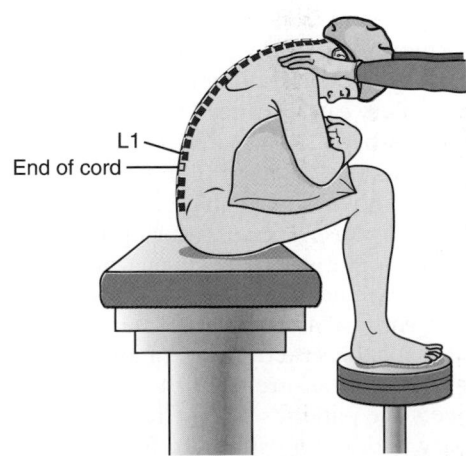

Figure 7.2 Spinal block—sitting position. (From Phillips, N. [2017]. *Berry and Kohn's operating room technique* [13th ed.]. St. Louis, MO: Elsevier.)

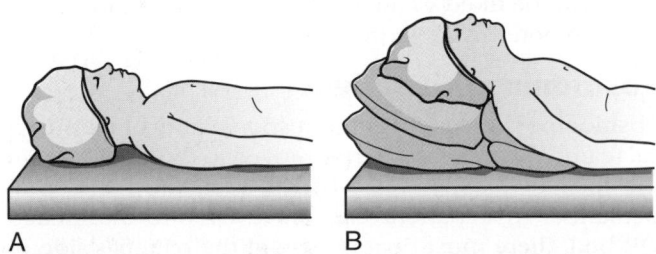

Figure 7.3 Short neck or morbid obesity. (A) Supine position. (B) Sniffing position. (From Phillips, N. [2017]. *Berry and Kohn's operating room technique* [13th ed.]. St. Louis, MO: Elsevier.)

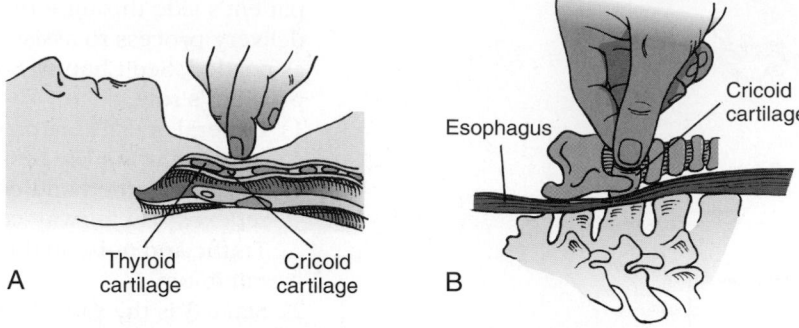

Figure 7.4 Cricoid pressure. (A) Index finger displaces cricoid cartilage posteriorly, thus obstructing esophagus. (B) Two-finger technique obstructs esophagus between body of sixth cervical vertebra and cricoid cartilage. (From Phillips, N. [2017]. *Berry and Kohn's operating room technique* [13th ed.]. St. Louis, MO: Elsevier.)

perioperative nurse may be asked to stabilize the anterior throat at the level of the cricoid cartilage to assist the anesthesia provider with intubation (Fig. 7.4).

b. **Awake intubation.** The patient's condition may necessitate intubation before general anesthesia can be performed. Topical anesthesia will be applied to the throat to suppress the gag reflex. As soon as intubation is established the general anesthesia is rapidly induced. This method is used if the patient is known to have a full stomach or is assessed to present a difficult intubation.

c. **Special circumstances during intubation.** Modification of intubation positioning and processes are individualized according the patient's need. **Pregnant patients** can have inferior vena caval and aortic pressure from the enlarging uterus in the supine position. This can cause a drop in blood pressure and a decrease of cardiac output. A small wedge can be placed under the right hip at the lumbar level to shift the uterine weight to the left 12 to 15 degrees. A left lateral tilt should be used for pregnant patients after 18 weeks of gestation.

If the pregnant patient's blood pressure suddenly decreases while in the supine position, the perioperative nurse can gently push the uterus to the left to relieve the venous pressure. The OR bed can be tilted to the left 15 to 45 degrees to relieve hypotensive syndrome.

Positioning the Patient

Positioning the patient is the responsibility of the surgical team. The patient is safely moved to the OR bed from the locked transport cart by an adequate number of personnel. If a patient can move over to the locked OR bed, there must be a person at the patient's side of the transport cart and a person at the receiving side of the OR bed.

1. **Incapacitated patients** require a minimum of four persons or more for a move between the transport

cart and the OR bed, or from the OR bed to the transport cart. Patient moving devices should be used as available. Both patient-bearing surfaces are locked before the move. Care is taken not to dislodge any catheters or IV tubing. Moving the patient between two surfaces is an organized effort. The person at the patient's head calls the count of three so all personnel work together.

When moving the patient, care is taken not to drag the patient's skin across the sheets. A friction injury to the skin can result. The motion of the patient's tissue beneath the skin is referred to as shearing force. This can cause vessel constriction and result in deep tissue necrosis (Fig. 7.5). Deep tissue injury may not be immediately apparent postoperatively.

2. Positioning the patient is safely done when the anesthesia provider indicates the patient is adequately anesthetized and physiologically stable. Prepping and/or urinary catheter placement is not started until the anesthesia provider states it is safe to do so.

Soft tissue and bony area padding is individualized by body size, physical condition, and type/duration of surgical procedure. Risk assessment for soft tissue pressure injury includes nutrition status, laboratory tests, comorbidities, preoperative skin condition, peripheral pulses, and body mass index. Positioning pressure injury can be caused by devices on or inside the patient's body. Items such as catheters, drains, prosthetic devices, jewelry, piercings, hair pins/clips, subsurface implants (pacemaker, etc.), and cosmetic implants can cause pressure during positioning.

The surgeon and the anesthesia provider determine whether the surgical position provides adequate surgical site exposure and the best approach for the safe delivery of anesthesia. The circulating nurse assures that the OR bed is locked and meets the patient's weight requirements, and necessary padding, positioning devices, and personnel are immediately available.

Vacuum positioning devices (e.g., bean bag) are used in some surgical procedures to minimize a shift

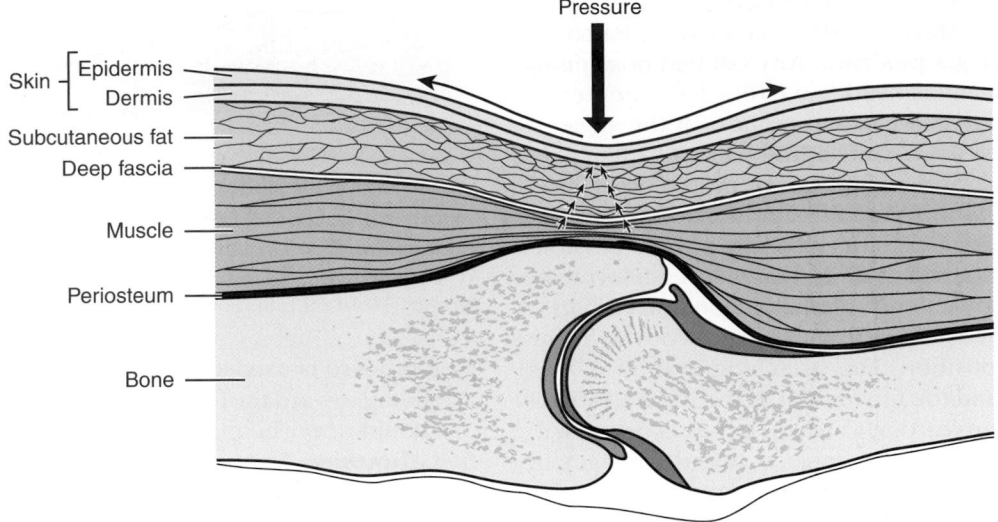

Figure 7.5 Tissues are affected by pressure, which causes deep tissue damage and necrosis. (From Phillips, N. [2017]. *Berry and Kohn's operating room technique* [13th ed.]. St. Louis, MO: Elsevier.)

in the patient's body. The vacuum positioner is padded with gel pads under the patient. The surface takes shape and becomes firm as air is suctioned into the room suction system. When the positioner is fully evacuated the stopper is placed in the suction port to maintain rigidity. Do not leave the room inline suction activated and attached. The connection could be detached and the patient could suddenly shift on the OR bed, causing injury.

3. **Supine.** The patient is positioned on the back facing up (Fig. 7.6). The OR bed surface should be pressure-reducing material and provide at least 1 inch of padding between the patient's body and the frame surface of the OR bed. The mattress should be thick enough and designed to support the patient's body weight. A blanket should not be placed over the OR bed sheet because that causes the pressure reductive surface to be less effective.

   a. Pressure-sensitive areas include the patient's occiput (back of head), scapulae (shoulder blades), olecranon (elbows), sacrum, coccyx (buttocks), and calcaneum (heels).

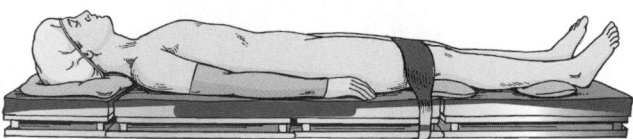

Figure 7.6 Supine position. Patient lies straight on back, face upward, with arms at sides, legs extended parallel and uncrossed, and feet slightly separated. Strap is placed above knees. Head is in line with spine. Note small pillow under ankles to protect heels from pressure. Arms are secured with lift sheet or placed on armboards. (From Phillips, N. [2017]. *Berry and Kohn's operating room technique* [13th ed.]. St. Louis, MO: Elsevier.)

   b. The patient's arms can be tucked in a neutral position (palms facing toward the body) with a drawsheet and elbow protectors. The drawsheet should extend from above the elbows (mid-upper arm) to the hand. The drawsheet is tucked under the patient and not under the mattress of the OR bed. Care is taken not to hyperextend the elbow and cause median nerve injury.

   If armboards are used, the padding should be even with the level of the OR bed mattress or the brachial plexus can be injured. The arms and hands are supinated and secured to protect the ulnar nerve. The armboard must not be abducted more than 90 degrees to prevent brachial plexus neuropathy.

   c. The patient's head should remain in a neutral position with a small pillow unless the anesthesia provider requires additional elevation to establish and maintain the airway (see Fig. 7.3).

   d. A small pillow can be placed under the patient's knees to reduce popliteal pressure and protect the peroneal and tibial nerves. This pillow can relieve lower back strain and prevent hyperextension of the knees.

   The safety strap is placed 2 inches above the knees over the blanket that covers the thighs. The perioperative nurse should be able to pass a hand between the safety strap and the patient's legs to assess that the strap is not too tight. The safety strap should not be obscured by a blanket. It should be visualized in place before the sterile drapes are applied.

   e. The patient's heels and Achilles tendons are protected with padding or heel cups. The padding also prevents the feet from flexing or hyperextending. The feet are uncrossed. The toes and the entirety of the patient's body must be protected from pressure caused by drapes and equipment (Mayo stand) placed over the body.

4. **Trendelenburg's position.** Any OR bed positioning can be moved into a head down tilt where the feet are higher than the head. The steepness of the angle allows a physiologic shift in the patient's internal organs. The subsequent pressure on the organ systems can be harmful to the patient, and the position should be maintained for the shortest time possible.

The intrathoracic and intracranial pressures can be complicated by using pneumoperitoneum carbon dioxide (CO_2) associated with laparoscopy in Trendelenburg's position. The stretching of the peritoneum and the movement of the internal organs can cause bradycardia. Cardiac output is decreased. Respiratory volume is decreased, and diaphragmatic pressure can cause stress on the alveoli. End-tidal CO_2 increases. The organ shift can cause a tracheal shift that could change the position of the endotracheal tube or laryngeal mask airway.

Typical Trendelenburg's position ranges between 15 and 39 degrees in a head down tilt. Cerebral blood flow and cerebral spinal fluid shift are increased, as well as intracerebral pressure. Venous outflow from the head is decreased. The patient may experience cerebral edema as a result. Intraocular pressure increases can cause ischemic pressure on the optic nerve. Steep Trendelenburg's position (between 30 and 45 degrees) can cause optic nerve neuropathy in susceptible patients.

The perioperative team must minimize the risk that the patient's body can slide cephalad, creating friction and shearing force. One method of preventing this is to lower the foot portion of the OR bed, causing the legs to flex at the knees for stability (Fig. 7.7).

Reverse Trendelenburg's. The opposite of the head down position is the head elevated position (Fig. 7.8). The head is 15 to 30 degrees higher than the feet and the hemodynamics shift to the lower body and legs. The elevation of 10 degrees may be adequate for the surgical procedure. Intracranial pressure is decreased, and venous pooling is increased in the lower body when the patient is in reverse Trendelenburg's position. A padded

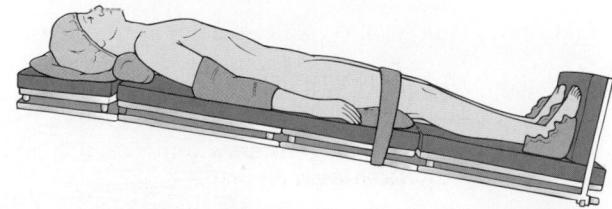

Figure 7.8 Reverse Trendelenburg's position, with soft roll under shoulders for thyroid, neck, and shoulder procedures. (From Rothrock, J. [2019]. *Alexander's care of the patient in surgery* [16th ed.]. St. Louis, MO: Elsevier.)

footboard is used to prevent the patient's body from sliding toward the feet. The patient's full body weight should never be placed against the footboard.

5. **Lithotomy.** The patient's legs are simultaneously raised and placed in leg holders (stirrups), and secured by two perioperative caregivers. The bottom part of the OR bed is lowered at the table break. The safety strap is not used over the abdomen or chest. The patient's hands should be protected from crush injury when the foot plate is raised and lowered (Fig. 7.9).

The lithotomy position can be modified by using Trendelenburg's and reverse Trendelenburg's position. The patient's buttocks should be even with the OR bed break and not extend over the end of the bed. Weight-appropriate leg holders are placed at even heights and should support the legs over the larger surface to minimize the risk for compression of soft tissue. The elevation of the feet positioning should be as low as possible to prevent a significantly decreased angle between the thighs and abdomen. A decreased

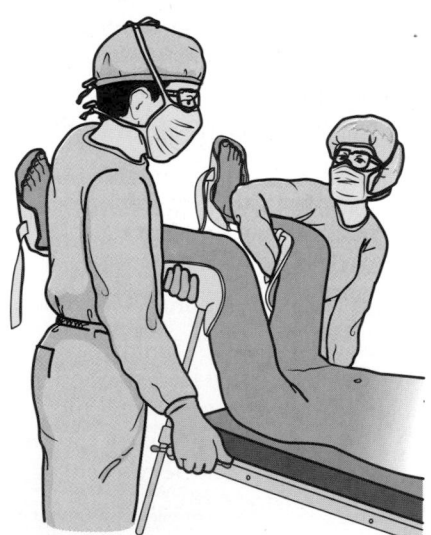

Figure 7.9 Lithotomy position. Patient is supine with foot section of OR bed lowered to right angle. Knees are flexed, and legs are elevated to the degree necessary for the type of surgical procedure. Note that buttocks are even with edge of the OR bed, and that sometimes a roll is needed under the buttocks to elevate the hips above the level of the bed. (From Phillips, N. [2017]. *Berry and Kohn's operating room technique* [13th ed.]. St. Louis, MO: Elsevier.)

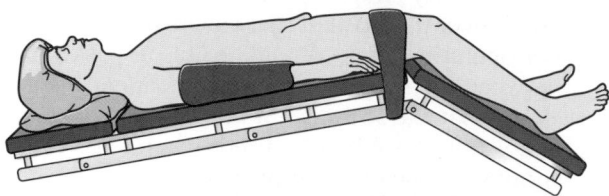

Figure 7.7 Trendelenburg's position. Note knees are over lower break in OR bed, with knee strap above knees. Arms are secured. Shoulder braces are not usually needed with this method of Trendelenburg's position. (From Phillips, N. [2017]. *Berry and Kohn's operating room technique* [13th ed.]. St. Louis, MO: Elsevier.)

angle can result in nerve (ilioinguinal nerve) and vascular compromise. At no time should members of the sterile team lean against the patient's legs.

Boot-style leg holders distribute the weight of the legs. **Knee-crutch leg holders** support the legs at the popliteal space and could cause compression of the peroneal nerve and the popliteal artery. Venous and lymphatic flow can be impeded. The weight and size of the patient's legs impact the effect of the pressure areas. **Sling-candy cane–style stirrups** support the weight of the legs with the feet and ankles. Padding is placed around the feet and ankles to minimize the risk for injury to the distal sural and plantar nerves. Care is taken to prevent the lateral aspect of the legs resting on the stirrup upright posts. The peroneal nerve could be damaged, causing paresthesia of the lower leg and foot drop.

Sequential compression devices (SCDs) or antiembolic stockings may be used with leg holders. When the legs are elevated, blood shifts from the venous system and increases blood in the central circulation.

The patient's arms can be positioned across the abdomen, tucked at the sides with a drawsheet, or secured on armboards. If the arms are tucked, the fingers should not extend beyond the break in the bed, to prevent a crush injury to the hand.

Removing the patient's legs from lithotomy leg holders is performed by two persons. The AORN Guidelines (2018) state that the patient's legs are removed from the leg holders in a flexed position simultaneously by supporting the feet and calves and slowly bringing the legs together. The legs are straightened slowly at the same time and lowered to the OR bed. Slow repositioning minimizes the hemodynamic shift from the central circulation to the legs. A blanket is placed over the patient's body, and a safety strap is placed over the thighs after the leg holders are removed from the OR bed.

a. **Levels of lithotomy** can range from low to exaggerated heights depending on the degree of access necessary to the perineal floor and genitalia. If an exaggerated level is used, the sacrum must be supported to decrease the weight of the torso on the legs. The higher the level used, the greater the risk for injury (Fig. 7.10).

b. **Hemilithotomy** is used when one leg is supported in a leg holder and the opposite leg is in traction or an arthroscopic leg positioner. The leg holder is positioned as low as possible to prevent strain on the patient's hip and lower back.

c. Potential complications of lithotomy position include nerve and vessel damage that may become permanent. The musculoskeletal system can be stressed and strained. Soft tissue injury can extend into compartment syndrome and rhabdomyolysis.

6. **Seated.** Fowler's position is when the patient's back is elevated to varied levels extending to full upright sitting posture (20–90 degrees). The foot section is

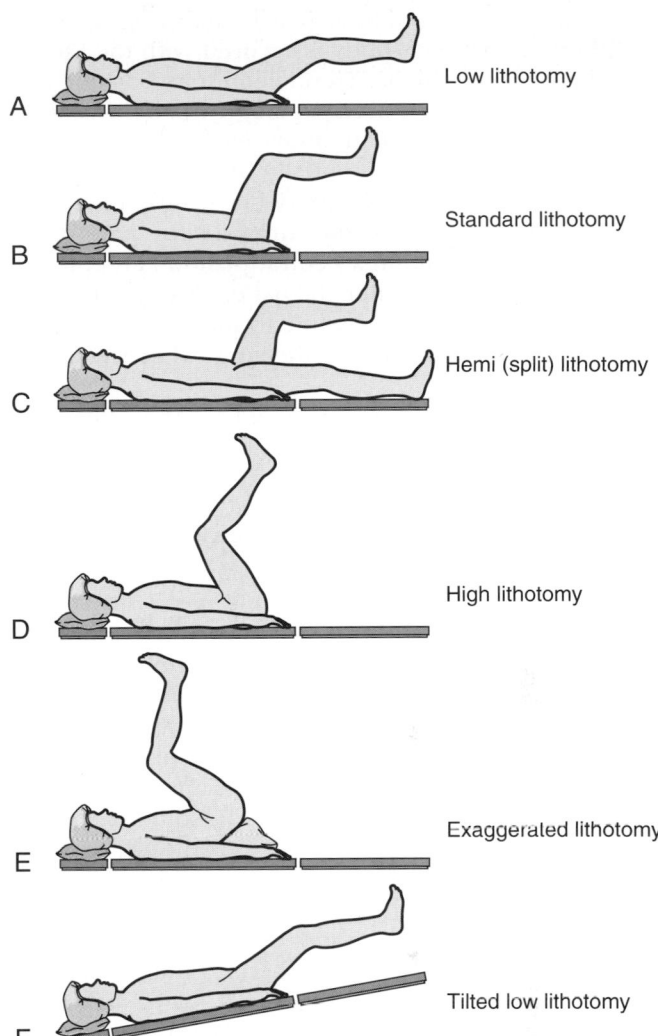

Figure 7.10 Commonly used lithotomy positions: (A) low lithotomy, (B) standard lithotomy, (C) hemilithotomy (split), (D) high lithotomy, (E) exaggerated lithotomy, and (F) tilted low lithotomy. (From Phillips, N. [2017]. *Berry and Kohn's operating room technique* [13th ed.]. St. Louis, MO: Elsevier.)

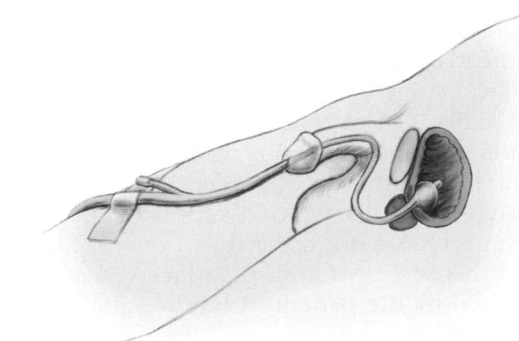

Figure 7.11 Secure the urinary catheter. (From Davis, J.H., et al. [1991]. *Essentials of clinical surgery*. St Louis, MO: Mosby.)

lowered to flex the knees 30 degrees. The arms are positioned across the abdomen on a pillow unless one of the shoulders is the operative site. SCDs can be applied to the legs to assist venous return. One variation is referred to as beach chair (Fig. 7.11). When the patient's body is secured with the safety strap over the thighs, Trendelenburg's position (10–20 degrees) may be used to place the patient's body at a working height and minimize elevation of the head. Seated patients are potentially bradycardic and hypotensive, and may experience cerebral ischemia.

When a shoulder is the surgical site, care is taken to secure the head in a neutral position and protect the patient's eyes. When the patient is draped and the face is covered, it is possible to injure the patient's eyes inadvertently during the surgical procedure on the shoulder.

Complications of positions where the head is elevated above the heart include pressure to the sacral area, venous pooling in the pelvis, venous thromboembolism (VTE), deep vein thrombosis (DVT), and venous air embolus (VAE). Pressure areas are padded with alternating pressure pads. SCDs may help with VTE and DVT prevention.

Treatment for VAE is removing air from the right atrium with a central venous catheter placed by the anesthesia provider. The OR bed is placed in steep Trendelenburg's position with the right side tilted up (left lateral). The air is withdrawn from the right atrium via syringe by the anesthesia provider. The surgical site is filled with irrigation solution, and the patient is administered 100% oxygen (O_2). In some situations, chest compressions can help break up the air bubble and push the air into the pulmonary vessels for disposal through the lungs.

7. **Lateral.** The patient is anesthetized in the supine position and repositioned laterally. Care is taken not to dislodge the urinary catheter, IV tubing, or endotracheal tube. Left lateral is when positioned on the left side. Right lateral is when the patient is positioned on the right side. Areas at risk for pressure injury when positioned laterally for greater than 4 hours include the ear, acromion process, olecranon, iliac crest, trochanter, lateral knee, and malleolus. The lateral position should be used for the shortest time possible.

The head should be positioned in alignment with the cervical spine on a head positioner (Fig. 7.12). A wide axillary-chest roll/support is placed longitudinally under the ribs to displace pressure from the lower arm and shoulder. Care is taken not to impinge the axillary blood supply or the long thoracic nerve. Do not use a rolled towel or blanket because this serves as a hard surface when compressed by the patient's body weight. Gel rolls are preferred.

The spine is kept in alignment. The breasts and abdomen are not permitted to lay dependent over the side of the OR bed and are not compressed by restraints or safety straps.

The arms are extended forward on armboards and secured with the upper arm parallel to the lower arm at a right angle to the torso. The upper arm must be

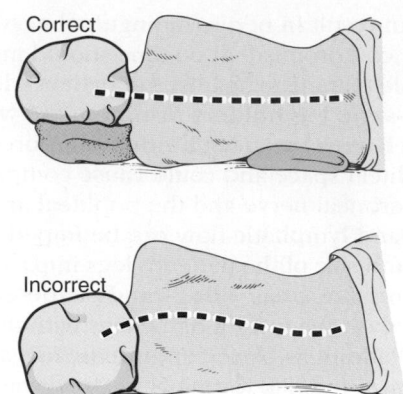

Figure 7.12 Proper alignment of spinal column in lateral position. (From Phillips, N. [2017]. *Berry and Kohn's operating room technique* [13th ed.]. St. Louis, MO: Elsevier.)

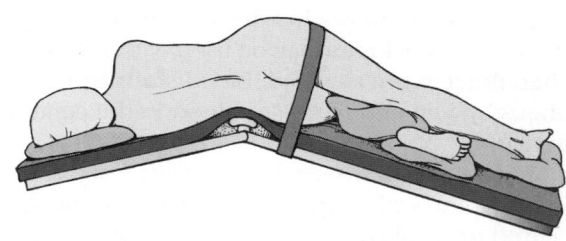

Figure 7.13 Right kidney position for a procedure on the right kidney. Patient is in lateral position with kidney region over OR bed break, or body elevation bar. The table is flexed. Note strap across hip to stabilize body, raised kidney elevator for hyperextending surgical site, and pillow between legs. The lower leg is flexed more than the upper leg. Patient's side is horizontal from shoulder to hip. The arm is supported with a double airplane armboard (not shown). (From Phillips, N. [2017]. *Berry and Kohn's operating room technique* [13th ed.]. St. Louis, MO: Elsevier.)

level with the shoulder. Both radial pulses should be monitored throughout the surgical procedure. A safety strap is used over the hip.

The dependent leg is flexed at the hip and knee. The upper leg is straight supported by a pillow between the knees. Bony prominences must not rest on each other. The feet and ankles are padded (Fig. 7.13).

The OR bed can be flexed to widen the angle between the ribs and the hip at the surgical site. If the kidney rest is used, the pressure of the patient's body against the OR bed is increased. If kidney braces are used, the longer brace is padded and positioned anterior, and the shorter brace is padded and positioned posteriorly at the level of the flank and not the iliac crest.

8. **Prone.** The patient is positioned facedown. The patient is anesthetized in the supine position on the transport cart. If a Foley catheter is necessary, it will be placed before moving to the OR bed. The anesthesia provider will indicate when it is safe to logroll the patient onto the OR bed. Adequate personnel are required. The transport cart must remain nearby at all

times in the event of an emergency and the patient must be rapidly positioned supine.

The move to the OR bed is done in steps, and care is taken to protect the catheter and IV tubing. Both surfaces are locked. The OR bed is level or slightly lower than the cart. The first move is to get the patient's body close to the edge of the cart. The next move is to roll the patient over to the facedown position on the OR bed with personnel to receive the upper body, middle body, and legs. The patient's arms are along the sides of the torso for this rolling move. Anesthesia personnel manage the patient's head and airway, and maintain the alignment of the cervical spine. The face is placed into a face positioning device by the anesthesia provider.

When the patient is received on the OR bed, the team lifts the torso, and chest rolls are positioned laterally from the clavicle to the iliac crest. The breasts and genitalia are positioned to prevent pressure. Abdominal pressure is reduced when the chest rolls are placed. Padding is placed under the knees and the dorsal aspect of the feet. The feet are high enough to prevent the toes from resting on the OR bed mattress or hanging over the edge. A safety strap is placed over the thighs (Fig. 7.14).

The arms are circumducted into a forward "diver's" position and pronated on armboards with elbows flexed. The abduction angle should be less than 90 degrees. The OR bed is placed in 5- to 10-degree reverse Trendelenburg's position to minimize the risk for facial edema and ocular pressure.

At the conclusion of the surgical procedure the moving process is reversed. The perioperative nurse must check to see that both the OR bed and the transport cart are locked and secure. The patient will be logrolled into the supine position. The arms are at the sides. Catheters, drains, and IV tubing are carefully protected.

Surgical Skin Preparation

The patient is in the desired position for the surgical procedure, and the anesthesia provider indicates the antiseptic skin preparation may begin. The perioperative nurse documents the condition of the site (before and after the prep), the antiseptic solution, and the person doing the prep in the patient's record.

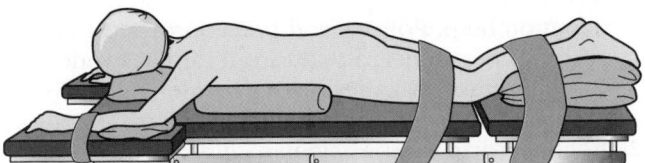

Figure 7.14 Prone position. Patient is placed on abdomen. Chest rolls are placed under axillae and sides of chest to the level of the iliac crest to facilitate respiration. Knees should be padded, and a pillow is placed under dorsum of feet. (From Phillips, N. [2017]. *Berry and Kohn's operating room technique* [13th ed.]. St. Louis, MO: Elsevier.)

Hair removal is done with clippers outside the OR as necessary, and hair near the surgical site can be coated with water soluble gel to minimize the risk for fire if using ESU or laser.

The act of prepping the skin is an aseptic process because the skin is never sterile, although sterile prep supplies and gloves may be used. The nonsterile person doing the prep must perform hand hygiene before donning gloves. Gloves are worn to prevent transfer of microorganisms from the prepping person to the patient. Examination gloves may be worn if prepping with an applicator. The surgical site marking must not be erased or obscured by the prepping process.

The choice of antiseptic solution is determined by the surgeon. Solutions used must be approved by the US Food and Drug Administration (FDA). Antiseptics are approved for external use only and are used according to manufacturer's instructions. Prep solutions are not permitted to pool under or around the patient. Sterile towels can be tucked in at the sides of the patient to catch any run off. Care is taken to prevent prep solutions from contacting electrocardiogram leads, tourniquets, or return electrodes. More information concerning antiseptic solutions can be found in Chapter 8.

Alcohol-based antiseptics are used with extreme caution and permitted to dry completely before drapes are applied. Draping before the alcohol-based prep is dry can allow flammable fumes to accumulate and become combustible in the presence of an ignition source (e.g., ESU or laser).

Patients susceptible to iodism can be prepped with non-iodine-based antiseptics. Examples include burn, thyroid, newborn, lactating, and pregnant patients. Any bloodborne iodine can adversely affect the thyroid function in these individuals. An alternative prep can be done with baby shampoo and saline.

Shellfish and seafood sensitivities are not indicators of iodine allergy. Care is taken to avoid detergent-based antiseptics and alcohol on mucous membranes. Detergents and alcohol can denude and irritate delicate tissues.

1. **Flat surfaces of the abdomen and back** should be squared off with sterile towels to minimize the risk for contamination from blankets and positioning devices during the prepping procedure.

   The umbilicus and areas considered contaminated are cleaned first, and the cotton-tipped applicators are discarded. If the surgical procedure requires perineal access, the perineum is prepped before the abdomen with a separate prep set and gloves. A stoma is covered with an adhesive drape. Prepping the contaminated area first minimizes the risk for contamination to the main abdominal surgical site by aerosolization or splash of contaminated prep solution.

   The abdominal skin prep starts at the incision line and moves outward. Do not pass back over the same area with a used sponge.

2. **Limbs** are prepped circumferentially while suspended up from the OR bed. Prep solution should not be permitted to run from the periphery back over the intended surgical site. Care is taken to clean the nails and between the fingers or toes during the prep.

3. **Vaginal preps** should be performed with povidone-iodine antiseptic solution unless contraindicated. An alternative prep is baby shampoo and saline. The American College of Obstetricians and Gynecologists supports the off-label use of 4% chlorhexidine (CHG) if povidone-iodine is contraindicated. Cesarean section patients may have fewer infections of the endometrium when povidone-iodine is used in the vagina.

   Povidone-iodine should not be used vaginally in pregnant women because the fetus may be exposed to the substance. Iodine crosses the placenta. Fetal skin may absorb the iodine, which could have an effect on the thyroid gland (iodism).

4. **Eyes** can be prepped with 5% povidone-iodine solution. Eyebrows are never shaved. Eyelashes may be trimmed with scissors coated with water-soluble gel to catch the hairs. CHG is unsafe to use around the face, ears, and eyes. It can cause blindness and deafness.

Specimen Management

Improper handling of specimens can result in additional surgery for the patient because of misdiagnosis. When a specimen is passed to the circulating nurse, it is important to verify the source site, label name, and method of processing requested (frozen or permanent section, fresh, culture, or smear). Notation of any orientation sutures or markings is included. The label is affixed only to the specimen container and not the lid. The container should be in a bag with a biohazard sticker attached. Additional information related to the specimen should be in the patient's medical record regarding antibiotics used, last menstrual period, or other details that could impact the results of laboratory studies.

1. Specimen containers are handled wearing gloves and personal protective equipment per Occupational Safety and Health Administration. Hand hygiene is required after removing gloves.

2. Specimens are kept moist unless otherwise indicated. Saline or preservative as appropriate may be added. Special solutions may be required for certain specimens. Add solution after the specimen is placed in the container to avoid splashing.

3. Stones and teeth should be sent dry.

4. Foreign bodies should be sent dry unless otherwise indicated. Forensic specimens require chain of evidence documentation and must never be left unattended. Metallic items (e.g., bullets, blade tips) should never have contact with other metals that could alter surface markings. Bloody clothes should be placed in paper bags and never in plastic bags. The plastic could cause degradation of DNA.

5. Surface cultures are taken before the skin is prepped. Prep solution can alter the culture results.

6. Tissue for hormonal studies may require special handling. Breast tissue must never dry out and is sent to pathology laboratory within 1 hour of removal. Testing for hormones can be altered if the tissue is permitted to dry.

Implants

The FDA requires tracking of implanted items used in patient care. The perioperative nurse is responsible for documenting data that would enable notification of surgeons and patients in the event of a recall of a defective device.

Universal Protocol requires verification of the correct type and size of the implant's availability as part of the time-out process before the surgical procedure begins. The composition of metallic implants should be considered if the patient has a metal allergy. The most common metal allergy is nickel. Documentation concerning implants used in patient care includes the following:

1. Patient's and surgeon's names and contact information

2. Device manufacturer and type/size of implant

3. Date of implantation, date of manufacture, and expiration if applicable

4. Lot number

5. Site/side of implantation

Explanted Devices

Any implanted device that is removed from the patient is documented in the patient's medical record. The reason for removal and the appearance/condition of the item is documented per facility policy and procedure. The item may be sent to the pathology laboratory for accession (identification) to document the actual removal.

Potential Emergency Situations

The perioperative nurse assures a clear path for emergency supplies and equipment throughout the surgical procedure.

Cardiac Event

The perioperative nursing actions. Keep in mind that most emergency drugs and treatments based on weight will be metered out according to body weight in kilograms. Many facilities refer to a cardiac event as "code blue."

1. Summon help. Policies and procedures must be in place for personnel roles during a cardiac event (e.g., cardiac arrest). An anesthesia provider is usually in charge of resuscitation and directs the resuscitation.

2. Begin cardiac compressions within 3 to 5 minutes. Implement BLS or ACLS protocol as appropriate. The ratio for chest compressions to breaths via ambu bag is 30:2 in the OR. Chest must be compressed at least 2 inches for an adult. For a child the chest is compressed one-third the diameter of the anterior-posterior depth of the patient's chest. Care is taken

not to displace the xyphoid process into the underlying organs. The carotid artery is assessed for a pulse with compressions.

3. Assist with defibrillation as appropriate. Assure that personnel stand clear during the application of the current. Transthoracic countershock (direct current 200–300 joules) is delivered to an adult patient. Child countershock is 2 joules/kg. Internal defibrillation is lower at 10 to 15 joules.

4. Assist with intubation and airway management as appropriate.

5. Assist with emergency drug administration and IV management as necessary.

   Blood may be drawn for electrolyte measurement. See Table 6.1 for normal blood chemistry values. An arterial line may be started and blood gases sent (Box 7.5).

6. Documentation is important for emergency management. One nurse should be assigned to record every step taken in the resuscitation process.

7. If the surgical procedure has begun, someone must remain as sterile as possible to control and protect the surgical site.

   Counts may be aborted, but every effort should be made for accountability to prevent RSI. X-ray may be required and may help with the accountability for surgical items or counts at the conclusion of the resuscitation activities.

Malignant Hyperthermia

Malignant hyperthermia (MH) is a hypermetabolic crisis stimulated in susceptible patients by halogenated anesthetics and depolarizing neuromuscular agents (succinylcholine) during general anesthesia. Local anesthesia drugs, nitrous oxide, and sodium pentothal are safe to use. **First signs of MH are unexplained tachycardia and an elevation of the end-tidal CO_2.** The blood in the surgical field looks dark and desaturated. As the symptoms increase, the patient's skeletal muscles go into sustained contraction and as a result, the body temperature rises rapidly as a later sign. The skin looks mottled and the patient is hypoxic. The contractions cause muscle breakdown, leading to rhabdomyolysis and the release of myoglobin in the urine. Myoglobin in the urine looks dark like cola.

1. First actions are to stop the anesthetic and oxygenate with 100% O_2. The anesthesia machine need not be changed. Safe agents may be used to sustain anesthesia as necessary. The surgeon should close the surgical site rapidly. The scrub person should remain sterile to help protect the sterile field. The circulating nurse will summon help.

2. **Dantrolene** is administered 2 to 3 mg/kg every 5 minutes up to 10 mg/kg. The anesthesia provider will need a central line if the peripheral veins are compressed by the rigidity of the skeletal muscles.

   Extremely large quantities of dantrolene are necessary, and the perioperative nurse will help by mixing the drug. Dantrolene is a yellow powdered drug in a 65-mL vial. Mannitol 3 g is included in the powdered drug. Only nonbacteriostatic sterile water (preferably chilled) is used to reconstitute the drug. Dantrolene administration continues postcrisis in a critical care unit for 24 to 48 hours postoperatively. More information about dantrolene is available in Chapter 8.

3. The patient is cooled by ice packs, cool irrigations by nasogastric and rectal tube. A cooling blanket may be used. A temperature probe Foley catheter may be inserted to measure core temperature. Temperature measurement is critical because the cooling process can lead to hypothermia. Active cooling can decrease when the body temperature decreases to 100°F.

   Do not irrigate the Foley catheter because the cool solution may distort the measurement of urine flow and color, which is critical. Urine may darken, thicken with myoglobin, and decrease in quantity. Additional mannitol and furosemide (Lasix) may be given to stimulate and sustain urine production.

4. Blood will be sent to the laboratory for frequent monitoring of electrolytes and blood gases. Electrolyte replacement and control is dependent on the results of these laboratory tests. Sodium bicarbonate may be needed.

5. The perioperative nurse documents all activities during an MH crisis.

6. Family history can reveal potential MH risk if family members had an unusual reaction or death during general anesthesia. MH is a familial genetic trait. It is autosomal dominant.

   Fresh muscle tissue is subjected to a caffeine contracture testing for diagnosis. Newer tests for MH are under development and investigation. More information can be found at the Malignant Hyperthermia Association of the United States website (http://www.mhaus.org).

7. Unexpected MH episodes are more common in patients with a known muscular disease such as muscular dystrophy and other muscular pathology.

Hand-Over to the Postoperative Nurse

Communication between the intraoperative nurse and the postoperative nurse mirrors most of the same patient information exchanged each time the patient's care is transferred to another caregiver. Refer to Chapter 6 for a description of the hand-over from the preoperative nurse to the perioperative nurse.

BOX 7.5   Arterial Blood Gases

pH	7.35–7.45
Paco$_2$	35–45 mm Hg
HCO$_2$	22–26 mEq/L
Base excess	−2 to 2
Pao$_2$	80–100 mm Hg
Sao$_2$	>95%

The anesthesia provider accompanies the patient to the postanesthesia care unit (PACU) and provides additional information specific to anesthesia delivery and the patient's responses. Some of the information shared will cross over into both the perioperative nurse's and anesthesia provider's hand over. Before the patient is taken to PACU, the perioperative nurse should inform the PACU if special equipment is needed, such as a ventilator or other special monitoring equipment.

The perioperative nurse hands over the care of the patient to the postoperative nurse (perianesthesia nurse) and provides the following information for the continuation of safe and efficient patient care.

1. Patient's name and identifying information
2. Surgical procedure and the surgeon's name: describes any features of the procedure that may have differed from the expected plan
   a. Location of incision(s) and closure
   b. Dressings and drains, casting, splints
3. The type of anesthesia used and the patient's physiologic responses: patient's level of consciousness, IV lines present, and any current or pending laboratory reports
4. The patient's vital signs and hemodynamic status including estimated blood loss
5. Allergies and sensitivities
6. Medications administered from the sterile field: the use of blood or blood products; quick review of SCIP measures performed preoperatively and any continuation or discontinuation of therapeutic activity (i.e., antibiotics)
7. Any physical limitations, appliances, or prosthesis; skin condition before and after the procedure (i.e., return electrode site, potential pressure areas from positioning); and any language or communication issues (i.e., deaf, blind, paralysis)
8. Specific physiologic expectations resulting from the surgical procedure including pain management
9. Location of the patient's family, who may be waiting in the facility

The perioperative nurse receives the patient in the OR and is accountable for patient safety. The perioperative nurse is responsible for all documentation of activities in the OR. At the completion of the procedure, the perioperative nurse gives a detailed report to the postoperative nurse for the hand-over.

LEARNING ACTIVITIES

MATCHING

INSTRUCTIONS: Match the term to the appropriate definition.

a. hand over
b. time out
c. LAST
d. final count
e. malignant hyperthermia (MH)
f. discarded
g. surgical checklist
h. FDA
i. Surgical Care Improvement Project (SCIP)
j. cavities or orifices
k. counts
l. shearing force
m. under right hip
n. Universal Protocol
o. x-ray
p. filter needle
q. Sellick maneuver (cricoid pressure)
r. National Patient Safety Goals (NPSG)
s. never event
t. after dispensing
u. decanter or pour spout
v. circumferentially
w. reverse Trendelenburg's
x. Trendelenburg's
y. lithotomy
z. venous air embolus removal

_____1. Designed to ensure the patient is having the correct surgical procedure and correct location
_____2. The information starting preoperatively to the completion of the procedure; initiated by WHO
_____3. Prevention of SSIs
_____4. Updated yearly by The Joint Commission to reflect current statistics and patient care trends
_____5. The surgical team and patient, if possible, discuss the details of the procedure
_____6. This is not reimbursable according to CMS
_____7. Shared responsibility between the circulator and scrub person
_____8. This should not be used as a substitute for counting because of radiation exposure
_____9. This process should begin at the sterile field, then Mayo stand, and instrument table; the surgeon is notified of the results
_____10. A count should be done for closure of all areas to prevent retained items
_____11. Drugs sealed in ampules should be drawn up with this device
_____12. Vials and IV bags should be dispensed to the sterile field by this device
_____13. Drugs in unlabeled containers on the sterile field should be handled in this manner
_____14. When should a medicine cup or basin be labeled?
_____15. Signs and symptoms a patient is having a reaction to the anesthetic
_____16. The occlusion of the esophagus to prevent regurgitation during intubation
_____17. The exchange of information from the perioperative nurse to the postoperative nurse (perianesthesia nurse)
_____18. Hypermetabolic crisis that causes skeletal muscle contractions and can lead to death if not immediately treated
_____19. This organization requires tracking of all implanted medical devices
_____20. Limbs should be prepped in this direction
_____21. A small wedge should be placed in this area for a pregnant patient experiencing a drop in blood pressure from vena caval or aortic pressure
_____22. The description of dragging a patient's skin across the sheets, causing friction or damage
_____23. OR bed tilted: positioning with head down, feet higher than the head
_____24. Head is elevated on the OR bed 15 to 30 degrees higher than the feet
_____25. The legs are removed from the leg holders simultaneously and slowly bringing them together and lowered slowly at the same time
_____26. OR bed is in steep Trendelenburg's position, right side tilted up (left lateral)

LEARNING ACTIVITIES ANSWERS

1. n
2. g
3. i
4. r
5. b
6. s
7. k
8. o
9. d
10. j
11. p
12. u
13. f
14. t
15. c
16. q
17. a
18. e
19. h
20. v
21. m
22. l
23. x
24. w
25. y
26. z

CHAPTER 8

Surgical Pharmacology and Anesthesia

Surgical pharmacology and anesthesia are an important part of patient care in the operating room (OR). The perioperative nurse must have good communication and assessment skills to evaluate patient information for safe medication delivery in the OR. The perioperative nurse continues the nursing process by verbally communicating with the preoperative nurse and introduction to the patient.

The perioperative nurse checks all documentation including laboratory data, radiology studies, NPO status, history and physical (H&P), pregnancy status, medication reconciliation data, and any other pertinent information. The perioperative nurse confirms the surgical procedure. Questions about the procedure can be answered at this time, or the perioperative nurse may need clarification about the current documentation. Any questionable topics will be referred to the anesthesia provider or the surgeon. The perioperative nurse can then relay information to the intraoperative staff.

The perioperative nurse should understand the importance of medication documentation, rights of medication administration, medication orders, known medication sources and types, transfer techniques to the sterile field, and anesthesia techniques for continuity of safe care.

Why Is Correct Medication Documentation Important?

1. Many patients take prescription drugs that may not be in the chart, or patients may not think over-the-counter medications (OTC), dietary supplements, lotions, creams, hormone or nicotine patches, birth control, home remedies, or herbal substances are considered medications. Some patients may be afraid to admit if they drink alcohol or use recreational drugs. Many of these items can cause complications if mixed with OR medications (Table 8.1).
   a. The OR uses antibiotics, anticoagulants, hemostatic agents, dyes, steroids, solutions, adhesives, gases, chemical implants (i.e., radiation seeds, pellets, chemotherapy, and implants with impregnated drugs), thrombolytic, closure materials, inhalers, and other agents that can react with medications.
   b. Some herbal and dietary substances can affect bleeding and the state of consciousness.
   c. Products given in the OR are dosed based on patient's weight in kilograms, vital signs, food and

drug sensitivity/allergy status, pregnancy, nutrition nutritional status, age, and organ function.
   d. Documentation of current medications and supplements prevents drug errors, adverse effects, or toxicity.
   e. **Use alert bracelet for allergies**. Patients should be asked about allergies to plant substances, food, and metals (i.e., nickel) because these substances can be used in the form of narcotics, prep solutions, hemostatic agents, and implants. Iodine allergy is extremely rare and is not related to seafood or shellfish allergies.

2. The perioperative nurse must be aware of all patient medications and **the seven rights of medication administration**. What are the seven rights of medication administration? Some medications can be administered differently in the OR.
   a. Right patient
      1) Obtain medications for one patient at a time.
      2) Acknowledge two forms of patient identification (name and birth date), and check identification band in the OR.
   b. Right drug
      1) Verify medications with the order (standing order, verbal order, or preference card). Confirm the drug and dosage verbally with the scrub person. Check the labeling on the sterile field.
      2) Can the medication be used safely for the patient's condition or comorbidity?
   c. Right route
      1) How is the medication going to be administered? Is the route planned correct and safe?
      2) Intravenous (IV), subcutaneous, irrigation, instillation, for packing, with implants, or closure: Is the route in the OR different from other applications?
   d. Right dose
      1) Is the dose appropriate for the patient's weight in kilograms and physical condition?
      2) Will subsequent doses be necessary after the surgical procedure?
   e. Right reason
      1) Why does the patient need the drug?
      2) Is there more than one reason to administer the drug?

TABLE **8.1**   Examples of Common Herbal and Dietary Supplements and Potential Complications

Herbal or Dietary Supplement	Action and Potential Complications	Notes on Patient Usage
St. John's wort	Prolonged sedative effect, photosensitivity, peripheral neuropathy, interferes with metabolism of some antibiotics, calcium channel blockers, and warfarin	Antidepressant, antiinflammatory, possibly antiviral
Ginkgo biloba	Bleeding, anticoagulant	Improves circulation and memory
Ginseng	Hypertension and tachycardia, hypoglycemia, bleeding	Boosts vitality, stimulant, enhances sexuality
Vitamin E	Bleeding, slows wound healing and collagen repair	Prevents heart disease
Vitamin A (beta carotene converts to vitamin A in the body)	Can cause complications in pregnancy	Reverses the adverse effects on wound healing caused by steroid use, enhances healing, boosts immune system, fights infection, fights inflammation
Vitamin C	Potential for kidney stones and anemia in toxic state; can interfere with vitamin B_{12}; water-soluble; excreted readily via kidneys	Enhances wound healing
Garlic	Bleeding, hypotension, hypoglycemia, antithrombotic, antiplatelet	Lowers cholesterol, prevents heart disease, fights infection
Fish oil	Bleeding, hypotension	Prevents heart disease
Bromelain (found in pineapple stems)	No known complications	Antiinflammatory, digestive aid
Echinacea	Liver complications, interferes with immunosuppression, can cause transplant rejection	Antiinfective, fights common cold, enhances wound healing
Ephedra (also known as ma huang)	Cardiovascular instability, palpitations, hypertension, seizures	Appetite suppressant, respiratory treatment, boosts energy
Kava	Prolonged sedative effect, liver toxicity	Sedative, antiepileptic
Valerian	Prolonged sedative effect, can go through withdrawal, potentiated by alcohol, nausea	Sedative, sleep aid, muscle relaxant
Black cohosh	Bradycardia, peripheral dilation, hypotension	Alternative to estrogen replacement
Ginger	Bradycardia, bleeding, hypotension	Antiemetic, digestive aid, cough suppressant, relieves menstrual cramps
Licorice	Hypokalemia and dysrhythmia, hypertension, bleeding, can affect electrolytes, edema	Digestive aid
Chaparral	Liver complications	Alternative anticancer therapy
Chamomile	Potential allergy, bleeding, can affect electrolytes	Digestive aid, antiinflammatory, antiinfective

From Phillips, N. (2017). *Berry and Kohn's operating room technique* (13th ed.). St. Louis, MO: Elsevier.

   f. Right time
     1) Is the timing appropriate for the drug to be effective (preoperative antibiotics)?
     2) Was the drug prepared immediately before the time of use?
     3) Does the drug or chemical need special timing for preparation?
   g. Right documentation
     1) Who prepared the medication, and who administered it?
     2) Document the administered dose and method or special circumstances for use.
     3) What is the patient's physical response to the drug or chemical?
3. Managing medication storage in the OR
   a. Medications are stored in secure areas such as emergency carts, anesthesia carts, or automated dispensing system (e.g., Pyxis). Mobile carts are locked when not in use. Only authorized personnel should have access. Emergency medications should be available for quick access.
   b. Medications must be stored in original containers and separated from sound-alike, look-alike, high-alert medications with dividers or bins. Some medications may require refrigeration or freezing.
   c. Use single-dose vials if possible or pharmacy prepared (compounded drugs), rotate stock, and check expiration dates.
   d. If a multidose vial is opened, it must be labeled and expires in 28 days (e.g., insulin). Care is taken to prevent contamination of the vial.

e. Policies must be in place for the return of medications obtained and not used during the surgical procedure.
4. Medication orders
   a. Standing orders
     1) Prewritten or printed orders should be double-checked against the patient's medical record.
     2) Orders must be legible, approved numbering and abbreviations.
     3) Written orders must go in the patient's medical record and include the prescriber's signature, date, and time when used.
   b. Verbal orders
     1) Use only if necessary, confirmed by read-back (spell medication and numbers). Avoid interruptions or loud areas.
     2) Can be written by the nurse with date and time, then reviewed, validated, and signed by the prescriber.
   c. Computerized documentation
     1) This type of documentation is standardized and easy to use. It must be kept up to date and password-protected.
     2) The Joint Commission (TJC) and the American Nurses Association (ANA) establish the standards of documentation. Perioperative Nursing Data Set (PNDS) uses the standardized language for perioperative nursing.

Drug Sources, Forms, and Routes

Sources of Drugs in the Operating Room

Drugs and materials used in surgery come from a variety of sources found in nature, chemicals, and manufactured by biotechnology. Sources can be plant based, biologic from human or animals, mineral based, or synthetically engineered. Care is taken if the patient has an allergy or sensitivity to a drug or chemical source.
1. **Plant-based drugs** come from leaves, flowers, roots, sap, oil, or pigment (Box 8.1).
2. **Biologic sources** are found in living creatures: humans, animals, reptiles, fish, microorganisms, and insects (Box 8.2).
3. **Mineral-based drugs** can be a combination of vitamins, minerals, salts, and metal compounds (Box 8.3).
4. **Bioengineered sources** can come from a combination of genetic and DNA technology.
5. **Synthetic drugs** are made from chemicals and semisynthetic drugs. They can start with a natural or biologic substance and be altered, or they can be combined with another material or chemical.

Forms of Drugs Used in the Operating Room

Surgical medications and materials come in a variety of forms dependent on the use and the necessary route of delivery. Most of these are pharmaceutical in origin.

BOX 8.1   Plant Sources of Drugs

- Leaves (atropine from belladonna leaves, indigo carmine)
- Blossoms (opium poppy, colchicine from crocus)
- Seeds (arabic)
- Fruit (cranberry)
- Tubers/roots (ginseng) and rhizomes (valerian, gentian)
- Oils (camphor, eucalyptus)
- Sap (aloe, gum arabic preservative)
- Bark (aspirin, quinine, cascara)
- Wood extract
- Resin (benzoin)
- Fungi (some antibiotics)
- Herbs (tranquilizers)
- Cellulose fibers (hemostatic)

From Phillips, N. (2017). *Berry and Kohn's operating room technique* (13th ed.). St. Louis, MO: Elsevier.

1. **Liquids.** Liquids are used on and off the sterile field during the surgical procedure. Solutions include IV solutions, antiseptic skin preps, irrigation, antibiotics, local anesthetics, hemostatic agents, contrast media, dyes, oils, adhesives, and stains.
2. **Solids.** Solid drugs (e.g., pills, tablets) may be given with a limited amount of water in the preoperative area or at home as directed (i.e., oral hypoglycemics). Other solid products may be powders that are reconstituted by the perioperative nurse or used dry on the sterile field. Care is taken to assure that correct diluent is used in reconstitution. Hemostatic agents can come in sheets, sponges, woven materials, wax, and granules. Time-released seeds, pellets, or beads may be used for continued therapies. Chemicals such as phenol are solid until warmed.
3. **Semisolids.** Semisolid products include lubricants, anesthetic gels, suppositories, ointments (i.e., antiseptic and antibiotic), creams, or jellies.
4. **Gases.** Medical-grade gases can be piped in or available in a tank. Gases such as anesthetic gas, oxygen (green tank), carbon dioxide (gray tank), medical air (yellow tank), and special equipment gases are used in many surgical procedures. Other forms of gas such as nitrogen (black tank) may be used to power high-speed instruments such as drills and saws, but not used as a drug. The perioperative nurse must know the differences in the gases and tank colors to prevent error during use.

Common Drug Routes Used in Surgery

1. **IV:** Used to administer fluids, sedation, antibiotics, pain relief, and treatments such as chemotherapy. The insertion can be a peripheral vessel or central line (port) in the chest.
2. **Hypodermic injection:** Used for local anesthetics, subcuticular (SQ).

BOX 8.2   Animal and Biologic Sources

Bovine
- Hemostatic agent
- Blood-based oxygen carrier (Hemopure)
- Insulin
- Serum albumin
- Heparin

Porcine
- Hemostatic agent
- Biologic dressing
- Insulin
- Heparin
- Pancreatic enzymes

Equine
- Serum vaccine
- Hormones (estrogen)
- Pericardial implant

Ovine
- Suture
- Lanolin
- Hyaluronidase ophthalmic

Rodents
Hamster
- Protein used in recombinant thrombin

Avian
- Viscoat for eye surgery

Microbes (Fungi and Bacteria)
- Antibiotics

Marine Animals
Snails
- Ziconotide (Prialt) for neuropathy

Fish
- Protamine

Reptilian
- Antivenom (antivenin)
- Ancrod
- Exenatide (Byetta)
- Blood pressure drugs (Captopril)

Human
- Blood
- Blood fraction
- Insulin from DNA technology
- Tissue:
    - Reconstruction
    - Biologic dressing
- Semen
- Hormones (growth hormone and insulin)
- Human source extraction:
    - Human skin equivalent
- Hemoglobin-based oxygen carrier (PolyHeme)

Insects
- Bee's wax: hemostasis as bone wax
- Spider antivenom

From Phillips, N. (2017). *Berry and Kohn's operating room technique* (13th ed.). St. Louis, MO: Elsevier.

BOX 8.3   Mineral Sources

- Multivitamins contain calcium, iron, copper, magnesium, selenium, and zinc.
- Potassium is replaced after diuretic administration.
- Iodine is used in contrast media and radioactive markers.
- Zinc is used for wound healing.
- Gold salts are used to treat rheumatoid conditions.
- Silver is used for antimicrobial action.
- Iron helps treat anemia.
- Tungsten compounds treat AIDS.
- Lithium is used for manic depressive disease.
- Sodium and chloride balance body fluids.
- Talc is powdered magnesium silicate.

From Phillips, N. (2017). *Berry and Kohn's operating room technique* (13th ed.). St. Louis, MO: Elsevier.

3. **Topical:** Used for prep solutions, transdermal creams, oral spray, anesthetic gels, and drug patches (i.e., estrogen or scopolamine).
4. **Intrathecal** (injection into the spinal canal or subarachnoid space): Used for spinal and epidurals. Skull ports can be used for intrathecal chemotherapy infusion.
5. **Intraarticular** (injection into a joint): Used for steroids, antiinflammatory drugs, and hyaluronic acid.
6. **Intramuscular** (injection into a muscle): Used for pain medication, sedation, and obstetrical drugs.
7. **Intraperitoneal or intrapleural** (instillation into the abdominal cavity or pleural space of the lungs): Used for irrigation, antibiotics, hemostatic agents, and powder pleurodesis (i.e., sterile talc or powdered antibiotic).
8. **Transmucosal:** Drugs can be absorbed directly through a mucous membrane via oral, vaginal, nasal, rectal, or urethral.

Pharmacokinetics

The drug route affects the four phases of pharmacokinetics. Pharmacokinetics is the study of how the body processes drugs through absorption, distribution, metabolism, and excretion.

1. **Absorption:** The process of how the drug is taken or administered. It varies based on how quickly it can enter the bloodstream.
2. **Distribution:** The circulatory process a drug goes through to reach its target.
3. **Metabolism:** The metabolic process of how the body breaks down the drug so it can be effective. Organ

disease can slow or accelerate how the drug is used in the body.

4. **Excretion:** The method on how the body removes the end waste products of the drug. Organ function (i.e., liver and renal) determines the excretion rate. Drugs can be excreted through bile, urine, sweat, feces, and respiration.

Common Drugs and Materials Used in Surgery

Examples of drugs used in surgery are listed in Table 8.2.

1. **Antibiotics.** Antibiotics may be ordered for patients who have known infections or for prophylactic reasons. Each class of antibiotic has a different mechanism of action and works on different microorganisms.
   a. Antibiotics can be given 1 hour before an incision, or up to 2 hours for vancomycin and fluoroquinolones (ciprofloxacin). Refer to Surgical Care Improvement Program (SCIP) measures in Chapter 7.
   b. Antibiotics should be discontinued within 24 or 48 hours after cardiothoracic surgery.
   c. Patients with an unknown type of infection should be cultured to find the exact microorganism. A specific antibiotic can then be given to treat the infection.
   d. Antibiotics can be given IV, mixed in irrigation, or used as a powder, slurry, or sclerosant. Antibiotic powder can be mixed into bone cement.

   Common antibiotics in irrigation can be polymyxin B (for gram-negative microorganisms). Bacitracin is mostly effective against gram-positive microorganisms, as well as some gram-negative. They are commonly used together.
   1) They can be broad spectrum, effective against both gram-positive and gram-negative microorganisms.
   2) They can be narrow spectrum, effective against a small range of microorganisms.
   3) Limited spectrum may be effective against one species of microorganism.
2. **Anticoagulants.** Anticoagulants are given to prevent the formation of blood clots by interfering with the clotting process or blocking thrombin. They are used for patients with high risk for pulmonary embolus (PE), deep vein thrombosis (DVT), or myocardial infarction. Anticoagulants do not dissolve preexisting clots.
   a. **Heparin** may be given in the preoperative area before surgery: 5000 units subcutaneously as a prophylactic measure to minimize the risk for clotting. Heparin may be given by the anesthesia provider 3 minutes before clamping an artery.
   b. Heparin is commonly used in irrigation on the sterile field for vascular cases (5000 units per 1000 mL of sterile saline) to maintain the patency of blood vessels and prevent clotting.

TABLE 8.2   Examples of Drugs Used in Surgery

Drug Category	Drug Classifications	Individual Drugs
Anticoagulants and Coagulants		
Antiplatelet agents	Anticoagulant	Aspirin
		Ticlopidine
Anticoagulants	Anticoagulant	Enoxaparin
		Heparin
		Protamine
		Warfarin
Coagulant hemostatics	Coagulant	Thrombin
Thrombolytics	Thrombolytic	Alteplase
		Streptokinase
		Urokinase
Antiinfectives and Antibiotics		
	Aminoglycosides	Gentamicin
		Kanamycin
		Neomycin
		Streptomycin
		Tobramycin
	Cephalosporins	Cefazolin
		Cefonicid
		Cefotaxime
	Lipopeptides	Daptomycin
	Macrolides	Erythromycin
	Oxazolidinones	Ketolides
		Linezolid
		Telithromycin
	Penicillins	Amoxicillin
		Ampicillin
		Carbenicillin
		Mezlocillin
		Penicillin G potassium
		Ticarcillin
	Quinolones	Ciprofloxacin
	Sulfonamide antimicrobials	Glycylcycline
		Sulfamethoxazole
		Tygacil
	Tetracyclines	Doxycycline
		Tetracycline
Autonomic Nervous System Agents		
Adrenergic agonists	Alpha- and beta-adrenergic agents	Epinephrine
Adrenergic antagonists	Antidysrhythmics	Isoproterenol
		Propranolol
Anticholinergics	Muscarinics	Atropine sulfate
		Glycopyrrolate
		Scopolamine

(Continued)

TABLE 8.2	Examples of Drugs Used in Surgery—cont'd	
Drug Category	**Drug Classifications**	**Individual Drugs**
Benzodiazepines		
Antianxiety medications	Sedative	Diazepam
		Lorazepam
		Midazolam
Central Nervous System Agents		
Analgesic agents	Narcotics	Fentanyl
		Meperidine
		Morphine
Surgical Dyes and Contrast		
Dyes		Bismarck brown
		Brilliant green
		Congo red
		Gentian violet
		Indian ink
		Indigo carmine
		Indocyanine green
		Isosulfan blue (radioisotopes)
		Methylene blue
		Trypan blue
Contrast media		Diatrizoate meglumine
		Iohexol
		Vasovist MRI contrast
Tissue stains		Lugol's iodine solution (Schiller's solution)
		Monsel's ferric solution

MRI, Magnetic resonance imaging.
From Phillips, N. (2017). *Berry and Kohn's operating room technique* (13th ed.). St. Louis, MO: Elsevier.

c. **Protamine** is an anticoagulant that may be administered to reverse the effects of heparin, 1 to 1.5 mg for every 100 units of heparin.

d. After surgical procedures such as total joints, patients may be placed on a low-molecular-weight heparin given daily subcutaneously to prevent DVT or PE. Examples include Lovenox, Enoxaparin, or Arixtra.

e. Oral long-term anticoagulants may be given for patients at risk for development of blood clots. The patient's prothrombin time (PT) and international normalized ratio (INR) should be checked frequently for bleeding disorders.

3. **Antiinflammatories.** Antiinflammatory agents may be given intraoperatively to reduce postoperative inflammation.

a. **Steroids** must be given with care because they can delay the healing process by suppressing the immune system.

b. **Corticosteroids** such as betamethasone, dexamethasone, prednisone, and triamcinolone acetonide (Kenalog) minimize edema in a localized area.

4. **Contrast media.** Contrast media is used as a diagnostic agent for radiologic studies. Common brands include Hypaque, Optiray, Omnipaque, Conray, Isovue, and Ultravist.

a. Check the patient's history for any reaction to iodized contrast media. Benadryl and prednisone may be given to patients with a history of sensitivity or allergic reactions.

b. Contrast media can be diluted with normal IV saline.

c. Contrast media is used with caution in patients with renal disease because it is excreted by the kidneys.

d. Certain types of contrast cannot be injected into the lumbar subarachnoid space (Hypaque).

e. Contrast media can be administered intraoperatively by hand with a syringe or an automatic injector device for large structures such as the aorta. All bubbles must be removed before administration, or they may show up on x-ray as an artifact.

5. **Surgical dyes.** Dyes are used to mark the skin, detect tissue damage, color the urine, or help with mapping of the lymph node system. Many types of dye are used during surgical procedures. Examples of common surgical dyes include the following:

a. **Gentian violet** is the purple dye in skin markers.

b. **Indigo carmine** is a blue dye usually given by the anesthesia provider to verify kidney function. The urine turns green.

c. **Isosulfan blue** (Lymphazurin) is used for sentinel lymph node biopsies. It can be traced with a Geiger counter.

d. **Methylene blue** is commonly used to detect bladder injuries, urinary anastomotic leaks, or lymph node removal, or observe patency of the fallopian tubes. The anesthesia provider can inject this dye IV to monitor urine production. The urine turns green.

e. **Fluorescein sodium** is a yellow indicator dye used in ophthalmic procedures to detect corneal injury. It is also used IV in conjunction with a Wood's lamp (black light) to confirm patency and viability of small vessels in the vascular system during skin flaps and certain bowel procedures. The dye glows yellow-green in the circulating blood under black light.

6. **Staining agents.** Staining agents are used to help visualize target tissue and distinguish normal from abnormal tissue.

a. **Lugol's solution** is used to perform the Schiller test on the uterine cervix. This iodine solution

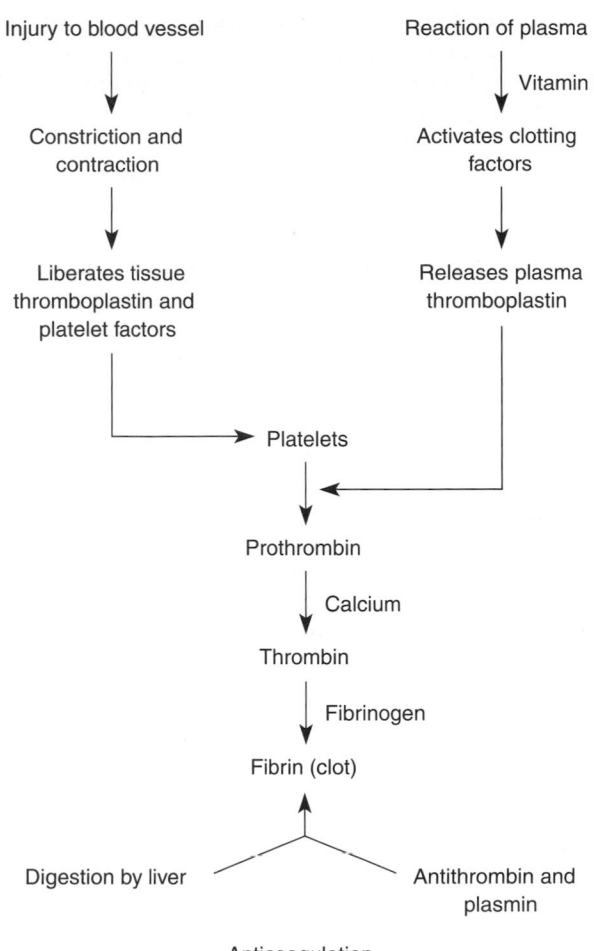

Figure 8.1 Mechanism of hemostasis. (From Phillips, N. [2017]. *Berry and Kohn's operating room technique* [13th ed.]. St. Louis, MO: Elsevier.)

stains normal tissue, but does not stain abnormal tissue.

b. **Acetic acid** is a white vinegar solution used as an indicator, but is not truly a stain. A vinegar solution of 3% to 5% is applied on the uterine cervix to detect human papillomavirus (condyloma or genital/venereal warts). Abnormal tissue will raise and appear white. If vinegar is used full strength, it will cause burns to the tissue.

7. **Hemostatic agents and solutions.** Chemical hemostatic agents are used to help accelerate clot formation (Fig. 8.1). Because many of the chemical agents are derived from different sources, such as bovine, porcine, or plant-based, the perioperative nurse should be aware of any patient sensitivities or allergies. Care is taken not to allow any form of hemostatic material to enter a blood salvage system. Hemostatic material in readministered blood would cause systemic clotting.

a. **Absorbable gelatin.** This is a porcine product that comes in a pad (Gelfoam), film, matrix (Floseal, Surgiflo), or powder. It is used for capillary bleeding and can soak up to 45 times its

weight in blood. It can be used dry or wet with saline, thrombin, or epinephrine. The powdered form can be made into a paste or slurry. It should not be used on infected tissue or encased within a closed space.

b. **Oxidized cellulose.** Oxidized cellulose is a cotton or rayon product. It is applied dry and can absorb 10 times its own weight. It can be placed on, sutured, or wrapped around an oozing area. It is not recommended for long-term use or for bone. Common products are Surgicel, NU-KNIT, and Fibrillar.

c. **Microfibrillar collagen.** This is a bovine product of powdered corium collagen. The collagen swells to form a clot by adhesion of the platelets. It is applied dry and held with pressure. Common products are Avitene, Surgiflo, and Instat.

d. **Absorbable collagen.** Absorbable collagen is a bovine product that comes in sponge form. It is used dry for oozing or bleeding. The sponge dissolves to help form a clot. It should be applied dry and not in an infected wound. It can absorb in 8 to 10 weeks. Common products are Helistat, Collastat, and SuperStat.

e. **Thrombin.** Thrombin is an enzyme that can be bovine or from humans. It is a topical solution that helps to accelerate the clotting process by converting fibrinogen to fibrin. The solution can be 5000 or 10,000 units. It should be in a shallow container on the sterile field and labeled correctly. It should never be drawn up in a syringe or injected. It is also available in a spray (Tisseel).

8. **Other forms of hemostatic agents.** There are other products with special uses to help control bleeding.

a. **Bone wax** is used as a mechanical barrier. It is sterile beeswax. It can be applied to bone with an instrument or with the fingers. It is used sparingly or removed because it can form a granuloma. It is used in cardiac (sternum), spine, orthopedics, and neurosurgery.

b. **Silver nitrate.** Silver nitrate is an antibacterial and astringent compound used for burns and sealing tissue. It is applied topically and comes in several forms including molded on sticks.

c. **Zeolite beads and Kaolin products.** These products may be seen in trauma patients who come into the OR. Zeolite beads are foil-wrapped 3.5-pound bags that can be packed into a wound. Koalin (QuickClot) is the same product but comes in a dressing form or pad. They are mainly used for severe hemorrhage.

d. **Monsel's solution or paste.** Monsel's solution is iron based and can be used for intrauterine bleeding at the placental site or used as a paste applied to the cervix or uterine biopsy sites.

9. **Antiadhesion agents.** Antiadhesion agents are used as a barrier to prevent scar tissue from attaching to organs. They come in a variety of materials such as bovine collagen sheets, cellulose,

and porcine. Some antiadhesion materials come in the form of a sheet, film, spray, or gel. Some antiadhesion agents may absorb over time, or some can be a permanent implant and sutured in place. Examples include:

a. **Seprafilm.** This is a clear thin translucent sheet composed of sodium hyaluronate carboxy-methylcellulose. It must be applied dry with dry gloves. It is used between the abdominal wall and internal organs to reduce postoperative adhesions in abdominal, pelvic, bowel, and other surgeries. It is an absorbable product.

b. **Sepragel.** Sepragel is a gel sheet of carboxy-methylcellulose that absorbs within 10 days. It should not be used in the presence of infection.

c. **Adept.** Adept is an icodextrin solution. It is used for endoscopic cases. It should be used at body temperature.

d. **Intercede.** Intercede is a knitted cellulose product that can be used wet or dry. It is used for laparotomy cases.

e. **DuraGen.** DuraGen is a bovine collagen product that is used as a dural patch. It can be used dry or moist, and sutured or glued in place.

f. **Preclude.** Preclude is a synthetic sheet of polytetrafluoroethylene. It is a permanent implant and can be sutured or stapled in place.

10. **Other medications and considerations**
    a. **Epinephrine.** Epinephrine (vasoconstrictor) is added to local anesthetics to decrease bleeding rate and slow the rate of the absorption of the anesthetic. Epinephrine should not be used in areas with reduced circulation, such as toes, fingers, penis, and tip of the nose. Doses of local medication can be increased because the epinephrine slows the absorption down and allows the drug to last longer. Concentrations come in 1:100,000 and 1:200,000 ratios. Always follow the recommended dosage.
        1) Epinephrine can cause tachycardia, palpitations, hypertension, diaphoresis, or other adrenergic reactions.
        2) Read labels of local medications carefully. Epinephrine may be incorporated within the drug at different ratios.
    b. **Eye medications.** Eye medications can be topical or for injection. The ophthalmic surgical procedure may require the use of one or many of the drugs.
        1) **Mydriatics** are used to dilate the pupil. They are commonly used to reduce the effect of trauma by paralyzing the sphincter muscle of the iris. Mydriatics include phenylephrine (Neo-Synephrine) and atropine.
        2) **Miotic** drugs constrict the pupil. They are used to reduce intraocular pressure and are commonly used for glaucoma. Miotic drugs include carbachol (Miostat), acetylcholine chloride (Miochol-E), and pilocarpine.

3) **Basic salt solution** is for irrigating and keeping the eye moist in the form of drops or bottles available in 250- or 500-mL increments. Examples include Blinx, Rinse, and Irrigate.

4) **Viscoelastic** drugs are thick, jelly-like drugs. They can be injected into the eye to keep the anterior chamber of the eye expanded and to protect tissue. They are commonly used during phacoemulsification. Some common drugs include Amvisc, Viscoat, Healon, and sodium hyaluronate. They usually come in sterile premeasured syringes.

5) **Ophthalmic viscosurgical device** is a new term for combination viscoelastic agents. An example is DuoVisc (Viscoat and Provisc).

c. **Benzyl alcohol.** Benzyl alcohol may be found as a preservative in some small vials of saline, sterile water, and medications. If large quantities of solution are needed, it is necessary to use IV quality fluids that do not contain preservative.

d. **Sodium bicarbonate.** This is a buffer that may be added to medications to reduce the stinging feeling when injected. It is also given to correct metabolic acidosis.

e. **Obstetric medications**
    1) **Magnesium sulfate** may be given to a pregnant patient to lower blood pressure in toxemia or as an anticonvulsant in preeclampsia. Dose is 4 to 5 g in 250 mL of fluid. Maximum dosage is 20 to 40 g/day.
    2) **Oxytocin** is a hormone that may be given as a uterine stimulant to stimulate labor contractions. It has vasoconstriction properties used to control hemorrhage by contracting the uterus after birth. Dose is 1 to 2 U/min IV. Maximum dose is 32 U/min. During cesarean sections, the surgeon may inject 10 units of oxytocin directly into the uterus to control bleeding after removal of the placenta.

f. **Pregnancy labeling.** The US Food and Drug Administration (FDA) changed the requirements for labeling drugs to include everyone who can be part of the reproduction process regardless of their sex. The former classifications were discontinued in 2015. More information can be found via the FDA website (http://www.fda.gov).
    1) Pregnancy (includes labor and delivery): information about dosing, risks to the fetus, information registry, clinical consideration, and effects of drugs
    2) Lactation (nursing mothers): lists the risks of the drug for actual nursing mothers, data collection, and clinical considerations
    3) Male and female individuals of reproductive potential: includes pregnancy testing, contraception, and the effects of drugs concerning infertility (spermatogenesis)

Anesthetics

1. Patients receiving a local anesthetic by the surgeon are monitored by a qualified nurse. Advanced Cardiac Life Support (ACLS) training is recommended for patient safety. An anesthesia provider is not present, and the patient does not have an IV access line. The perioperative nurse may not monitor the patient and circulate simultaneously.
   a. The perioperative nurse must be able to use all monitoring equipment. This includes blood pressure, electrocardiograph (ECG), oxygen saturation, pulse, respirations, and available suction. Any change in the patient's baseline vital signs should be reported to the surgeon immediately.
   b. Documentation should include vital signs every 5 to 15 minutes, observation of reaction during injection of local medication and during incision. When epinephrine is added to the local drug the patient's heart rate may increase.
   c. The perioperative nurse must know the signs of medication toxicity and the necessary emergency steps.
2. **Signs of local medication allergy or toxicity.** Local anesthetic systemic toxicity is a serious condition that must be recognized and treated immediately (Table 8.3).
   a. The patient may complain of dizziness, metallic taste, ringing in the ears, and numbness of the tongue or around the mouth.
   b. The patient may become confused, restless, or agitated, or respiratory rate might increase.
   c. The patient may develop an arrhythmia (tachycardia or bradycardia).
   d. The patient may develop seizures, coma, respiratory arrest, and/or asystole.
3. What actions should the monitoring nurse take if toxicity is suspected?
   a. Notify the surgeon immediately and call for an anesthesia provider.
   b. Maintain the airway and administer oxygen.
   c. Place an IV for medication administration.
   d. Continue monitoring and documenting the patient's vital signs.
4. **Local use in regional anesthetics** interfere with nerve conduction and the body's ability to feel pain. The same drugs are used in different dosages and concentrations for regional anesthesia. Epinephrine may be added for vasoconstriction and prolonged effect. Local anesthetics directly injected into target tissues are used for a small area, whereas regional anesthetics cover a larger neurovascular area such as a pain block for a limb.

   The drugs differ in the way they are metabolized by the body and how they react. The larger the blood supply, the quicker local anesthetics are absorbed and broken down. Local anesthetics are hydrochloride salts in solution; they can affect the heart and central nervous system.

TABLE 8.3 Comparison of Toxicity and Allergy Caused by Local Anesthetics

Toxic Reaction	Allergic Reaction[a]
Symptoms vary depending on the drug	Immediate localized reaction followed by generalized body reaction
Subjective	
Dizziness, somnolence, paresthesia, nausea, visual/speech problems	Sense of uneasiness, pruritus, agitation, paresthesia
Objective	
Decreased breathing rate and depth, muscle twitches, tremors, slurred speech, seizures, vomiting unconsciousness, coma	Erythema, urticaria, wheals
Vasovagal	
Dysrhythmias, bradycardia, vasodilation, hypotension, myocardial depression, cardiac arrest	Coughing, wheezing, bronchospasm, hypotension, hypovolemia, vasodilation, cardiovascular collapse, cardiac arrest
Treatment	
Supportive airway management; need intravenous (IV) line; Trendelenburg's position; muscular contractions are treated with diazepam (Valium)	Especially with amino ester type: airway management, IV fluids, epinephrine, diphenhydramine, and steroids as needed

[a]Not common with amino amide.
From Phillips, N. (2017). *Berry and Kohn's operating room technique* (13th ed.). St. Louis, MO: Elsevier.

Selection of drugs is determined by procedure, area of the body, extent of pain relief, and the patient's overall health. Very ill patients, geriatric patients, children, and anyone with liver or vascular disease may require lower individualized doses (Table 8.4). Local anesthetic drugs can be classified into two groups: amino esters and amino amides.
   a. **Amino esters** are rapidly broken down in plasma by pseudocholinesterase enzymes produced by the liver. The by-product, paraaminobenzoic acid, can stimulate allergies in some patients.
      1) **Cocaine** can be used as a topical vasoconstrictor in ENT surgery. It is available in 4% and 10% solutions. The 10% solution is not used

TABLE 8.4   Local and Regional Anesthetic Agents

Generic Name	Trade Name(s)	Uses	Concentration	Duration of Effect (h)	Maximum Dosage
Amino Amides					
Bupivacaine	Marcaine Sensorcaine	Local infiltration[a] Regional block[a] Surgical epidural	0.25%–0.50%	2–3	400 mg
Dibucaine	Nupercaine Percaine Cinchocaine	Local infiltration Peripheral nerves	0.05%–0.1%	3–3{1/2}	30 mg
Etidocaine	Duranest	Peripheral nerves Epidural	0.5%–1%	2–3	500 mg
Lidocaine	Xylocaine Lignocaine	Topical Infiltration[a]	2%–4% 0.5%	{1/2} to 2	200 mg or 4 mg/kg 500 mg or 7 mg/kg when mixed with vasoconstrictor
		Peripheral nerves[a] Nerve block[a] Spinal Epidural	1%–2%		
Mepivacaine	Carbocaine	Infiltration Peripheral nerves Epidural	0.5%–1% 1%–2%	{1/2} to 2	500 mg
Prilocaine	Citanest	Infiltration Peripheral nerves Regional block Epidural	1%–2% 2%–3%	{1/2} to 2{1/2}	600 mg
Ropivacaine	Naropin	Infiltration	0.2%	2{1/2} for surgical analgesia; 6–10 for surgical nerve block	200 mg for analgesia; 300 mg for nerve block
		Field block Nerve block Epidural Postoperative pain management Not used for Bier block	0.5% 0.75% 1%		
Amino Esters					
Chloroprocaine	Nesacaine	Infiltration[a] Peripheral nerves[a] Nerve block[a] Epidural Topical	0.5% 2% 2% 2%–3% 4%–10%	{1/4} to {1/2} {1/2}	1000 mg 200 mg or 4 mg/kg body weight
Cocaine		Topical anesthesia and vasoconstrictor in ENT surgery	4%	2	1 mg/kg
Procaine	Novocain	Infiltration	0.5%	{1/4} to {1/2}	1000 mg or 14 mg/kg body weight
		Peripheral nerves Spinal	1%–2%		
Tetracaine	Cetacaine Pontocaine	Topical Spinal	2% 1%	2–4	20 mg

[a]Epinephrine may be used.

From Phillips, N. (2017). *Berry and Kohn's operating room technique* (13th ed.). St. Louis, MO: Elsevier.

very often anymore because of toxic reactions. The fatal dose is 1.2 g.

2) **Tetracaine** a common topical ophthalmic solution. It is available in a 2% solution. It is effective for 2 to 4 hours. Maximum dose is 20 mg.

3) **Procaine** (Novocaine) is used for infiltration, dental procedures, nerve blocks, or spinals. It has a short duration time of up to 30 minutes. Maximum dose is 14 mg/kg.

b. **Amino amides** are stable drugs metabolized by the liver. Patients with liver disease should be monitored closely and given a low starting dose. Toxicity can occur if the drug builds up in the bloodstream.

1) **Lidocaine** (Xylocaine) is one of the most commonly used amides for local anesthesia and blocks. It works quickly and can last up to 2 hours. It comes in concentrations of 0.5% to 2% and is available with epinephrine. It can be used to treat arrhythmias and pulseless ventricular tachycardia. Lidocaine is also available in a topical form for mucous membranes. Maximum dose is 200 mg (4 mg/kg) with epinephrine, the maximum dose is 500 mg (7 mg/kg).

2) **Bupivacaine** (Marcaine, Sensorcaine) is four times stronger than lidocaine. It takes longer to work, but can last up to 3 hours. It comes in concentrations of 0.25% to 0.75% and is available with epinephrine. It can be used for some blocks. Maximum dose is 400 mg in 24 hours.

3) **Ropivacaine** (Naropin) is used for nerve blocks, epidurals, and postoperative pain. It comes in concentrations of 0.2% to 0.75%. Test dose is recommended; follow instructions for dosage for procedure.

4) **Mepivacaine** (Carbocaine) works quickly and comes in concentrations of 0.5% to 2%. It can be used for local areas and peripheral nerve blocks. Maximum dose is 400 mg.

5. **Moderate sedation and general anesthesia.** A combination of drugs may be given for moderate sedation and general anesthesia. These drugs relieve the patient's anxiety and may make them drowsy so they do not remember the procedure. Other drugs such as narcotics keep the patient pain free. Muscle relaxants and anesthetic gases are also used when appropriate (Table 8.5).

a. **Benzodiazepines.** This class of drugs is given to reduce anxiety and provide sedation. They produce drowsiness and can have an amnesic effect in larger doses. They can cause respiratory depression and changes in blood pressure and heart rate in some patients.

1) **Midazolam** (Versed) is a sedative and anxiolytic. It is contraindicated in patients with narrow-angle glaucoma.
   a) Commonly used for preoperative sedation and moderate sedation; can last up to 2 hours
   b) Works quickly, 3 to 5 minutes given IV; initial dose: 1 to 2 mg (2.5–5 mg over 1 hour)

2) **Diazepam** (Valium) is sedative, anxiolytic, skeletal muscle relaxant, and anticonvulsant.

TABLE 8.5 **Depth of General Anesthesia and Pupil Reactions**

From	To	Patient's Responses	Patient Care Considerations
Induction of general anesthesia by IV or inhalant gas	Begins to lose consciousness; will have recall Bispectral state 100	Drowsy, dizzy, amnesic	Close OR doors. Keep room quiet. Stand by to assist. Initiate cricoid pressure if requested.
Loss of consciousness: excitement phase	Relaxation, light hypnosis; low probability of recall Bispectral state 70-50	May be excited, with irregular breathing and movements of extremities; susceptible to external stimuli (e.g., noise, touch)	Restrain patient. Remain at patient's side, quietly, but ready to assist anesthesia provider as needed.
Surgical anesthesia stage of relaxation	Loss of reflexes: depression of vital functions Bispectral state 40: maintenance range	Regular respiration; contracted pupils; reflexes disappear; muscles relax; auditory sensation lost	Position patient and prepare skin only when anesthesia provider indicates this stage is reached and under control.
Danger stage: vital functions too depressed	Respiratory failure; possible cardiac arrest Bispectral state 0	Not breathing; little or no pulse or heartbeat	Prepare for cardiopulmonary resuscitation.

IV, Intravenous; *OR,* operating room.
From Phillips, N. (2017). *Berry and Kohn's operating room technique* (13th ed.). St. Louis, MO: Elsevier.

it is contraindicated in patients with narrow-angle glaucoma.

    a) Works quickly, 1 to 5 minutes given IV; dose: 5 to 10 mg (over 2–4 hours); can last up to 4 hours

    b) May be given orally with a small amount of water

  3) **Romazicon** (Flumazenil) is a reversal agent for all benzodiazepines.

    a) Works within 60 seconds. Initial dose is 0.2 mg IV (over 15 seconds). Dose can be repeated every 1 minute, up to 1 mg; duration: 10 to 15 minutes

    b) Romazicon can cause heart palpitations, nausea, and vomiting. Use with caution in patients with renal disease

    c) Monitor patient for 1 hour after dose

b. **Narcotics.** Narcotics can be given at any time during the perioperative period to produce analgesia. They are used in many procedures and can be given in small doses, bolus, or continuous infusion. Patients given narcotics are monitored closely because they affect the central nervous system, resulting in respiratory depression. Patients with head injuries, breathing problems, obesity, or age older than 60 years are at an increased risk for complications. Common narcotics include:

  1) **Morphine (Astramorph, Duramorph):** fast-working analgesic used for moderate to severe pain (1–3 minutes)

    a) Dose: 1 to 2 mg, up to 0.1 mg/kg. May last 3 to 4 hours. Can cause respiratory suppression, constipation, or urinary retention.

    b) Morphine is commonly used for conscious sedation and epidurals.

  2) **Fentanyl (Sublimaze):** fast-working analgesic (1–3 minutes), also provides sedation. Fentanyl is 100 times more potent than morphine.

    a) Dose: 25 mcg (up to 2 mcg/kg); may last 30 to 60 minutes.

    b) Causes delayed respiratory depression and can interact with monoamine oxidase inhibitors.

  3) **Meperidine (Demerol):** fast-working analgesic (1–5 minutes)

    a) Dose: 10 to 20 mg (up to 1 mg/kg); may last 1 to 2 hours.

    b) Use with caution in patients with head injuries, liver and kidney damage, and monoamine oxidase inhibitors.

  4) **Narcan (Naloxone):** is a reversal agent for narcotics (opioids)

    a) Initial dose: 0.4 to 2 mg IV, intramuscularly (IM), subcutaneously, or nasal spray 4 mg; may last 30 to 60 minutes. Redose every 2 minutes up to 10 mg.

    b) Can cause tachycardia, stroke, and hypertension. It is metabolized by the liver and excreted by the kidneys.

c. **Neuromuscular blockers.** Muscle relaxants are administered as part of general anesthesia to patients before insertion of an endotracheal tube (ET) or during procedures where skeletal muscle relaxation is necessary, such as abdominal surgery. The neuromuscular blockers work on all skeletal muscle including the diaphragm and respiratory muscles.

The anesthesia provider must use mechanical ventilation and watch the patient closely. A nerve stimulator may be used to measure the degree of relaxation. Muscle relaxants can be short, intermediate, or long acting. They also fall into two categories: nondepolarizing and depolarizing muscular blockers.

  1) **Nondepolarizing neuromuscular blockers** prevent muscle contraction by binding to cholinergic receptors. Nondepolarizing muscle relaxants do not cause fasciculation and are not malignant hyperthermia (MH) triggers.

    a) **Atracurium** (Tracrium) is an intermediate-acting agent lasting up to 30 minutes. It is used for intubation and relaxation maintenance. The dose for intubation is 0.3 to 0.5 mg/kg. It can cause hypotension, vasodilation, and histamine release.

    b) **Vecuronium** (Norcuron) is an intermediate-acting agent lasting up to 30 minutes. It is used for intubation and relaxation maintenance. The dose for intubation is 0.08 to 0.1 mg/kg. It has no cumulative cardiovascular or histamine effects.

    c) **Rocuronium** (Zemuron) is an intermediate-acting agent lasting up to 30 minutes. It is used for intubation and relaxation maintenance. It must be refrigerated. The dose for intubation is 0.6 mg/kg. It can cause tachycardia and possible reaction with some antibiotics. Patients recover quickly with no lasting cardiovascular effects.

    d) **Pancuronium** (Pavulon) is long onset, potent, and long lasting up to 1 hour or longer. The initial dose is 0.04 to 0.1 mg/kg. It is used for relaxation maintenance. It can cause histamine release, hypotension, tachycardia, and bronchospasm, and is contraindicated in neonates and children because it contains the preservative benzyl alcohol.

    e) **Neostigmine** (Prostigmin) is the reversal agent for nondepolarizing neuromuscular blockers and is usually given with atropine. The dose is 0.5 to 2 mg. It is a cholinergic and inhibits the destruction of acetylcholine. It is contraindicated in patients with asthma, seizure disorders, arrhythmias, coronary artery disease, bowel obstruction, and urinary retention.

2) **Depolarizing neuromuscular blockers** stimulate the autonomic system. It acts like the neurotransmitter acetylcholine and causes depolarization (contractions). These involuntary muscle contractions are fasciculations that result in flaccidity. Depolarizing neuromuscular blockers are Malignant hyperthermia (MH) triggers.

a) **Succinylcholine** (Anectine, Quelicin, Sucostrin) is a very rapid-onset depolarizing neuromuscular blocker, 30 to 60 seconds. It lasts only 4 to 6 minutes. It is usually used for intubation. The dose is 0.5 to 1.5 mg/kg. It can cause increased intracranial and intraocular pressure, muscle pain, muscle rigidity, changes in potassium levels, and paralysis. There is no reversal agent. Succinylcholine is the only depolarizing neuromuscular blocker used in the United States.

6. **Inhalation anesthetic gases and vapor** are inhaled through the face mask, ET, or laryngeal mask airway (LMA) to induce unconsciousness. Oxygen is supplied to the gas machine and delivered in measurements of liters. The anesthetic gases are mixed with oxygen through the breathing circuit. Halogenated inhalants can trigger MH.

The inhaled agent and oxygen fill the lungs; it is transported to the circulatory system and then into tissue. The depth of anesthesia is determined on the concentration of the agent in the brain. Several different inhalation agents are available; they each have their own advantages and disadvantages (Table 8.6).

a. **Nitrous oxide.** Nitrous oxide is a nonflammable, nonhalogenated gas mixed with oxygen. It provides rapid induction and quick recovery.

TABLE 8.6   Commonly Used General Anesthetic Agents

Generic Name	Trade Name	Administration	Characteristics	Uses
Inhalation Agents				
Nitrous oxide	None	Inhalation	Inorganic nonvolatile gas; slight potency; pleasant, fruitlike odor; nonirritating; nonflammable but supports combustion; poor muscle relaxation	Rapid induction and recovery; short procedures when muscle relaxation unimportant; adjunct to potent agents. Should be mixed with 30% oxygen to prevent hypoxia.
Halothane	Fluothane	Inhalation	Halogenated volatile liquid; potent; pleasant odor; nonirritating; cardiovascular and respiratory depressant; incomplete muscle relaxation; potentially toxic to liver	Rapid induction; wide spectrum for maintenance; depth of anesthesia easily altered; rapid reversal Rarely used
Enflurane	Ethrane	Inhalation	Halogenated ether; potent; some muscle relaxation; respiratory depressant	Rapid induction and recovery; wide spectrum for maintenance Rarely used
Desflurane	Suprane	Inhalation	Halogenated liquid with low solubility; desflurane has faster uptake by inhalation and elimination	Not used for induction with children. Can be used for maintenance in adults and children.
Sevoflurane	Ultane	Inhalation	Volatile liquid form, nonflammable and nonexplosive; noted for its rapid induction and rapid emergence qualities	Used for adults and children Rapid elimination
Isoflurane	Forane	Inhalation	Halogenated methyl ether; potent; muscle relaxant; profound respiratory depressant; metabolized in liver	Rapid induction and recovery with minimal aftereffects; wide spectrum for maintenance

(Continued)

TABLE

8.6   Commonly Used General Anesthetic Agents—cont'd

Generic Name	Trade Name	Administration	Characteristics	Uses
Intravenous Agents				
Thiopental sodium	Pentothal sodium	Intravenous	Barbiturate; potent; short acting with cumulative effect; rapid uptake by circulatory system; no muscle relaxation; respiratory depressant	Rapid induction and recovery; short procedures when muscle relaxation not needed; basal anesthetic
Methohexital	Brevital	Intravenous	Barbiturate; potent; circulatory and respiratory depressant	Rapid induction; brief anesthesia
Propofol	Diprivan	Intravenous	Alkyl phenol; potent short-acting sedative-hypnotic; cardiovascular depressant	Rapid induction and recovery; short procedures alone; prolonged anesthesia in combination with inhalation agents or opioids
Ketamine	Ketaject, Ketalar	Intravenous, intramuscular	Dissociative drug; profound amnesia and analgesia; may cause psychologic problems during emergence	Rapid induction; short procedures when muscle relaxation not needed; children and young adults
Fentanyl	Sublimaze	Intravenous	Opioid; potent narcotic; metabolizes slowly; respiratory depressant	High-dose narcotic anesthesia in combination with oxygen
Sufentanil	Sufenta	Intravenous	Opioid; potent narcotic, respiratory depressant	Premedication; high-dose narcotic anesthesia in combination with oxygen
Fentanyl and droperidol	Innovar	Intravenous	Combination narcotic and tranquilizer; potent; long acting	Neuroleptanalgesia
Diazepam	Valium	Intravenous, intramuscular	Benzodiazepine; tranquilizer; produces amnesia, sedation, and muscle relaxation	Premedication; awake intubation; induction
Midazolam	Versed	Intravenous, intramuscular	Benzodiazepine; sedative; short-acting amnesic; central nervous system and respiratory depressant	Premedication; conscious sedation; induction in children

From Phillips, N. (2017). *Berry and Kohn's operating room technique* (13th ed.). St. Louis, MO: Elsevier.

It is administered along with other IV drugs to maintain general anesthesia. It is safe to use for MH-susceptible patients.

1) Advantages include pleasant odor, delivered by face mask, and provides amnesia and analgesia for short procedures with few after effects.
2) Disadvantages include poor muscle relaxation and can cause hypoxia. It should not be used in bowel, laparoscopy, or inner-ear procedures, or for pregnant patients.

b. **Desflurane** (Suprane) is a halogenated liquid turned into a vapor in the anesthesia machine. It requires a special vaporizer to heat the liquid. It is used for induction and maintenance for adults. Desflurane is an MH trigger.

1) Advantages include rapid recovery. It is commonly used for bariatric surgeries.

2) Disadvantages include a bad odor and can cause hypotension. It is not used for induction in children.

c. **Sevoflurane** (Ultane) is a halogenated liquid that turns into vapor in the anesthesia machine. It is nonflammable and nonexplosive. It is used for both children and adults. Sevoflurane can trigger MH.

1) Advantages include rapid emergence, elimination quickly by the lungs, and can be used for patients with increased intracranial pressure.
2) Disadvantages include that it can cause glycosuria and proteinuria during the surgical procedure.

d. **Isoflurane** (Forane) is a halogenated liquid that is turned into a vapor in the anesthesia machine. It causes muscle relaxation and slows the heart rate.

Cardiac output is unchanged. It is metabolized by the liver, so it is safe to use in renal disease. Isoflurane can trigger MH.
1) Advantages include less cardiac depression and less organ toxicity.
2) Disadvantages include respiratory depression and vasodilation of peripheral and coronary vessels.

7. **IV anesthetic agents**
   a. **Propofol** (Diprivan) is a common IV anesthetic that produces sedation and amnesia in small doses, but unconsciousness in larger doses. It is supplied in a thick white milky soybean and egg lecithin emulsion. It is available only in IV form. Propofol is not used in a patient with egg or soybean allergies. Dose for induction is 1.0 to 2.5 mg/kg. Dose for sedation is 0.5 to 1 mg/kg.
      1) Advantages include a rapid onset in less than 45 seconds. It can be used for moderate sedation, general anesthesia, for patients on ventilators, and for procedures such as magnetic resonance imaging. Emergence is very rapid without side effects. Propofol is used in neurosurgery where patient response is needed.
      2) Disadvantages include a burning sensation when injected. It can cause hypotension, respiratory depression, or cardiovascular depression.
   b. **Ketamine** (Ketalar) is a phencyclidine derivative. It causes dissociative anesthesia. The patient is awake and may not realize what is happening. Dose for induction is 0.5 to 2.5 mg/kg. Dose for sedation is 12.5 to 50 mcg/kg/min.
      1) Advantages include rapid onset, less than 30 seconds. It can be given IV, IM, and orally. Low dose does not cause respiratory depression. It can be used alone or with other medications. It is used frequently for children and short procedures.
      2) Disadvantages include hallucinations and delirium on emergence. Room noise should be kept at a minimum as the patient begins to emerge from the drug.
   c. **Pentothal** (thiopental sodium) can be used as a sedative-hypnotic in patients with sensitivity to other IV anesthetic drugs. It can be used in combination with regional anesthesia. The dose for induction is 3 to 5 mg/kg. The dose for sedation is 1.5 to 5 mg/kg.
      1) Advantages include rapid action and cerebral protectant properties.
      2) Disadvantages include lowered arterial pressure and decreased cardiac output. It is not used in chronic renal or hepatic disease.

8. **Adjunct medications used during anesthesia for nausea and gastric reflux**
   a. **Antiemetic**
      1) **Ondansetron** (Zofran) is an antiemetic drug used to prevent nausea and vomiting. It can be administered preoperatively. It can last 12 to 24 hours. The dose is 4 mg before induction.
      2) **Metoclopramide** (Reglan) is an antiemetic drug used to reduce gastric fluid volume and nausea and vomiting. The dose is 10 mg at the end of the procedure. It can last about 6 hours.
      3) **Scopolamine** is considered a sedative and antiemetic. It can be placed behind the patient's ear in the form of patches before surgery. The dose is 1.5 mg over 72 hours. The IV dose is 0.6 mg, 3 to 4 times a day.
   b. **Antacid**
      1) **Omeprazole** (Prilosec) is a proton pump inhibitor. It may be given orally before surgery to prevent the release of gastric acid. The dose is 60 mg.
      2) **Pantoprazole** (Protonix) is a proton pump inhibitor. It is given IV to reduce gastric acid release. It can work within 20 minutes. The dose is 4 mg/mL.

9. **Emergency medications** are available to the anesthesia provider based on the patient's symptoms. Drug reversal agents were previously mentioned. See Chapter 7 for intraoperative emergency situations. Some common emergency medications include:
   a. **Cardiac medications** may be needed for tachycardia, bradycardia, or cardiac arrest.
      1) **Adenosine** is an antiarrhythmic administered when a patient has tachycardia. It restores the heart to normal sinus rhythm. Dose: 6 mg IV bolus. Repeat in 1 to 2 minutes if needed. It produces brief asystole followed by restoration of normal sinus rhythm.
      2) **Amiodarone** is a class III antiarrhythmic used for life-threatening ventricular arrhythmias. It has a high survival rate. Dose: IV push, 300 mg in 20 to 30 mL of normal saline (NS) or dextrose 5% in water (D5W). The dose can be repeated in 150 mg doses every 3 to 5 minutes.
      3) **Atropine** is an anticholinergic agent used for bradycardia (heart rate <60). It is also used for asystole and atrioventricular nodal block. Dose: 1 mg IV, repeat every 3 to 5 minutes.
      4) **Epinephrine** (Adrenalin) is an adrenergic drug. It is used in emergency asystole, pulseless ventricular tachycardia, asthma, and allergic reactions. It can be given through an ET (inhalant), subcutaneously, IM, and IV. Dose for asystole: 1 mg IV push every 3 to 5 minutes.
      5) **Vasopressin** (Pitressin) is an antidiuretic hormone. It is used for pulseless arrest. It raises blood pressure by constricting blood vessels, restricts renal excretion, and increases peristalsis. Dose: 40 units IV push.
      6) **Dopamine** (Intropin) is an adrenergic agonist and antiarrhythmic. It is used for hypotension, increased cardiac output, and renal failure.

Doses vary based on intended use and symptoms.

7) **Nitroglycerin** is a smooth muscle relaxant. It increases coronary blood flow by dilating arteries, reduces blood pressure, and relieves angina. It comes in many forms: sublingual, buccal, oral, ointment, patch, and IV. Dose for IV: 5 mcg/min, up to 20 mcg/min. IV nitroglycerine solutions are protected from light that would affect the stability of the drug.

b. Diuretic drugs

1) **Furosemide** (Lasix) is a diuretic. It is used to treat edema and hypertension caused from heart failure and renal disease. Dose IV: 20 to 40 mg. It can be given intraoperatively to lower intracranial pressure.

2) **Mannitol** (Osmitrol) is a form of diuretic used to treat increased intracranial pressure and intraocular pressure. It is not used in complete anuria. A test dose given at 0.2 g/kg for urinary output of 30 to 50 mL/h. Dosage may range between 50 and 100 g/24 h. The average dose is 100 g/24 h.

c. Additional drugs available for the anesthesia provider

1) **Phenytoin** (Dilantin) is used to prevent or treat seizures after neurosurgery and head trauma. Dose: 10 to 15 mg/kg.

2) **Dantrolene sodium** (Dantrium, Revonto, Ryanodex) is used for the treatment of an MH crisis. It works by blocking the accumulation of calcium in the skeletal muscles. A central line is used because a large quantity of the drug is needed quickly and the peripheral circulation is unreliable. Dose: 2 to 3 mg/kg IV bolus. Repeat dose every 5 to 10 minutes.

   Dantrium and Revonto are supplied in 65-mL vials of dry powder. Mannitol is included with the drug as a diuretic to increase renal function. Each vial must be reconstituted with 60 mL of preservative-free sterile water. If water with preservative is used, the amount of preservative would be toxic. Saline is never used to mix this drug. Each vial requires vigorous shaking to dissolve the powder. See Chapter 7 for team activities during MH crisis.

   Ryanodex is a form of dantrolene supplied in 250-mg vials. It must be reconstituted with 5 mL of nonbacteriostatic sterile water. This variety of dantrolene mixes rapidly. It must be used within 6 hours of mixing.

Role of the Anesthesia Provider in the Administration of Anesthesia

1. Anesthesia is the art of administering drugs safely in a balanced manner so the patient does not feel pain and does not recall the procedure. The anesthesia provider, surgeon, and patient decide which type of anesthesia is the safest method with maximal benefit. Patient safety is the number one priority in deciding which type of anesthesia to administer. The perioperative nurse should understand the preanesthesia evaluation and the types of anesthesia, equipment, stages, and safety measures.

   a. The preanesthesia evaluation is done by a qualified anesthesia provider. The anesthesia provider looks at all data in the patient's medical record. Information includes the intended surgical procedure and H&P, laboratory values, radiology reports, and comorbidities.

   1) The anesthesia provider questions the patient regarding past surgical procedures, medical history, and family anesthetic history.

   2) The anesthesia provider assesses the patient's age, weight in kilograms, baseline vital signs, history of gastric reflux, sleep apnea, and any other comorbidities.

   3) The anesthesia provider classifies the patient according to one of the six categories of the American Society of Anesthesiologists patient risk classification system (Box 8.4).

   b. The anesthesia provider is not present during local anesthesia given by the surgeon.

BOX 8.4 American Society of Anesthesiologists Classification

- Class I theoretically includes relatively healthy patients with localized pathologic processes. An emergency surgical procedure, designated E, signifies additional risk. For example, a hernia that becomes incarcerated changes the patient's status to class I-E.
- Class II includes patients with mild systemic disease (e.g., diabetes mellitus controlled by oral hypoglycemic agents or diet).
- Class III includes patients with severe systemic disease that limits activity but is not totally incapacitating (e.g., chronic obstructive pulmonary disease or severe hypertension).
- Class IV includes patients with an incapacitating disease that is a constant threat to life (e.g., cardiovascular or renal disease).
- Class V includes moribund patients who are not expected to survive 24 hours with or without the surgical procedure. They are operated on in an attempt to save their lives; the surgical procedure is a resuscitative measure, as in a massive pulmonary embolus. The patient may or may not survive the surgical procedure.
- Class VI includes patients who have been declared brain dead but whose organs will be removed for donor purposes. Mechanical ventilation and life support systems are maintained until the organs are procured.

From Phillips, N. (2017). *Berry and Kohn's operating room technique* (13th ed.). St. Louis, MO: Elsevier.

A perioperative nurse monitors the patient's vital signs, but no sedation is given. Patients receiving moderate sedation are administered local anesthesia by the surgeon and are sedated and monitored by a qualified perioperative nurse.

2. Anesthesia administered by the anesthesia provider.
   a. Monitored Anesthesia Care (MAC)
      1) The anesthesia provider administers IV sedation drugs. All monitoring devices are in place and the patient may be given oxygen by nasal cannula. The patient is not completely unconscious.
      2) The anesthesia provider documents all vital signs at regular intervals and the patient's level of consciousness is tested by the response of verbal commands.
      3) The surgeon administers local medication at the incision site.
      4) The anesthesia provider must be able to perform emergency resuscitation if necessary.
   b. **Regional anesthesia.** Regional anesthesia is a sterile procedure performed by the anesthesia provider to a certain area of the body. A selected anesthetic drug is injected into a certain area or dermatome to numb the surrounding nerves (Fig. 8.2). Examples include the following:
      1) **Spinal.** Spinal anesthesia is an intrathecal block used to numb the body below the waist. Spinal anesthesia can be used for many procedures, such as cesarean sections, orthopedics, bowel, bladder, prostrate, vascular, and other lower body procedures.

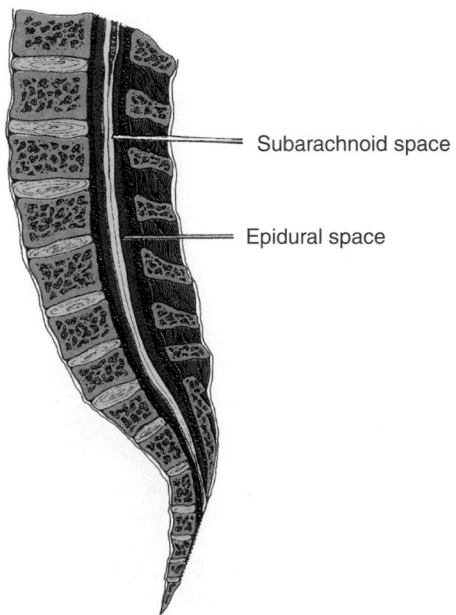

Subarachnoid space

Epidural space

Figure 8.2 Agent is injected into the subarachnoid space for spinal anesthesia or into the epidural space for epidural anesthesia. (From Phillips, N. [2017]. *Berry and Kohn's operating room technique* [13th ed.]. St. Louis, MO: Elsevier.)

A spinal needle is placed in the subarachnoid space at the desired spinal lumbar level below L2. The stylet from the spinal needle is removed and cerebral spinal fluid should leak out if the needle is in the correct position. A syringe with the selected local medication is attached to the spinal needle and injected into the subarachnoid space.
   a) The nurse may assist the anesthesia provider in the positioning of the patient for regional anesthesia (see Chapter 7).
   b) The patient should be monitored for complications, including hypotension, hypothermia, hematoma, neurologic changes, postdural headache, venous stasis, and migration of the anesthetic above L2, which can cause respiratory paralysis.

2) **Epidural.** An epidural is similar to the spinal in positioning and procedure. The epidural differs in the injection area of the medication. The anesthetic is injected into the space above and surrounding the dura mater. A single injection can be administered or a catheter may be left in place for continuous dosing to relieve postoperative pain. Epinephrine may be used to slow down the absorption of the anesthetic for longer pain management results.

3) **Nerve blocks.** Nerve blocks can be done during any phase of surgery (preoperatively, intraoperatively, postoperatively). A nerve block can be done on many body parts to block the pain in a group of nerves or plexus. Examples of blocks include brachial, axillary, vertebral, cervical, intercostal, arm and hand, celiac, retrobulbar, femoral, and others. Nerve blocks can be used with other forms of anesthesia and can be used for short- or long-term pain relief. Nerve blocks can last from 4 to 24 hours depending on the anesthetic agent and plexus.

4) **Bier block.** A Bier block is very common for upper extremity procedures lasting less than an hour. A double tourniquet is placed on the upper arm, but not inflated. An IV catheter is placed in the hand. The arm is elevated, prepped, and wrapped with a sterile Esmarch to exsanguinate the limb. The proximal cuff is inflated, and the wrap is removed. The local anesthetic is then injected into the catheter, and the anesthesia provider waits for it to take effect. Once the limb is numb, the distal cuff is inflated and the proximal cuff is deflated. The proximal cuff must be let down very slowly at the end of the procedure so that the patient does not receive a bolus of medication. Fast release can cause central nervous system toxicity, such as respiratory depression, cardiac events, neurologic changes, seizures, or hypotension.

c. **General anesthesia.** General anesthesia is the art of balancing a combination of drugs: oxygen, benzodiazepines, narcotics, inhalant gas, and muscle relaxants. General anesthesia purposely results in an unconscious patient who needs ventilation assistance and does not recall the surgical procedure.

The anesthesia machine has everything the anesthesia provider will need to maintain the patient. It includes oxygen, anesthesia gas, mechanical ventilator, breathing circuit, monitoring devices, safety alarms, and an attached anesthetic waste gas hose (purple tubing at the rear of the machine). Supplies and necessary drugs may be kept alongside the anesthesia machine (Fig. 8.3).

Steps to achieve safe general anesthesia include complete physical and airway assessment, risk assessment, procedure knowledge, drug dose knowledge, and extensive training. General anesthesia is supervised by an anesthesiologist, who is present for induction and emergence at the conclusion of the surgical procedure.

3. **Airway management.** The perioperative nurse may assist with intubation and provide cricoid pressure (Sellick's maneuver) to prevent regurgitation of stomach contents into the airway. See Chapter 7 for

perioperative nursing interventions in airway management.

a. The airway is visually assessed for potential intubation difficulty using the Mallampati classification system. Patients with a history of sleep apnea have redundant pharyngeal tissue that may cause difficulty during intubation (Fig. 8.4).

b. Awake intubation may be necessary using a fiber-optic or rigid laryngoscope for direct visualization of the vocal cords if there is a possibility of airway obstruction.

c. The ET is inserted into the trachea. After confirming placement by listening to the lungs, the balloon cuff is inflated (Fig. 8.5).

d. Uncuffed ET tubes are used for children younger than 8 years. An inflated cuff causes pressure over the redundant tissue of the pharynx.

e. LMA is placed over the larynx and inflated to hold it in place (Fig. 8.6).

f. A nasotracheal tube can be used if an oral tube is not possible. McGill forceps can be used to place it into the trachea (Fig. 8.7).

4. **Stages of general anesthesia** (Fig. 8.8)

a. **Stage 1** (induction): The patient is administered drugs and loses consciousness. All monitors and vital signs are closely watched. Airway is established and maintained for the patient. The induction phase begins with oxygenation of the patient. Then the patient is given a combination of drugs such as a benzodiazepine, inhalation agent, propofol, and/or neuromuscular relaxation. The combination of agents is customized to

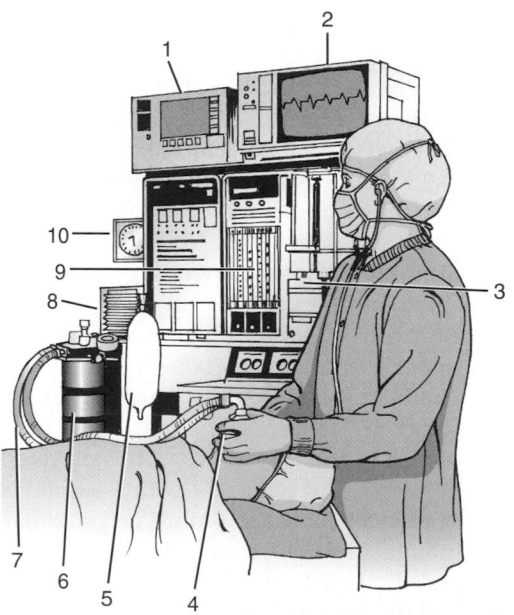

Figure 8.3 Anesthesia machine for maintenance of general anesthesia. *1*, Anesthetic and respiratory gas monitor; *2*, physiologic monitor (channels include electrocardiograph, blood pressure, temperature, heart rate, and pulse oximeter); *3*, flow-through vaporizers; *4*, face mask; *5*, reservoir "breathing" bag; *6*, carbon dioxide absorber canister; *7*, patient breathing circuit; *8*, ventilator; *9*, flowmeters for gases; *10*, sphygmomanometer for manual blood pressure. (From Phillips, N. [2017]. *Berry and Kohn's operating room technique* [13th ed.]. St. Louis, MO: Elsevier.)

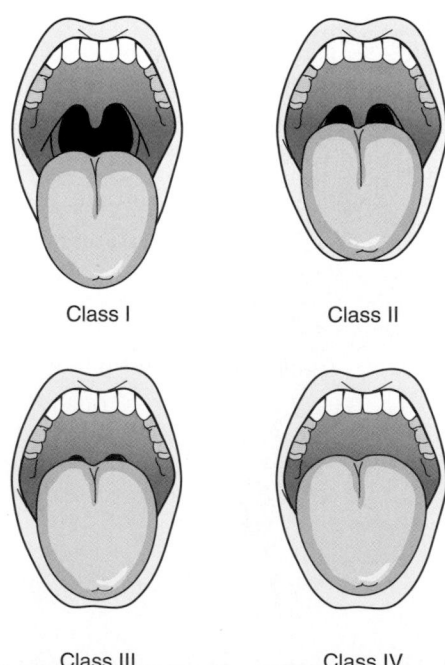

Class I   Class II

Class III   Class IV

Figure 8.4 Mallampati classification for difficult intubation. (From Phillips, N. [2017]. *Berry and Kohn's operating room technique* [13th ed.]. St. Louis, MO: Elsevier.)

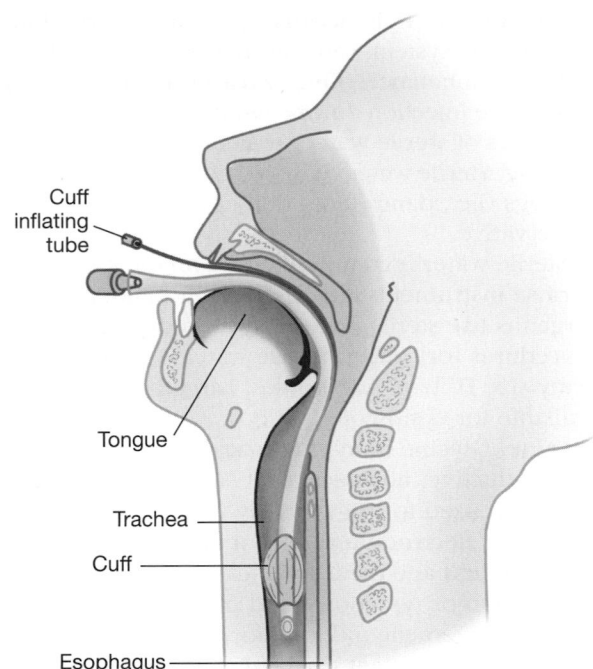

Figure 8.5 Endotracheal tube in position. (From Rothrock, J. [2019]. *Alexander's care of the patient in surgery* [16th ed.]. St. Louis, MO: Elsevier.)

STAGE	PUPIL		RESP	PULSE	BP
1st Induction	Usual size	Reaction to light		Irregular	Normal
2nd Excitement	or			Irregular and fast	High
3rd Operative				Steady and slow	Normal
4th Danger				Weak and thready	Low

Figure 8.8 Levels of unconsciousness associated with general anesthesia. *BP*, Blood pressure; *RESP*, respirations. (From Phillips, N. [2017]. *Berry and Kohn's operating room technique* [13th ed.]. St. Louis, MO: Elsevier.)

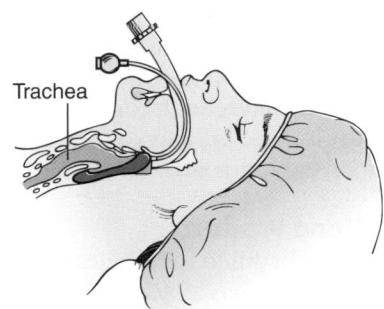

Figure 8.6 Laryngeal mask airway. (From Phillips, N. [2017]. *Berry and Kohn's operating room technique* [13th ed.]. St. Louis, MO: Elsevier.)

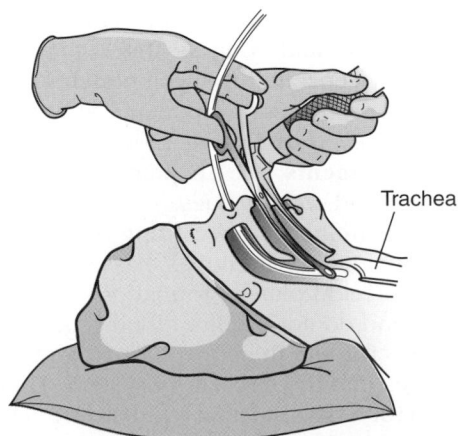

Figure 8.7 Nasotracheal intubation with Magill forceps. (From Phillips, N. [2017]. *Berry and Kohn's operating room technique* [13th ed.]. St. Louis, MO: Elsevier.)

the patient's needs. The room should be quiet during the induction phase; hearing is the last sense of patient awareness.

b. **Stage 2** (excitement): Vital signs may be slightly unstable. The patient is unconscious but still has reflexes.

c. **Stage 3** (maintenance): This is the stage where it is safe to begin positioning and prepping after anesthesia gives permission. The maintenance phase may include the administration of narcotics to keep the patient pain free. During this stage the anesthesia provider keeps the patient in an unconscious state and uses monitoring devices for vital signs. Some additional monitoring devices may be added, such as a bispectral index (BIS) monitor. This is like an EEG; the monitor pad is applied to the forehead. The BIS monitor sends a readout from 0 to 100 (0 is no brain activity, 100 is wide awake). The patient is usually maintained near 40 throughout the procedure. A temperature probe or skin sensor may be added. Critical patients may have an arterial line or central venous pressure monitor. The patient is maintained and carefully monitored until the procedure is complete.

d. **Stage 4:** This is the **danger stage**. The patient overdoses or reacts to the medications. The cardiovascular and respiratory systems begin to fail because the medulla in the brain is depressed.

e. The **emergence phase** takes place when the procedure is complete. The anesthesia provider allows the maintenance drugs to wear off, or may administer reversal agents for a quicker recovery. The patient is administered oxygen along with IV pain medication.

The patient must have laryngeal reflexes before extubation can take place. Extubation takes place once the patient can breathe without risk for aspiration or laryngospasm. Patients with a history of sleep apnea may remain intubated for a longer period. An oral or nasal airway may be inserted to keep the oropharynx clear and facilitate breathing.

Intravenous and Bottled Fluids

IV and bottled fluids are used regularly as part of many surgical procedures. Fluid therapy is used to maintain daily fluid balance, replace lost fluids, expand hollow organs for visualization, or irrigate surgical sites. Blood and blood products are given to patients in the event of hemorrhage or dangerously low blood counts. Fluid replacement is determined based on the patient's vital signs, current blood work, or hemodynamic status. Crystalloids are often given for volume expansion. Colloids contain protein and are given to create a fluid shift into the vascular compartment.

Common Fluids and Solutions Used During the Surgical Procedure

1. **NS** 0.9% NaCl. Normal saline (NS) is an isotonic solution used for irrigation, fluid replacement, maintaining fluid balance, and treating metabolic acidosis. NS is a crystalloid used to balance electrolytes, for irrigation, and for reconstitution of many medications. NS is run IV with packed red blood cells (PBRCs). NS is similar to blood plasma so there is no shift in fluids between the vascular compartment and the interstitium. NS is conductive and can interfere with monopolar ESU during irrigation. It is available in many size IV bags, vials, and bottles (1000, 500, 250, and 50 mL). Smaller NS vials may contain preservative and could be toxic if used in large quantities.
2. **D5W.** Dextrose 5% in water Dextrose solutions are used to hydrate patients, provide extra calories, enhance liver function, and spare protein. D5W is a crystalloid. D5W is available for IV use in 2.5%, 10%, 20%, and 50%. IV bags are supplied in 1000, 500, and 250 mL.
3. **Dextrose 5% in NS** (D5NS). This solution is used for burn patients, shock, and circulatory insufficiency. D5NS is a crystalloid. IV bags are supplied in 1000, 500, and 250 mL.
4. **Lactated Ringer's** (LR). LR is also known as Hartmann's solution. It is a crystalloid salt solution used to rehydrate patients from burns and severe diarrhea, replace electrolytes, and stimulate renal activity. IV bags are supplied in 1000, 500, and 250 mL.
5. **Sterile water.** Sterile water is a hypotonic solution. It is nonconductive crystalloid and does not interfere with electrocautery. Sterile water is not used

routinely for IV fluid because it can be absorbed into the vascular system, causing hypervolemia and acid-base imbalances. One IV use exception is during dantrolene injection during an MH crisis where large quantities of sterile water are necessary for IV use of the drug. Sterile water vials (60 mL) for reconstitution of drugs (i.e., dantrolene) do not contain preservative.

Sterile water is commonly used on the sterile field to rinse instruments and fill catheter balloons. Some surgeons use sterile water irrigation during surgical procedures for cancer. Sterile water is available in many size IV bags and bottles. Large bags are available for cystoscopy.

6. **Glycine.** Glycine is an amino acid solution. It is a nonconductive, nonelectrolytic, and nonhemolytic fluid. It is used to irrigate body cavities and can be used with electrocautery. It can be used in hysteroscopy to expand the uterine cavity, bladder expansion for tumor resections, and prostate resections. Fluid management and monitoring (intake and output) are important to avoid water intoxication. Glycine is available in large sterile bags and bottles.
7. Other IV solutions such as **Isolyte E** and **Plasma-Lyte** are crystalloids available to treat water loss and dehydration because the pH is similar to blood.
8. **Colloid volume expanders. Hetastarch** (Hespan) is used to increase blood volume to keep the circulation moving. It is made with cornstarch. It is not used in patients with corn allergies. It comes in a 6% solution in NS. **Albumin** is also a colloid volume expander. It comes in a 5% and 25% solution in NS. Blood is a colloid.

Blood and Blood Products

Patients who are scheduled for surgical procedures may sign a consent form to have blood or blood products if needed. Patients who wish to refuse blood and blood products will sign a declination form. The patient's blood type is determined by antigens. Blood contains clotting factors, carries O_2 to organs and tissue, removes waste CO_2, maintains acid-base balance, carries nutrients, transports hormones and enzymes, controls body temperature, and controls water content. Whole blood is usually separated into components for specific needs. Blood types, blood components, and replacement options are all necessary factors in fluid replacement.

1. **Blood components.** See Chapter 6 and Table 6.2 for complete blood count values.
   a. **Platelets** influence the clotting process and are given when the patient has massive blood loss or has a defect in platelet formation. They are universal and do not require blood type matching. Platelets form in the bone marrow and migrate in particles into the circulatory system. They can be stored for 5 days at room temperature. They come supplied in 50-mL bags.
   b. **White blood cells (WBCs):** Leukocytes protect the body from disease; they are part of the

immune system produced by the patient's body. There are five types of WBC that are measured individually by the laboratory differential. WBCs can be an indicator of infection, inflammation, or histamine release.

c. **Red blood cells (RBCs):** Erythrocytes contain hemoglobin that carry O_2 and remove waste CO_2 from tissues. Normal RBCs have no nucleus. PRBCs are supplied in 1-unit bags or 350 mL/unit. One unit can raise a patient's hemoglobin by 1 g/dL. They are blood type specific. PRBCs can be refrigerated for 42 days.

d. **Plasma** is composed of water and dissolved proteins (albumins, globulins, fibrinogen), clotting factors, glucose, hormones, and electrolytes. It is given to restore clotting factors. Plasma makes up 55% of the total blood volume. It can be stored frozen up to 1 year. It should be used within 6 hours after thawing. It is type specific. **Cryoprecipitate** is the plasma portion of blood. It is usually administered in combination with other blood products. Cryoprecipitate alone may be given in multiple units. It contains the clotting factors but is given mainly for the clotting factor VIII. It can be frozen for up to 1 year.

2. **Blood type review.** Rh compatibility means only an Rh-positive donor is compatible with an Rh-positive recipient of each type. Rh negative is more compatible with each blood type. Antigens that cause reactions can be present in any blood type and require testing before use.

   a. **Type A** is compatible with AB blood type. Rh factor must match.

   b. **Type B** is compatible with AB blood type. Rh factor must match.

   c. **Type AB** is the universal recipient. Rh factor must match. Type AB plasma is a universal donor.

   d. **Type O** has no antigens and can be donated to any type if the Rh factor matches. Type O negative is a universal donor to all blood types regardless of the Rh factor of the recipient in an emergency situation.

3. **Considerations for the perioperative nurse concerning blood transfusion.**

   a. Patients at risk for significant blood loss will be typed and cross-matched for a potential blood transfusion to minimize the risk for transfusion reactions. Any signs of reaction require immediate cessation of the transfusion. Reactions in an anesthetized patient include:

      1) Hyperthermia and skin flushing may occur as the patient's body breaks down red cells.

      2) Dark urine is caused by hemoglobin from the kidneys.

      3) Awake patients may complain of back or flank pain and chills. The patient may report dizziness and bloody urine.

   b. Blood and blood products must be checked for correct patient ID, correct blood type and Rh, and identifying numbers on the unit and matching patient number.

   c. A large-bore needle (18–20 gauge) is used with NS IV to run blood.

   d. Blood is refrigerated, and transfusion must be completed within 4 hours of removal from the refrigerator.

   e. The perioperative nurse must check to determine whether the patient has autologous blood in storage for use in the OR if needed. Some patients will donate blood for their own use during a surgical procedure and have the blood bank store it. The process of autologous blood storage is isolated from other blood stored for general use. If not used, the blood will be discarded because it is not tested for suitability for use in other patients.

   Blood salvage devices are another form of autologous transfusion. The suction apparatus used for blood salvage is not used to evacuate anything other than blood. Great care is taken to prevent any hemostatic material from entering the blood salvage unit. The blood in the unit would be rendered useless and, if administered, could cause serious systemic clotting.

   f. Documentation includes all of the identifying information for the patient and the type of blood product administered. The anesthesia provider will record all the vital signs, observation of the infusion site, and duration of the infusion. The perioperative nurse documents who gave the infusion and the identification data of the blood product used in the medical record and on the comprehensive surgical checklist. This information is shared with the postoperative (perianesthesia) nurses in the hand-over report in the PACU.

Perioperative nurses should be aware of the drugs and anesthesia procedures used in the surgical environment. Although the nurse does not administer the drugs, a practical knowledge of what they are and how they work is a benefit to the patient's care. In the event of an emergency in the OR, the nurse is capable of assisting the anesthesia provider in treating the patient.

Surgical pharmacology is more than anesthesia drugs. Medications and pharmaceutical preparations, such as intraoperative treatments (e.g., antiadhesion chemicals/sheets, irrigations), are commonly used in the sterile field. Responsibility for careful usage requires the knowledge and skill for proper handling and preparation of every pharmaceutical used in patient care.

LEARNING ACTIVITIES

INSTRUCTIONS: Complete the crossword puzzle. Use the clues to help identify the words.

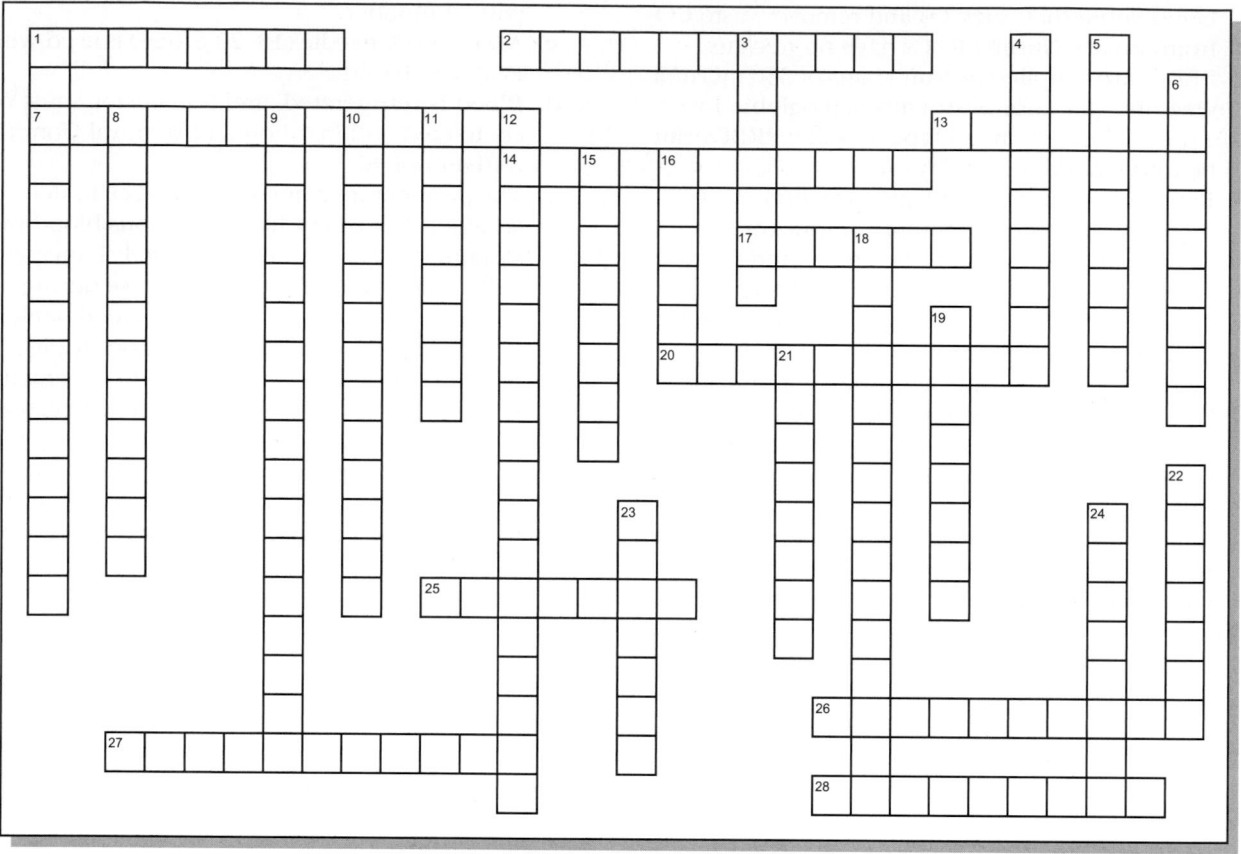

ACROSS

1. Antiinflammatory used intraoperatively or postoperatively to reduce inflammation; can delay the healing process
2. Reversal agent for nondepolarizing neuromuscular blockers
7. Used as a diagnostic agent for radiologic studies
13. A topical hemostatic agent that is available in a film, spray, or powder
14. Amino amide four times stronger than lidocaine; it is the generic name for Marcaine and Sensorcaine
17. Reversal agent for narcotics and opioids
20. Used to treat malignant hyperthermia
25. Absorbable gelatin, comes in powder or sponge form; powder can be mixed with saline to make a paste; the sponge can be moistened in saline, thrombin, or epinephrine
26. Antibiotic commonly used in irrigation that is effective against mostly gram-positive microorganisms
27. A vasoconstrictor added to local anesthetics to decrease bleeding
28. Antiadhesion agent available in a clear thin sheet and applied dry; composed of sodium hyaluronate carboxy-methylcellulose

DOWN

1. Depolarizing neuromuscular blocker that has no reversal agent and is a malignant hyperthermia trigger
3. Amino acid irrigation used for hysteroscopy and bladder resections; it is nonconductive and nonelectrolytic
4. The antidote for heparin
5. A double tourniquet is used for this upper extremity anesthetic
6. Given for massive blood loss to influence the clotting process
8. Inhalation agent that is safe for use if malignant hyperthermia is suspected
9. Buffer added to medications to reduce stinging upon injection

10. Given IV to detect bladder injuries, urinary leaks, and uterine tube observation
11. Furosemide is what category of drug used to treat edema and hypertension?
12. Includes Helistat, Collastat, and SuperStat hemostatic sponges; when applied, the coagulation mechanism forms a clot
15. Common IV anesthetic that produces sedation and amnesia; emergence is rapid without side effects
16. Quick-acting sedative and anxiolytic; contraindicated in patients with narrow-angle glaucoma
18. Plasma portion of blood given in multiple units to restore clotting factor VIII
19. Solution used to hydrate patients, provide extra calories, spare protein, and enhance liver function
21. Topical hemostatic solution that accelerates the clotting process by converting fibrinogen to fibrin
22. Most commonly used parenteral anticoagulant measured in units
23. During induction of anesthesia, which sense is the last of patient awareness
24. Oxidized cellulose applied dry, made of cotton or rayon fabric; not recommended for use on bone

LEARNING ACTIVITIES ANSWERS

Across

- 1. STEROIDS
- 2. NEOSTIGMINE
- 7. CONTRAST MEDIA
- 13. FLOSEAL
- 14. BUPIVACAINE
- 17. NARCAN
- 20. DANTROLENE
- 25. GELFOAM
- 26. BACITRACIN
- 27. EPINEPHRINE
- 28. SEPRAFILM

Down

- 1. SUCCINYLCHOLINE
- 3. GLYCOPYRROLATE
- 4. PROTAMINE
- 5. BIBLOCK
- 6. PLATELETS
- 8. NITROUS OXIDE
- 9. SODIUM BICARBONATE
- 10. METHYLENE BLUE
- 11. IURETIC
- 12. ABSORBABLE COLLAGEN
- 15. PROPOFOL
- 16. ERSEY
- 18. DRY
- 19. DEXTROSE
- 21. THROMBIN
- 22. HEPARIN
- 23. HEARING
- 24. SURGICAL

CHAPTER 9

Surgical Site Management

SCIP (Surgical Care Improvement Project) measures are employed to minimize the risk for surgical site infection (SSI). The administration of antibiotics 1 hour preoperatively allows for circulatory distribution of the drug before the surgical incision is made. Vancomycin can be administered 2 hours before the incision is made. Intraoperative redosing is based on the duration of the surgical procedure. The determination about the use of antibiotics is made by the surgeon after checking for allergies. Documentation on the comprehensive surgical checklist confirms SCIP measures were followed.

Anatomy and Physiology of the Skin and Tissues

1. As the largest organ of the body, the skin thickness varies according to the location on the body. The intact skin is the best barrier to infection for the patient and the caregiver. Injury to specific tissue layers manifests differently depending on the area and underlying structures affected, and the cause of the interruption of the integrity (Table 9.1). Healing is impaired if the dermal layer is lost (Fig. 9.1).
2. Physiologic properties of the skin to consider throughout the perioperative care period
   a. **Thermoregulation.** One goal of patient care is **normothermia**. The patient's body responds to the surrounding temperature by vasodilation in response to heat, and vasoconstriction in response to cold. The vasculature of the skin regulates body temperature by constricting to conserve heat and moisture, and sweating to release excess heat. Perspiration is sensible fluid loss that works like a cooling system. The perioperative nurse assures the room temperature is between 68°F and 75°F for the average adult. Pediatric operating rooms (ORs) may be as warm as 85°F.
      1) Overheating with excess blankets combined with drapes causes the patient to sweat and lose fluids. Overall, this can lead to imbalance in fluids and electrolytes. As the fluids evaporate, the patient may shiver because of a cooling effect.
      2) Loss of body heat and sustained cool temperatures leads to **hypothermia**. Exposure of the surgical site causes loss of body heat. Hypothermia predisposes the patient to potential SSI. Using warming devices, warm

intravenous (IV) solutions, and warm solutions helps minimize the risk for SSI.
   b. Interface with the environment
      1) Tactile sense is stimulated by touch. The patient can be reassured by gentle handling.
      2) Dermal medications can be absorbed through the skin (i.e., hormones, nicotine patch, nitroglycerine).
   c. General health indicator
      1) During the assessment the patient's skin may appear pale, flushed, cyanotic, or other color indicator of a potentially serious health condition.
      2) The skin may feel clammy, dry, rough, or other than soft, supple, and warm.
3. Essential anatomy to review
   a. *Arterial supply* is critical for tissue perfusion (O_2) and successful application of the SCIP protocol. Hypoxia of tissue can cause ischemia followed by tissue necrosis. Arterial anatomy is critical, because problems with the arterial supply affect organ systems and can lead to death.
   b. *Venous drainage* is important for removing waste products of metabolism (CO_2). Venous stasis ulcers can develop and lead to infection and eventually loss of a limb. Obstruction of the venous drainage in tissue can create a buildup, leading to complications such as compartment syndrome and rhabdomyolysis. The resultant myoglobinemia can cause multisystem organ failure.
   c. *Innervation* is important for vascular function, muscle motion, and sensation. Injury during positioning can cause nerve damage that could be temporary or permanent. Surgical procedures and anesthesia involving the nervous system (i.e., brain and spinal cord) can cause death.
   d. *Lymphatics* follow the path of the venous system. An obstruction of one affects the other. Nodes are located near joints or organs. Node samples are serious diagnostic surgical procedures for cancer staging. The perioperative nurse must have knowledge of lymphatic pathways and nodal locations. The thoracic duct in the chest and the cisterna chyli of the intestines play a major role in lymphatic drainage and distribution of nutrition. Lymphedema can result from obstruction of the lymph system in a limb.

TABLE 9.1   Anatomic Tissue Types

Histologic Tissue Type	Description	Implications to Surgical Team
Epithelial Tissue		
A. Types		
1. Simple	Single layer of cells (endothelium) that lines the blood vessels, heart, and lymphatics	Delicate tissue that is easily damaged by rough handling
2. Stratified	Several layers of cells that form the skin, gastrointestinal tract, genitourinary (GU) tract, reproductive tract, and oropharynx; lines area that serves as a passage; reduces friction with mucus; can convert into keratin	Superficial layer of body cover; surface modifications are performed here; forms hair and nails
3. Transitional	Combination of simple and stratified layers found in ureters and bladder	Encountered during GU reconstruction and neoconstruction
B. Cellular Surface Structure		
1. Squamous	Flat	
2. Columnar	Tall, cylindric	
3. Cuboidal	Square	
Connective Tissue		
A. Fluid	Blood, lymph, chyle, cerebrospinal fluid, synovium vitreous and aqueous, and mucinous material	Care with body substance isolation and provision of hemostasis
B. Fibrous		
1. Areolar	Loose network forming the frame for subcuticular tissue	Reorganized during liposuction and fat transplantation procedures
2. Adipose	Fat that fills the loose network; visible in fetus at 14 weeks' gestation; not found in eyelid, penis, scrotum, labia minora, cranium, or lung tissue	
3. Reticular	Forms firmer framework for organs and vessels	
C. Supportive		
1. Cartilage	Avascular, no lymphatics or nerves	Structural integrity is altered during rhinoplasty and otoplasty; cartilage may be used as graft material; radical neck reconstruction may involve tracheal rings or laryngectomy for multidisciplinary treatment
a. Hyaline	Translucent, articular, and rubs against other articular surface; forms the epiphyseal line in long bone, portions of the nose, and tracheal rings	
b. Costal elastic	Becomes fibrous with age; found in ribs, nose, trachea, and larynx	
c. White	fibrocartilage	Forms circular menisci in joints and between vertebrae
d. Yellow elastic	Found in auricle of ear, eustachian tubes, and epiglottis	
2. Erectile	Found in corpus cavernosa, clitoris, and nose	
D. Hard	Bony surfaces covered with periosteum except at articulations and cartilaginous areas of circulating nurse insertion points	Reconstruction requires framework of underlying bone or graft material; autologous bone may be harvested from graft site for neoconstruction; donor bone may be used as transplant material

TABLE 9.1   Anatomic Tissue Types—cont'd

Histologic Tissue Type	Description	Implications to Surgical Team
1. Cancellous bone	Spaces are filled with red marrow; erythroblasts and smaller vessels	
2. Compact bone	Hollow center filled with yellow marrow (higher fat content) and larger vessels	
Muscle Tissue		
A. Visceral	Smooth, involuntary muscle; hollow organs, vessels, glands, areola, scrotum, iris of eye	Skeletal muscle may be used to replace bulk lost to debridement; vascularized flaps replace radical tissue excisions
B. Skeletal	Cylindric, striated, voluntary cells	
C. Cardiac	Branching cells, nonnucleated, less fibrous connective tissue	
Nerve Tissue		
A. Types		
1. Neuron	Cells generate and conduct nerve impulses; has multiple cytoplasmic fibers on one side (dendrites) and a single myelinated extension from the other side (axon)	Nerves may be injured during any procedure
2. Neuroglia	Insulate and support neurons in central nervous system	
B. Classification by Activity Type		
1. Afferent	Sensory	
2. Efferent	Motor	

From Fortunato, N. M., & McCullough, S. M. (1998). *Plastic and reconstructive surgery.* St. Louis, MO: Mosby.

4. Planning the surgical incision site can be a complicated process. The surgeon will use physical landmarks to determine where the incision(s) will be made. Abdominal landmarks delineate quadrants and include the xyphoid, iliac crests, pubis, and umbilicus. Laparoscopic port access will be planned for creating a pneumoperitoneum, manipulating internal structures, and removing or working on a target organ.

   Stomas (ureterostomy, ileostomy, or colostomy) are preplanned to avoid appliance interference with the patient's activities of daily living (i.e., sitting, standing, walking, or physical exercise) (Fig. 9.2).

   Specific landmarks are associated with other body parts, such as limbs, the spine, and head/neck. The surgeon marks the area of the incision with indelible ink to indicate the area that provides the best surgical site exposure. Considerations include:
   a. Nearest approach to target organ without damaging vessels and nerves
   b. Avoid muscle cutting as appropriate
   c. The best method for closure that supports healing; if the circulation and circulatory drainage are impaired, it will not heal and can lead to SSI
   d. Aesthetics: follow the natural lines of the skin (Langer's lines, maximal lines of tension) as much

as possible so approximation and closure of edges match evenly without undue tension

Preventing Surgical Site Infection (SSI)
Perioperative nurses can help minimize the risk for infection.
1. Preoperatively, the surgeon may order the patient to have a shower or bath with 2% chlorhexidine gluconate (CHG)-impregnated cloths. Instruct the patient to wash before the procedure and to avoid the head, neck, and face. CHG is not safe for use around the eyes and ears, and could cause serious damage (i.e., blindness or deafness).
2. The preoperative antibiotics as ordered are given on time. SCIP protocol should be followed (IV antibiotics are administered 1 hour before incision unless vancomycin is ordered, then it may be given 2 hours before the incision). The SCIP protocol applies to antibiotics given before tourniquet inflation blocks the circulatory system in a limb or clamp time on an artery.
3. Maintaining aseptic and sterile techniques during the patient's care throughout the perioperative period minimizes the risk for SSI.
4. Surgical skin prep is aseptically performed without contamination. Foley catheter is inserted using sterile

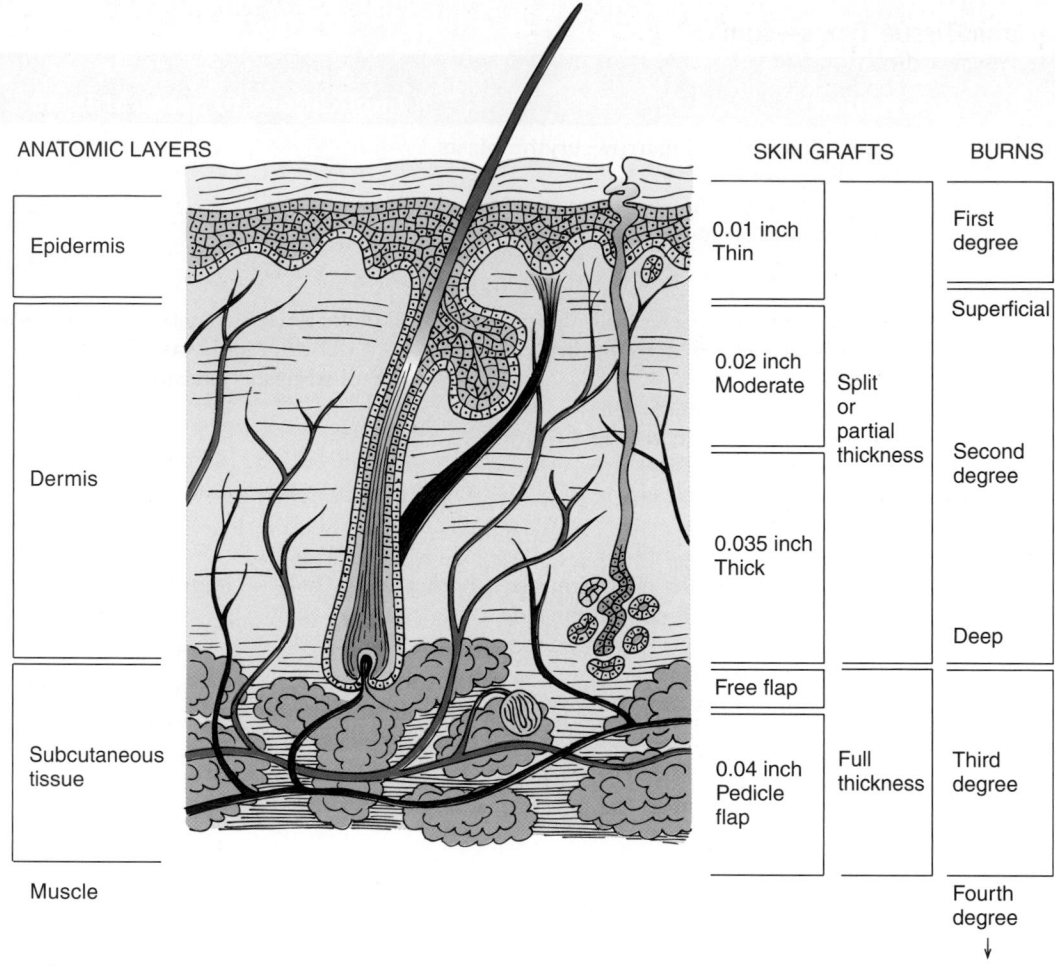

ANATOMIC LAYERS

Epidermis

Dermis

Subcutaneous tissue

Muscle

SKIN GRAFTS

0.01 inch Thin

0.02 inch Moderate

Split or partial thickness

0.035 inch Thick

Free flap

0.04 inch Pedicle flap

Full thickness

BURNS

First degree

Superficial

Second degree

Deep

Third degree

Fourth degree
↓

Figure 9.1 Cross section of skin and subcutaneous tissue, relative thickness of skin grafts, and categorization of burn injury. (From Phillips, N. [2017]. *Berry and Kohn's operating room technique* [13th ed.]. St. Louis, MO: Elsevier)

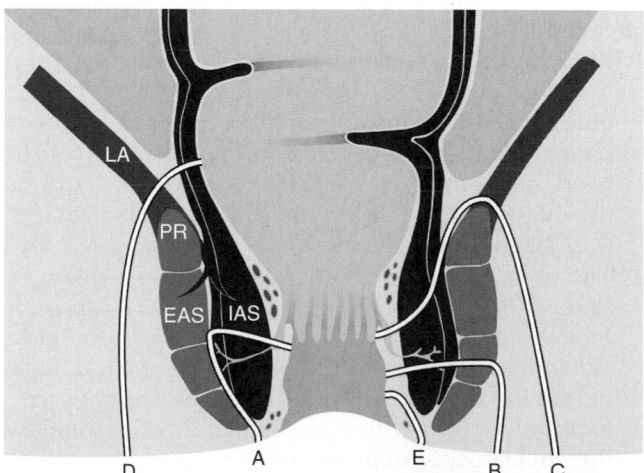

Figure 9.2 Pathways of perianal fistulae. Parks classification: (*A*) intersphincteric, (*B*) transsphincteric, (*C*) suprasphincteric, (*D*) extrasphincteric, and (*E*) superficial. *EAS*, external anal sphincter; *IAS*, internal anal sphincter; *LA*, levator ani; *PR*, puborectalis. (From Yassin, N. A., Day, N., & Phillips, R. [2014]. Imaging of anal fistulas. *Seminars in Colon & Rectal Surgery*, *25*(4), 176–182)

technique (if ordered). Hair is removed with clippers outside the OR if necessary. A child's hair should be saved for the parents.

Influences on Surgical Site Healing

1. **Wound class** is assigned by the perioperative nurse at the end of the surgical procedure. The Centers for Disease Control and Prevention developed the wound classification system to predict the patient's risk for SSI (Box 9.1).
   a. *Class I:* clean (infection rate 1%–5%). The primary incision is made in the OR under sterile technique. No breaks in technique. No inflammation or infection at the time of incision. No gastrointestinal leakage, primary closure, and may have a closed drainage system if necessary.
   b. *Class II:* clean-contaminated (infection rate 8%–11%). No infection or inflammation at the time of incision. Alimentary, genitourinary, or respiratory system entered under controlled circumstances. Primary closure and may be drained. No major break in sterile technique.

BOX 9.1 Wound Classifications

Clean Wound (Expected Infection Rate: 1%–5%)
- Elective procedure with wound made in ideal OR conditions
- Primary closure; wound not drained
- No break in sterile technique during surgical procedure
- No inflammation present
- Alimentary, respiratory, and genitourinary tracts or oropharyngeal cavity not entered

Clean-Contaminated Wound (Infection Rate: 8%–11%)
- Primary closure; wound drained
- Minor break in technique occurred
- No inflammation or infection present
- Alimentary, respiratory, and genitourinary tracts or oropharyngeal cavity entered in controlled conditions without significant spillage or unusual contamination

Contaminated Wound (Infection Rate: 15%–20%)
- Open fresh traumatic wound of less than 4 hours' duration
- Major break in technique occurred
- Acute nonpurulent inflammation present
- Gross spillage/contamination from gastrointestinal tract
- Entrance into genitourinary or biliary tracts with infected urine or bile present

Dirty and Infected Wound (Infection Rate: 27%–40%)
- Old traumatic wound of more than 4 hours' duration from dirty source or with retained necrotic tissue, foreign body, or fecal contamination
- Organisms present in surgical field before procedure
- Existing clinical infection: acute bacterial inflammation encountered, with or without purulence; incision to drain abscess
- Perforated viscus

From Phillips, N. (2017). *Berry and Kohn's operating room technique* (13th ed.). St. Louis, MO: Elsevier.

---

  c. *Class III:* contaminated (infection rate 15%–20%). Nonpurulent inflammation is present. Open, fresh traumatic wound, major break in technique, or gastrointestinal spillage is present.

  d. *Class IV:* dirty and infected (infection rate 27%–40%). Infection is clinically present before the incision is made. Old traumatic wound with necrotic and devitalized tissue. Perforated viscera.

2. **Mechanisms of surgical site closure and healing**

  a. **Primary closure** (primary intention, primary union)

    1) No tissue is lost, and the edges approximate evenly without dead space underneath. Fluids could accumulate in dead space allowing for microbial growth. Sterile technique is observed.

    2) There is minimal scarring.

    3) Healing takes place in phases.

      a) *Lag phase:* inflammatory response. Tissue fluids accumulate, and local blood cells deposit fibrin to seal the edges that meet. Epithelial cells migrate to bridge the incision over the first 5 days.

      b) *Proliferative phase:* fibroblasts complete the bridging of the incision. Collagen is secreted from the fibroblasts to form fibers that strengthen the incision. Reepithelialization is completed over 20 days.

      c) *Maturation phase:* begins at day 14 and the scar tissue is established. As vascularity changes, the scar turns pale. Maturation can take several weeks to several months.

  b. **Secondary closure** (second intention)

    1) The wound edges are not approximated and are left open. Secondary closure is common in chronic wounds and takes longer to heal.

    2) The wound heals by granulation forming from the bottom up if the dermal base is present. The wound may need a full-thickness skin graft (See Chapter 12). Types of grafts that might be used to fill a defect include:

      a) Autograft: from patient's own tissue (permanent)

      b) Allograft: cadaver graft (not permanent)

      c) Isograft: from an identical DNA match (twin)

      d) Bioengineered: from biologic source

    3) As the wound heals, the edges soften and may need some debridement as the base granulates upward. The risk for infection is high.

    4) The wound heals slowly. The edges marginate toward the center as the wound contracts.

    5) The scar is not as strong as the surrounding tissue. The scar can be very tight and need surgical release.

  c. **Tertiary closure** (delayed primary closure)

    1) The wound cannot be closed immediately. It is cleaned, debrided, and packed for closure after 3 days or more.

    2) The risk for infection is high, and multiple debridements may be necessary. Many wounds requiring delayed primary closure are septic to start.

    3) When the infection clears and the edges are clean and clear, a type of primary closure may be utilized to approximate the edges. Retention sutures may be necessary.

    4) Usually a wide scar forms as the surrounding skin contracts. Scar revision may be needed at a later date.

3. **Other factors that affect tissue healing**

  a. Surgical technique, hemostasis, and prevention of retained surgical items (RSIs) affect tissue healing.

1) The method of tissue handling contributes to best practices for incisional healing. Incisional creation method can affect the way the edges heal when primary closure is used. The differences in using sharp dissection versus opening with the electrosurgical unit (ESU) may be apparent postoperatively if the edges are devitalized.

2) Hemostasis is important to prevent hematoma and clot formation. Excess blood in a surgical site can support the growth of microorganisms. The method of hemostasis can cause tissue trauma and impair healing. Eschar from ESU use can accumulate, causing a mechanical barrier for the healing process. Interruption of the blood supply causes tissue ischemia and necrosis. Devitalized tissue cannot heal.

3) RSIs are a nidus for infection. The body will try to encapsulate the foreign object, but cannot resorb it. Healing does not take place.

4) SSI is a main cause of poor tissue healing. Bacteria produce a persistent biofilm that is resistant to antibiotic therapy.

b. Patient comorbidity and nutrition status affect tissue healing.

1) Patient circulatory and respiratory health play a large role in healing. If circulation and oxygenation are deficient, the tissues cannot repair themselves through regeneration.

2) Nutritional status is critical for the provision of proteins and minerals for tissue growth and health.

3) Wound healing is complicated by diabetes and its vascular and neurologic effects. Individuals with diabetes have a higher incidence of chronic wounds caused by lowered immunity and decreased angiogenesis.

4) Obesity can cause wound healing complications by circulatory disease and poor nutritional intake.

5) Nutrition deficit of vitamins and minerals in obesity and alcoholism negatively affects tissue regeneration.

c. Medication regimens preoperatively, intraoperatively, and postoperatively affect tissue healing when in the patient's system.

1) Anticoagulants, aspirin, and some herbs can cause delayed clotting and may promote the formation of hematoma and seroma.

2) Nicotine patches cause vasoconstriction that decreases blood flow to the tissues.

3) Immunosuppressants prevent the body from naturally fighting infection. Infection is the leading cause of failure to heal.

4) Corticosteroids and nonsteroidal anti-inflammatory drugs (NSAIDS) delay healing by minimizing the inflammatory process necessary for the three processes leading to collagen deposition.

5) The hormones estrogen and androgen can affect tissue healing. Androgens in older male patients can negatively affect mucosal wound remodeling and angiogenesis. Estrogen and testosterone in older females have faster mucosal tissue healing.

d. Radiation and chemotherapy affect tissue healing.

1) Antineoplastic drugs slow the process of fast-growing cells.

2) Radiation causes tissue and vessel destruction.

e. The psychosocial aspects of healing include the following:

1) Smoking negatively affects wound healing.

2) Stress reduces the inflammatory response necessary for healing and causes cortisol levels to rise. Cortisol is a glucocorticoid class of hormones produced by the adrenal glands.

Postoperative Wound Care

1. Dressings are applied with tape that does not cause the patient skin irritation (Table 9.2). Patients with tape sensitivity may have other material in place to secure the dressing. Circumferential wraps, like Coban, ACE, Elastoplast, or roller gauze (Kerlix or Kling), staples, or sutures can be used to keep a dressing in place. Tape can be used to secure the edges of wrapped dressings. Latex-free products are used to secure the dressing by the perioperative nurse at the conclusion of the surgical procedure. Many types of dressings and materials are available in many forms and offer support for wound healing (Table 9.3).

a. A single primary layer is applied directly to the surgical site by the sterile team. The primary dressing can be an impregnated mesh (Vaseline, Betadine, or other antimicrobial material), cotton, rayon, porous plastic, or other fabric.

b. A secondary layer is applied over the primary layer for additional support and absorption. Thicker cotton or synthetic material is used.

c. Negative pressure dressing may be used for wounds subject to second intention healing and other larger traumatic incisions. Also known as Wound Vac, the negative pressure removes excess serous drainage and promotes granulation of the wound base. Sterile technique is critical.

A thicker, porous, foamlike dressing is placed directly over the wound, and a perforated drain is placed over top. The drain and foam pad are covered with a clear adhesive dressing that seals the edges. The drain is attached to a receptacle in a vacuum device that helps remove excess fluids and facilitate healing. Contraindications to using Wound Vac include:

1) Untreated infected wound

2) Underlying organs are exposed beneath the wound

3) Necrotic tissue that is poorly debrided

4) Malignancy in the wound

TABLE **9.2**   Dressing Materials

Dressing Material	Composition and Properties	Indications for Use	Advantages	Disadvantages	Notes
Alginate	Originates from brown seaweed; highly absorbent; becomes a gel when exposed to exudate, creating a moist environment	Used for infected and noninfected wounds with moderate to heavy drainage; some are used for tunneling wounds	Can absorb 20 times its own weight in fluid; rehydrates wound and facilitates debridement; requires secondary dressing cover	Contraindicated for use with light exudate or dry eschar; can promote bacterial growth if used with occlusive dressing cover; not used with third-degree burns	Packaged as ropelike fibers or pad; do not use with alkaline solutions; packaged sterile; remains in place 2–4 days
Composite	Composed of two or more moisture-enhancing materials in combination with absorbent material	Used for partial-thickness or full-thickness wounds with moderate to heavy exudate; can also be used over fresh granulation or necrotic tissue	Facilitates debridement and allows for moisture/vapor exchange; safe for use over healthy or infected tissue; easy to apply and remove	Should be placed in area with border of healthy intact tissue for anchoring; should not be used for light exudate; may cause excess moisture loss; can become very adherent	Check manufacturer recommendations about use with adjunct topical medications
Exudate absorber	Added to wound surface to eliminate dead space and absorb exudate; minimizes odors	Used for full-thickness wounds with moderate to heavy exudate; can be used with necrotic wounds; some can be used as lining material before packing and surface dressing	Can absorb five times its own weight in fluid; rehydrates wound and facilitates debridement; requires secondary dressing cover	Contraindicated for use with light exudate or dry eschar	Supplied in bottles or packets; clean wound and irrigate before use; fill the wound cavity to eliminate dead space and line the defect
Foam	Semipermeable, either hydrophilic or hydrophobic	Creates a moist environment and affords thermal insulation	Nonadherent; repels contaminants and is easy to apply and remove; absorbs light to moderate exudate; can be used with compression dressings; requires secondary dressing cover	Not used for dry wounds; can cause maceration of adjacent skin	Some erythema or itching may occur during the first 24 hours; not used with occlusive dressings; change more frequently if exudate is heavy
Gauze	Composed of woven or nonwoven materials; can be impregnated; used as primary or secondary dressing; can be natural or synthetic material; nonocclusive	Used for wound protection, wicking, and absorption; can be used wet or dry; packaged in rolls, pads, or strips	Moderately absorbent; less expensive to use and can be used in combination with other material; can be used as packing	Needs to be changed frequently; can leak or strike-through; can dry out, causing injury to healing tissue	If applied wet and allowed to dry, gauze can be debridement agent; may be saturated with oils, iodophor, bismuth, petroleum jelly, scarlet red

(Continued)

9.2 Dressing Materials—cont'd

Dressing Material	Composition and Properties	Indications for Use	Advantages	Disadvantages	Notes
Hydrocolloid	Occlusive, adhesive wafer; the contact layer may differ in composition; creates a moist environment; supplied in packets, tubes (paste), oral discs, and wafers; can be cut to fit	Clean wounds granulate, and necrotic wounds debride autolytically	Impermeable to contaminants; self-adhesive and can remain in place for 3–5 days without tissue damage; slight to moderate absorption	Not used with heavy exudate, sinus tracts, or infection; not intended for full-thickness wounds exposing bone; visualization of the wound not possible; occlusive properties inhibit air exchange; can injure fragile tissue at wound edges	Safe to use under compression devices and wraps; can be used at ostomy sites or areas affected by incontinence
Hydrogel	Water- or glycerin-based gel, gauze, or sheet dressing that has high moisture content; supplied in tubes, packets, spray, liquid	Used for partial-and full-thickness wounds; good for burns, necrosis, and radiated tissue	Very soothing; can rehydrate dried tissues; used to fill dead space and facilitate debridement	Not used for absorption of exudate because of inherent moisture content; can dry out easily; not a bacterial barrier; may be difficult to secure to wound	Keep covered after application to prevent evaporation of the gel
Transparent film	Adhesive, semipermeable membrane; bacterial and water barrier permeable to oxygen	Waterproof, but permeable to air and moisture vapors; bacterial barrier	Promotes a moist environment for new granulation and autolysis of necrotic tissue	Not used for infected wounds; periphery of wound needs to be intact to apply the film; may be hard to apply	Used for superficial and partial-thickness wounds with minimal exudate
Skin sealant	Barrier film applied in liquid form that dries to form a plastic like barrier coating; supplied in liquid form and individual wipes	Used on intact skin surrounding a wound, ostomy site, or over a surgical incision closed by primary intention	Waterproof barrier	Can sting raw skin when applied; has alcohol base to cause drying by evaporation	Some have vapors that may be harmful to inhale as product evaporates

From Phillips, N. (2017). *Berry and Kohn's operating room technique* (13th ed.). St. Louis, MO: Elsevier.

TABLE 9.3   Wound Care Materials

Product and Examples	Description	Indications for Use	Instructions for Use
Antimicrobial: antiseptics, cadexomer iodine, honey, Hydrofera blue, mupirocin ointment, silver cream, silver dressings	Inhibits growth and replication of microorganisms	Partial- or full-thickness wound Critical colonization, infection, or biofilms Odorous wound	Cleanse wound Avoid saline in nanocrystalline silver products Apply to wound Apply appropriate secondary dressing as needed and secure in place
Calcium alginate: Restore CalciCare (Hollister), SeaSorb (Coloplast), Algisite (Smith & Nephew)	Polysaccharide derived from brown seaweed Highly absorbent Converts to viscous, hydrophilic gel Provides moist environment Hemostatic properties	Partial- or full-thickness wound with or without depth Moderate to heavily exudative wound Contraindicated in third-degree burns	Cleanse wound base Place or lightly pack into wound Apply appropriate secondary dressing and secure in place Change as needed, usually every 24–48 hours
Charcoal: CarboFlex odor control (ConvaTec), Lyofoam C (Mölnlycke, ConvaTec)	Activated carbon (charcoal) Absorbs toxins and wound degradation products Absorbs volatile amines and fatty acids responsible for odor	Malodorous wound (e.g., infected, fungating) Fecal fistula Pressure ulcer	Apply as a "filter" for odor control If absorbing exudate, may need to be changed daily; weekly if no exudate Can be reused if filter only
Collagen: Puracol collagen (Medline), Biostep (Smith & Nephew), Cellerate gel (Hymed Group), CollaSorb (Hartmann)	May enhance deposition of organized collagen fibers Chemoattractant to granulocytes and fibroblasts Bioresorbable Hemostatic properties Most processed from bovine or porcine sources	Full-thickness wound with or without depth Noninfected wound Minimal to moderate drainage Contraindicated in bovine sensitivities and third-degree burns	Packaged as gels, alginates, sheets, powders Cleanse wound as appropriate Apply to wound base Apply appropriate secondary dressing Secure as necessary
Promogran (Systagenix Wound Management)	Some collagens also inactivate matrix metalloproteinases	Chronic wound free of necrotic tissue	Read manufacturer's instructions carefully; some may need to be moistened with saline if wound bed dry
Composite: Tegaderm absorbent clear acrylic dressing (3M), Alldress (Mölnlycke), Covaderm Plus (DeRoyal)	Combine physically distinct components into single dressing Functions as bacterial barrier Absorptive layer distinct from alginate, foam, hydrocolloid, hydrogel Semiadherent or nonadherent	Partial- or full-thickness wound without depth Dry to heavy exudate (depends on dressing components) Product selection varies based on wound characteristics	Cleanse wound as appropriate Dressing application dependent on product selected Can function as either primary or secondary dressing May be used with topical medications

Modified from Bryant, R. A., & Nix, D. P. (Eds.). (2016). *Acute and chronic wounds: current management concepts* (5th ed.). St. Louis, MO: Elsevier.

5) Untreated osteomyelitis in a contaminated wound

6) Allergy to any of the dressing components, including the adhesive layers

2. **Drains.** Monofilament, nonabsorbable suture can be applied around the drain to secure it in place. Most active drains have radiopaque markings along the length of the tubing for radiographic depth measurement. Drains help minimize dead space in the wound.

a. *Passive drains* allow fluid, blood, and exudate to flow from the wound by gravity. Passive drains do not have applied suction to promote evacuation. Foley catheters are passive drains for urine, but can be placed securely in a wound by inflating the balloon.

b. *Active drains* have a suction reservoir or mechanical apparatus that pulls fluids from the wound by negative pressure. The tips of active drains have perforations along the end. Closed suction is activated on the sterile field after the incision is closed. Receptacles can be activated by compression to drain fluids from the wound. Chest tubes as a form of active drainage are discussed in Chapter 12.

Potential Complications of Wound Healing

Circulation is key to the prevention and treatment of wound healing complications.

1. **SSIs** are commonly localized, but can become systemic, leading to sepsis and multisystem organ failure. SSIs can be superficial or deep. Primary superficial or deep SSI is usually caused by microorganisms introduced into the site during the surgical procedure. Secondary deep SSI after the surgical procedure is uncommon because fibrin forms a seal within the wound within hours of closure (Box 9.2).

2. **Wound disruption** is caused by failure of the surgical site to close properly between the 5th and 10th postoperative day. Predisposing factors can precipitate wound closure failure. Infection or other factors,

such as diabetes, immunosuppression, poor tissue handling during the surgical procedure, steroid use, radiation, or chemotherapy can cause failure to heal after surgery.

a. *Dehiscence* is the separation of the superficial layers. The edges fail to unite. Infection may be present, or the tissue edges are devitalized and cannot approximate. If a serous exudate is present a culture should be obtained to determine the presence of microorganisms. Delayed primary closure may be possible if the wound is debrided and the infection is cleared.

b. *Evisceration* is the separation of the deep layers of tissue over the organs that extends to the surface of the body. The viscera protrude and create a surgical emergency. The organs must be repositioned and the layers closed. Infection may be present and must first be treated and debrided before reapproximating the separated edges.

3. **Compartment syndrome** is most common in a limb, but can happen in other areas, such as the abdomen. Arterial flow is usually present, but venous and lymphatic drainage is obstructed. Fluids build up in fascial compartments, causing pressure within the muscle/fascial layers. Rhabdomyolysis causes myoglobin to release into the blood and accumulate in the kidneys. Multisystem organ failure can follow and cause death.

4. **Adhesions and scar formations** are abnormal fibrous bands that bind organs and tissues together. Adhesions can cause bowel obstruction, female infertility, and other blocked passages within the body. Surgical intervention is usually necessary for adhesions.

a. *Hypertrophic scars* form when there is an excess of fibrin deposited on the edges of the incision. The remodeling stage is prolonged. This can be caused by tension on the incision, poor approximation of the wound edges, infection, burns, or inflammatory response to a foreign body, such as suture. Suture knots can form

---

BOX 9.2 Identification of Surgical Site Infections

Adhesions: Adherence of serous membranes to one another, causing fibrous tissue to form; sometimes occur in healing and inflammatory processes; commonly occurs in or around gastrointestinal tract, where adhesions may form bands and cause obstructions and subsequent surgical emergencies.

Chemotaxis: A cellular function, particularly of neutrophils and monocytes, whose phagocytic activity is influenced by chemical factors released by invading microorganisms.

Dead space: Air or empty space between layers of tissue or beneath wound edges that have been approximated.

Dehiscence: Separation of layers of surgical wound.

Evisceration: Extrusion of internal organs or viscera through gaping wound.

Gangrene: Anaerobic infection process that may occur instead of healing; implies necrosis (death of tissue) and putrefaction (decomposition); usually caused by failure of nutriment or blood to reach a part.

Keloid: Dense, unsightly connective tissue or excessive scar formation that is often removed surgically.

"Proud flesh": A mass of excessive granulation formed when a wound shows no other sign of healing or excessive cicatrization.

From Rothrock, J. (2019). *Alexander's care of the patient in surgery* (16th ed.). St. Louis, MO: Elsevier.

granulomas if excessively large. The hypertrophic scar is large, but the scar does not extend beyond the borders of the wound. The scar is red, but later becomes lighter and flatter.

Hypertrophic burn scars can become less elastic and cause contractures that may require surgical intervention to release to increase flexibility and mobility.

b. *Keloids* form in response to an overactive proliferation of fibroblasts. Keloid scars extend beyond the borders of the wound and can continue to grow and become painful. Keloids are more common in darker skinned individuals and are more prominent over the neck, upper shoulders, and back.

Keloids can be vascular and bleed easily when injured or scratched. Silicone sheeting can be applied to reduce the size of the scar. Keloids can be injected with an antiinflammatory medication or excised and closed with an inert material (i.e., staples or monofilament, nonabsorbent suture).

5. **Hematoma and seroma** cause a nidus for microbial growth and form a barrier to healing. Neovascularization is blocked. The buildup of blood and serum can support deep abscess formation. Draining a serous wound and controlling hemostasis during the surgical procedure can prevent this complication.

Prevention of surgical site complications is a desired outcome in perioperative patient care. Perioperative nurses should be able to identify factors that could influence wound healing. A knowledge of skin anatomy and physiology is important for the process of surgical site care during and after the surgical procedure. Postoperatively, early recognition of potential complications can prevent serious injury to the patient and effect prompt treatment.

LEARNING ACTIVITIES

INSTRUCTIONS: Complete the crossword puzzle. Use the clues to help identify the words.

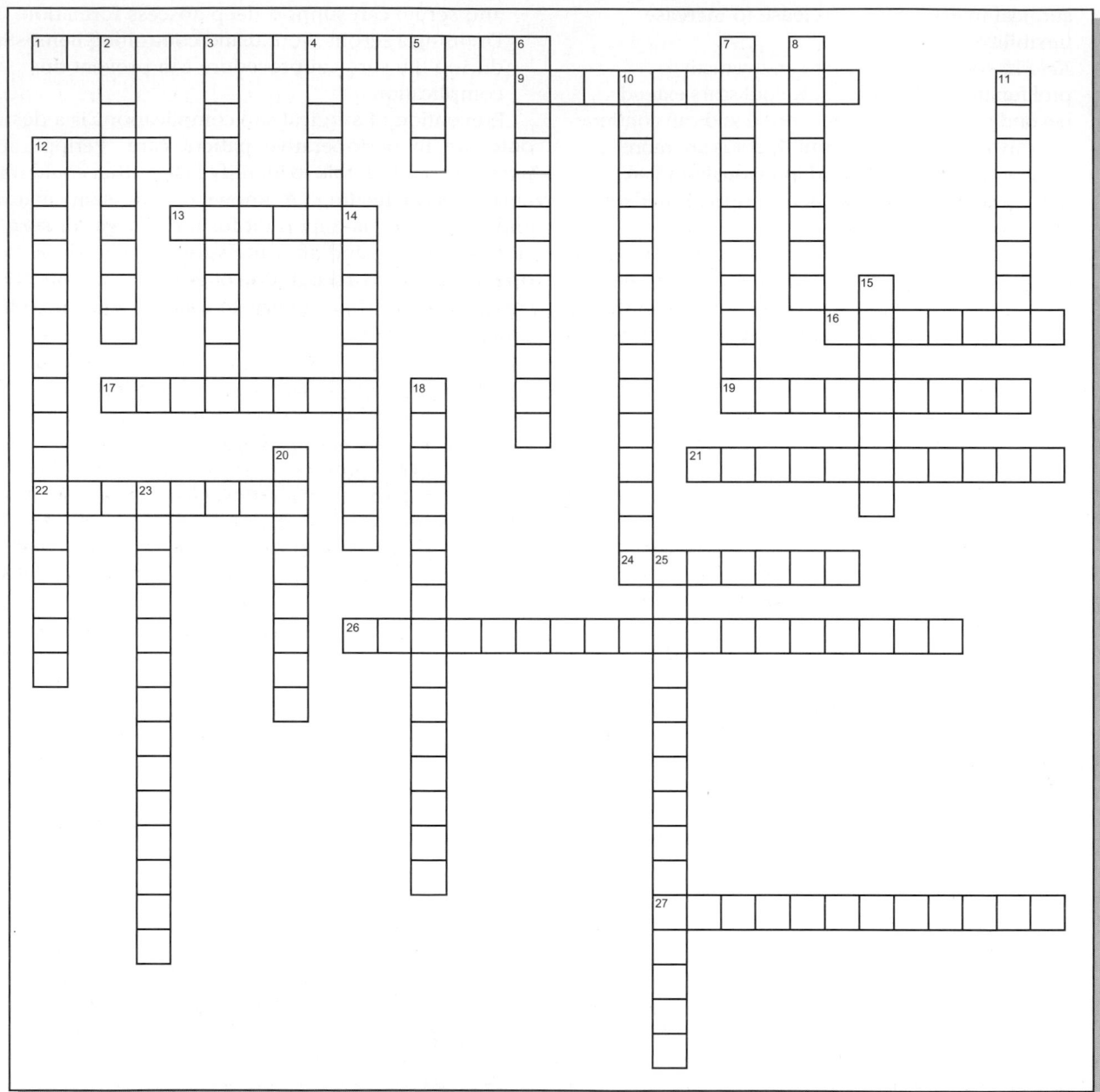

ACROSS

1. Wound cannot be closed immediately; it may need to be cleaned, packed, and debrided; infection may be present
9. This antibiotic may be administered 2 hours before incision
12. Measures employed to minimize the risk for SSI (use abbreviation)
13. Overactive scar formation beyond the incision border; it continues to grow; common in darker skinned individuals
16. Dirty or infected wound; old or necrotic wound
17. This type of dressing uses a sponge and negative pressure to remove serous drainage; it may be attached to a vacuum device
19. Abnormal fibrous bands form and bind tissue or organs together; surgery is usually needed
21. The administration of this drug should be 1 hour preoperatively for distribution through the circulatory system before incision

22. This phase of healing is from the inflammatory response; occurs within the first 5 days
24. Affects wound healing by vasoconstriction
26. Collagen is secreted to form fibers that strengthen the incision; it is completed over 20 days
27. Allows fluid and blood to flow from the wound by gravity

DOWN

2. This type of cancer treatment can damage tissue and blood vessels
3. This type of drain is attached to a suction reservoir and placed after the incision is closed
4. Clean wound with no break in technique
5. The largest organ of the body and barrier to infection
6. The deep layers separate, exposing organs; this is a surgical emergency
7. Loss of body heat; puts patient at a greater risk for SSI
8. This disease complicates healing because of poor circulation
10. This nonsteroidal medication can delay the healing process
11. Contaminated wound, open or traumatic; major break in technique such as gastrointestinal spillage
12. Wound is left open; the wound heals by granulation from the bottom up
14. Separation of the superficial layers; edges do not unite; it may be closed by delayed primary closure
15. Clean contaminated wound; alimentary, genitourinary, or respiratory system is entered
18. Wound healing can be affected if vitamins, minerals, and protein are lacking for tissue growth
20. Collection of blood or serum; it is formed by neovascularization blockage
23. No tissue loss, edges approximate evenly; minimal scarring
25. This phase begins at day 14 with the formation of scar tissue; it can take weeks to months

LEARNING ACTIVITIES ANSWERS

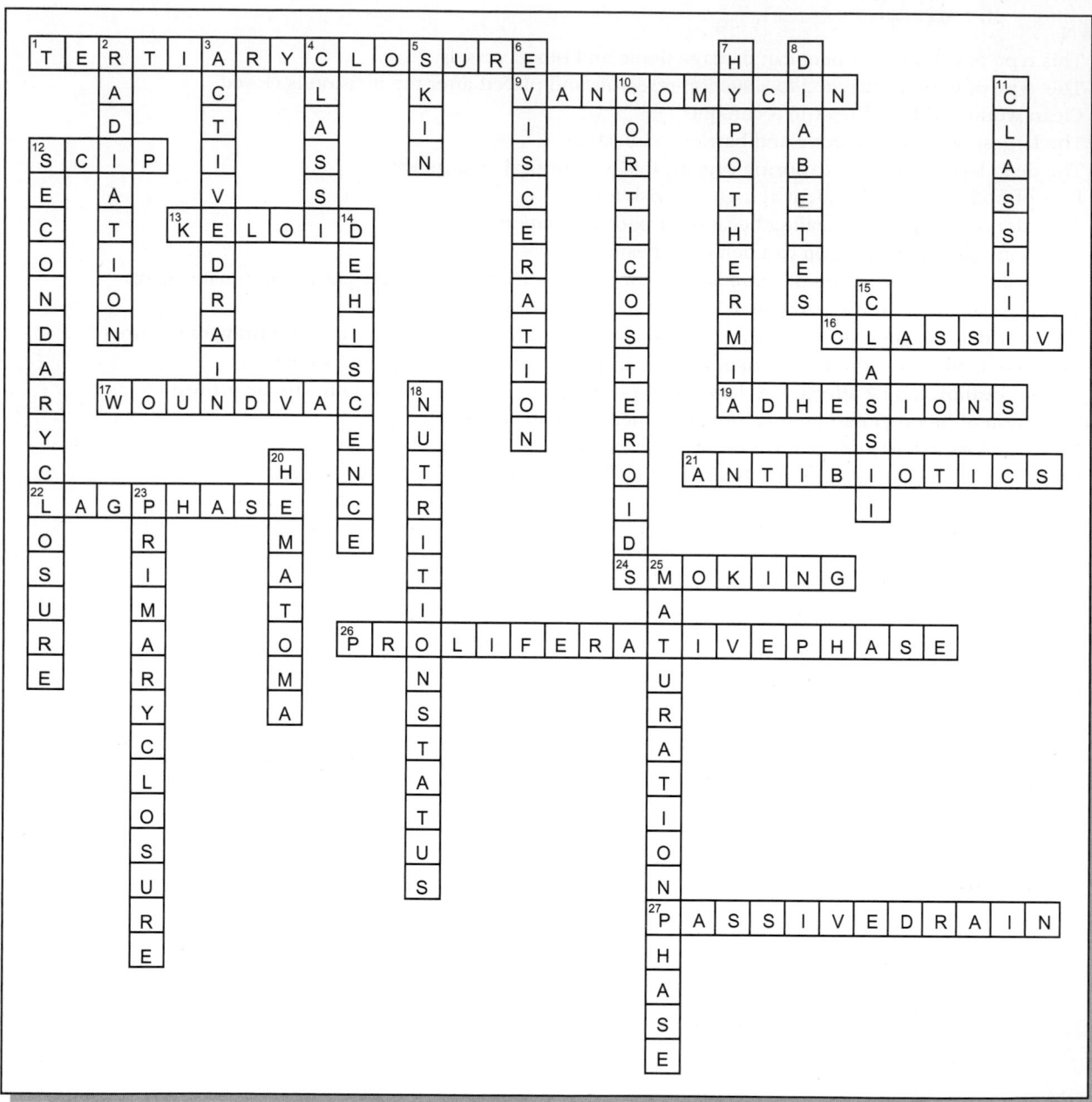

CHAPTER 10

Care of Surgical Instruments

Patient care items in the operating room (OR) are either disinfected or sterile. Before actually processing for patient use, each item must be decontaminated so disinfection or sterilization is most effective. After decontamination, the method of processing depends on the manufacturer's instructions for use (IFU) and how the item will be used in patient care in the perioperative environment. The perioperative nurse demonstrates knowledge of the different processes of decontamination, disinfection, and sterilization to keep patient care items safe from microbial contamination.

The Centers for Disease Control and Prevention (CDC) has adopted Spaulding's Level of Care, which classifies the importance of patient care items based on the level of infection risk. The items are classified as critical, semicritical, and noncritical. Each level requires different processing and handling to achieve the reduction of microorganisms rendering the item safe for use in patient care.

The Three Levels of Spaulding's Classification of Patient Care Items

1. **Critical items** must be **sterile**. These items are used on sterile tissue and entry into the vascular system. The process of sterilization is confirmed and documented by the use of biologic indicators. Examples of sterile items include surgical instruments, invasive catheters, implants, endoscopes, or any item that penetrates body tissue and contacts the vascular system (i.e., biopsies with an endoscope).
2. **Semicritical items** require high-level disinfection (HLD). These items are used on intact skin and mucous membranes. Examples of items include vaginal probes, laryngoscope blades, respiratory equipment, and anesthesia equipment.
3. **Noncritical items** require intermediate to low disinfection. These items are used on intact skin; examples are blood pressure cuffs, tourniquets, or stethoscopes. Items are disinfected with a facility-approved cleaner at the point of use and can be used outside the restricted area. Other noncritical items can be environmental, such as furniture or linens.

Decontamination

Items used in patient care must be decontaminated before processing for patient use. Decontamination renders items safe for handling by processing personnel, but not safe for patient care. Appropriate personal protective equipment (PPE) is worn. PPE for decontamination may include heavy-duty gloves, aprons, waterproof shoe covers, special mask or respirator, hair cover, eye protection or shield, or other chemical-specific PPE.

1. **Point of use cleaning in the surgical field.** All surgical instrumentation on the sterile field should be cleaned during and after the surgical procedure at the point of use with sterile water (saline can be corrosive to the finish of certain materials). Some facilities require the application of an enzymatic precleaner to soiled instruments before transporting to the processing area.

   Keep instruments moist until processing to minimize the formation of biofilm. Disassemble all instruments with all jaws and ports open. Flush lumens. Secure sharp items according to facility policies to prevent injuries to processing personnel.
2. **Transporting contaminated items to the processing area.** Transport in closed or covered carts for decontamination.
3. **Preparing items for disinfection or sterilization.** Effective cleaning (washed with nonfilm soap), rinsing, purging, and drying are all critical steps in the preparation of instruments for disinfection or sterilization. All instruments should be processed according to IFU.
   a. Manual cleaning or ultrasonic cleaning (cavitation) is done in the decontamination area. Mechanical cleaning has shown to remove more debris. Mechanized washer-disinfectors or washer-sterilizers are used at most facilities to decontaminate instrumentation and render it safe for the processing personnel to handle and prepare trays.
   b. Some instruments require lubrication or sharpening to keep them in working order before processing.

Disinfection

There are three levels of disinfection, but they do not classify an item as sterile. Disinfection kills or inhibits the growth of most microorganisms with the exception of endospores.

1. **Three levels of disinfection.** Different chemicals and times are used for each level of disinfection. Disinfectants are chemical solutions of different

strengths specific for the type of processing desired. Some items must soak for a certain period and be rinsed with sterile water before use in patient care. IFU are followed to achieve the necessary level of disinfection. Each level of disinfection is classified by the intended use of the item in safe patient care.

a. **HLD.** HLD is used for semicritical items. Chemical agent kills all microorganisms (bacteria, fungi, and viruses) except endospores. HLD is not effective for prion contamination. IFU must be followed to achieve the desired results. Chemicals used for HLD must be US Food and Drug Administration (FDA) approved and in compliance with local, state, and federal regulations.
   1) HLD requires specific exposure time, chemical strength, and documentation.
   2) Chemicals used in HLD are toxic and require special training, Standard Precautions, and task-specific PPE.

b. **Intermediate-level disinfection.** Chemical agent kills most bacteria, viruses, and fungi on noncritical items.
   1) Process inactivates tuberculosis (TB), but does not kill endospores.
   2) Chemical agents are approved by the Environmental Protection Agency (EPA) as hospital-grade germicides.

c. **Low-level disinfection.** Chemical agent kills most vegetative bacteria and some fungi on noncritical items.
   1) Process inactivates some viruses, such as HIV, but is not effective against TB
   2) Chemical agents differ in the concentration and time of contact to be effective
   3) Point of use manual wipe down for patient care items
   4) Nontoxic, detergent-based, odorless, mixes easily with water, and leaves no residue

2. **Chemical disinfectants.** Chemical disinfection agents must be facility approved by the FDA and EPA, and have the safety data sheet available in case of exposure. All chemical disinfection agents must be labeled, including chemical ingredients, dilution, date mixed, special handling, warnings, list of microorganisms or viruses it is effective against, safety information, storage temperatures, PPE, and specific use.

   Manual and chemical disinfection requires a separate area away from clean items, wrapping, and sterilization supplies. The CDC requires at least 3 feet separating clean work areas from decontamination areas.

a. **Common chemical disinfectants** (Table 10.1)
   1) **Alcohol 70% to 95%** (ethyl, isopropyl): works by breaking down cell protein
      a) Fast acting, used to wipe down surfaces and equipment, bactericidal, fungicidal, pseudomonacidal, and kills many viruses

   b) Highly flammable, skin irritant, can be corrosive
   c) Evaporates quickly and may not provide a long enough exposure time to kill microorganisms

   2) **Chlorine compounds** (i.e., bleach, sodium hypochlorite): works by oxidation of enzymes
      a) Housekeeping disinfectants (surfaces, beds, floors); low-level disinfectant, when diluted with water
      b) Bactericidal, tuberculocidal, fungicidal, most viruses
      c) Can be a respiratory irritant if not diluted correctly; can be corrosive on instrumentation

   3) **Glutaraldehyde** (Banicide, Cidex): works by altering cell protein
      a) HLD use kills most bacteria and endospores.
      b) Processing methods and time depend on the item and the material; follow IFU. Average shelf life after reconstitution is limited.
      c) Cold, noncorrosive sterilant and sporicidal after 10 hours of exposure; minimum of a 2% solution is needed for sterilization.
      d) Used on endoscopes, plastics, rubber, and heat-sensitive items. Must be rinsed thoroughly with sterile water. Endoscopes for HLD require a longer soaking time per IFU.
      e) Must be handled by personnel with training, knowledge, and proper PPE.

Sterilization With Chemicals

Each load of sterilized supplies is assigned a load number. The lot number is used to recall loads if any item processed is questionable for sterility. Each load parameter is documented in the processing department records.

1. **Hydrogen peroxide gas plasma and hydrogen peroxide vapor.** STERRAD or vapor sterilization uses radio frequencies to create gas that maintains a low, 104°F temperature. Gas plasma sterilization works by oxidation. Aeration is not necessary. Items in packaging can be stored after processing.
   a. Sterilization can take between 35 and 75 minutes depending on the item and model of the machine. It is highly sporicidal at low temperatures.
   b. This is a dry, nontoxic method used for metal- and moisture-sensitive items requiring low temperature. Items with lumens should be approved for processing by length and diameter.
   c. Nonwoven polypropylene wrappers, Tyvek envelopes, or perforated trays are used to package instruments processed with this method.
   d. A biological indicator is run daily in the machine with a *Geobacillus stearothermophilus* endospore strip or vial. A chemical indicator is placed on the inside and outside of each package.

TABLE 10.1   Common Liquid Chemical Disinfectants

Disinfectant Agent	Level of Disinfection	Timing	Virucidal	Fungicidal	Sporicidal	Mycobacterium (Tuberculocidal)	Hazards	Notes
Alcohol, 70%–95%								
Ethyl	Intermediate level	10–30 minutes for both	Yes, but not all lipid viruses, HAV	Yes	No	Yes	All forms are flammable	Bactericidal but not bacteriostatic. Ineffective against spores. Noncorrosive.
Isopropyl	Intermediate level		Yes, but not enteroviruses	Yes	No	Yes		Denatures proteins. Harms rubber and plastic. Combined with other disinfectants to form a tincture that can extend the bactericidal action. Rapid evaporation. Used in skin antisepsis.
Aldehyde, Toxic: skin, eye, and respirator irritant								
Aqueous acidic 2%	High level	20–90 minutes at 68°F–77°F (20°C–25°C)	Yes	Yes	No	Yes; very slow	OSHA exposure limit is 0.05 ppm. Can cause respiratory irritation. Carcinogenic.	Excellent materials compatibility. Local regulations may restrict disposal of used product. Inexpensive to use. Use in well-ventilated area. Reduced effect in detergent.
Glutaraldehyde								
Banicide 3.5%	Sterile	10 hours at 77°F (25°C)	Yes	Yes	Yes	Yes		30-Day reuse period. Absorbed by neoprene or PVC gloves.
	High level	45 minutes at 77°F (25°C)						
Cidex activated alkaline 2.4% dialdehyde	Sterile	10 hours at 77°F (25°C)	Yes	Yes	Yes	Yes		Coagulates blood and tissue. Activated alkaline form has shelf life of 14–30 days. Concentration level must be monitored.
	High level	45 minutes at 77°F (25°C)	Yes	Yes	Some	Yes		

(Continued)

TABLE 10.1　Common Liquid Chemical Disinfectants—cont'd

Disinfectant Agent	Level of Disinfection	Timing	Virucidal	Fungicidal	Sporicidal	Mycobacterium (Tuberculocidal)	Hazards	Notes
Cidex OPA (0.55%) ortho-phthal-aldehyde	High level	12 minutes at 68°F (20°C)	Yes	Yes	Some, but improves when the pH is increased to 8. Scopes pass sporicidal test at 32 hours at 20°C	Yes; superior action	No known irritations	Requires no activation and remains more stable over a wide range of pH (3–9). Stains protein gray; 14-day reuse period. Concentration level must be monitored
Cidex OPA (5.75%) ortho-phthal-aldehyde concentrate	High level	5 minutes at 122°F (50°C)			Scopes pass sporicidal test at 32 hours at 122°F (50°C)			Used in an automated endoscope high-level disinfector by EvoTech Integrated Endoscope Disinfection System.
Phenol Compound								
1.64% with 0.95% glutaraldehyde (Sporicidin)	Sterile	12 hours at 77°F (25°C)	Yes	Yes	Yes	Yes	Skin and eye irritant. Carcinogenic. Toxic to animals.	Effective in presence of organic matter. Leaves an active residue. Effective in detergents.
	High level	20 minutes at 77°F (25°C)	Yes, but limited	Yes	No	Yes		Maximum reuse period of 7 days.
Quaternary Ammonium Compounds (Quats)								
C0.1%–2% concentration	Low	10 minutes	Limited; lipophilic only	Yes	No	No	No odor and low toxicity	Easily inactivated by organic debris. Effective in temperatures up to 212°F (100°C). Most effective in alkaline solution. Neutralized by detergents and hard water. Nonirritating and noncorrosive. Inexpensive. Inactivated by use with gauze pads. Surface disinfection.

Halogens Chlorine and chlorine compounds such as sodium hypochlorite	Low to high based on concentration and pH	10–30 minutes	Yes	Yes	Limited	Yes	Toxic and corrosive. Do not autoclave chlorine solutions; will vaporize and cause free chlorine gas inhalation hazard. Dangerous gas forms if mixed with ammonia.	Ethyl alcohol 60% can be added to increase kill potential. Oxidizes metallic objects. 1:10 dilution of 6% chlorine bleach (household bleach) contains 6000 ppm available chlorine. Combines with protein and decreases in effectiveness. Premixed solution can be stored in cool place in a light-proof container.
Iodophors (Wescodyne)	Low at a wide range of pH	10–30 minutes	Yes	Yes	No	Yes		Alcohol can be added to extend effectiveness in a solution of 1:10 in 50% ethyl alcohol. Vaporizes in hot water (120°F–125°F [48°C–51.6°C]). Reduced action in presence of protein. Inactivated iodophor loses brown-yellow color. Becomes clear when deactivated.
Peracetic Acid STERIS 0.2%	Sterile	12–30 minutes at 122°F–133°F (50°C–56°C)	Yes	Yes	Yes	Yes, even at low temperatures. Can be a fire hazard at high temperatures when dry	Wear PPE if risk of contact to skin, eyes, or mucous membranes	Used in STERIS processing as a single-use liquid chemical sterilant. No residue. Uses filtered tap water for rinse. Can corrode metallics. Approximately $6 per cycle. No special disposal requirements. Protect from light and heat.

(Continued)

10.1 Common Liquid Chemical Disinfectants—cont'd

Disinfectant Agent	Level of Disinfection	Timing	Virucidal	Fungicidal	Sporicidal	Mycobacterium (Tuberculocidal)	Hazards	Notes
Sporox Hydrogen Peroxide 7.5%	Sterile	6 hours at 68°F (20°C)	Yes	Yes	Yes	Yes	Wear PPE to protect eyes	Requires no activation. Has no special disposal instructions.
	High level	30 minutes at 68°F (20°C)	Yes	Yes	Some	Yes		Must monitor minimal effective concentration. Maximum reuse period of 21 days. May enhance removal of organic debris. Not effective as a disinfectant in presence of organic matter.

HAV, Hepatitis A virus; *OSHA,* Occupational Safety and Health Administration; *PPE,* personal protective equipment; *ppm,* parts per million; *PVC,* polyvinylchloride.
From Phillips, N. (2017). *Berry and Kohn's operating room technique* (13th ed.). St. Louis, MO: Elsevier.

2. **Peracetic acid.** Used on heat-sensitive, moisture-stable equipment. STERIS is used for HLD and sterilization. The solution is heated between 122°F and 131°F, then internally rinsed with filtered tap water that passed through ultraviolet light to render it sterile. It works by oxidation, and is a broad-spectrum antimicrobial. Peracetic acid is not hazardous. It leaves no residue. Items are processed for immediate use, not stored. The STERIS machine has an internal documentation log that records each load.
   a. Effective against bacteria, fungi, TB, and endospores.
   b. The item(s) for processing must be completely disassembled before processing.
   c. A biological indicator is used daily to test the machine with a *G. stearothermophilus* endospore strip.
   d. A chemical indicator is used for each load to document the sterilization process was completed.
3. **Ethylene oxide gas sterilizer (EO, ETO).** It is used on heat- and moisture-sensitive items, low-temperature sterilization 85°F to 145°F, and has no residue. It disrupts DNA and protein to kill microorganisms and endospores. It is flammable, toxic, and requires long sterilization and aeration time.
   a. It can be used on solutions in glass ampules and plastics except polyvinylchloride (PVC). PVC can absorb EO gas.
   b. Items must be clean and completely dry (including lumens) before processing. Wet items can form ethylene glycol, which causes hemolysis of red blood cells.
   c. It requires special handling and PPE (rubber, neoprene, or nitrile gloves). Occupational Safety and Health Administration (OSHA) regulations, personnel monitoring (dosimeter badges), and exposure limits are set by OSHA. Exposure cannot exceed an 8-hour work shift (0.5 ppm). Employee health records must be kept for 30 years because it is carcinogenic.
   d. Requires a chemical indicator (outside of package) and biologic indicator (*Bacillus atrophaeus*) for every load.
4. **Considerations for chemical disinfection and sterilization.** Personnel should be educated in the health risks, first aid, exposure measures, infection control safe practices, equipment safety, standards, guidelines, instrument processing, maintenance of equipment, and quality assurance testing.
   a. Processing areas should be located away from patient areas and have limited personnel access, proper ventilation systems, covered soaking containers, and warning signs.
   b. Eyewash stations and showers should be immediately available in case of exposure.
   c. Before processing, verify compatibility of the item with the processing method according to the IFU.
   d. Disinfectant and sterilant solutions should be checked for expiration date, discoloration, contamination, and concentration. Items should be fully immersed in solution and meet the time requirements for the level of processing desired.
   e. Documentation should include load number, physical monitors, chemical, time, temperature, and confirmation for sterility with a chemical, biologic, and internal mechanical indicator. Include printouts, digital readings, gauge readings, graphs, and personnel signatures in the permanent department records.
   f. Contaminated PPE and expired chemical solutions should be disposed of according to facility policy and EPA regulations.

Thermal Sterilization

Sterilization of patient care items and instrumentation is dependent on the material of the item, how it will be used, and the IFU. Steam under pressure or dry heat is used in thermal sterilization.

1. **Steam under pressure.** Thermal destruction of microorganisms and endospores is done with steam under pressure for heat- and moisture-stable items in an autoclave. Steam is cost-effective, easy to use, time effective, reliable, residue free, and has computerized settings for accurate documentation.

   The steam denatures protein, and living microorganisms cannot survive for more than 15 minutes. The 30 pounds of pressure (psi) enables the steam to penetrate endospores. Certain instruments and devices may have longer exposure times; see manufacturer recommendations. The two types of steam sterilizers are gravity displacement and prevacuum (Dynamic air removal).
   a. **Gravity displacement** sterilizers consist of two parts: an outer jacket and an internal chamber. The steam enters the chamber near the top of the back of the sterilizer. Ambient air is heavier than steam and is forced downward by gravity to the bottom of the chamber to the steam discharge area at the lower front.

      A thermometer measures the steam temperature when the chamber is full of steam. When the temperature reaches the desired setting, the sterilization timing process begins. The contents in the sterilizer are positioned so that steam reaches all surfaces as the steam is displaced downward. Ambient air pockets prevent sterilization of all surfaces.
      Wrapped Instruments/Packaged Instruments
      250°F exposure time of 30 minutes
      270°F exposure time of 15 minutes
      275°F exposure time 10 minutes
   b. **Prevacuum sterilizer** (dynamic air removal) uses a high power pump system to remove the ambient air before the steam is injected into the chamber. A prevacuum period of 8 to 10 minutes removes the air so the steam can easily penetrate all

surfaces of the chamber contents. A **Bowie-Dick** air removal test must be done daily for all prevacuum sterilizers to confirm the air pump is functioning properly. A postvacuum cycle shortens the drying time. Temperature is controlled around 270°F (132°C) at a pressure of 27 psi. A completed sterilization cycle including the dry time can take from 15 to 30 minutes. Wrapped Instruments/Packaged Instruments 270°F exposure time of 4 minutes 275°F exposure time of 3 minutes

  c. **Immediate-use steam sterilization (IUSS).** IUSS is not a preferred method of sterilization and is used only in emergency situations. Instruments should be decontaminated and cleaned in the processing area before immediate-use sterilization.

      IUSS is also known as "flash sterilization." Flash sterilization is the process of sterilizing unwrapped items that are needed quickly for the sterile field. The process takes between 3 and 10 minutes with no dry time or cooldown.

      Gravity or prevacuum sterilizer can be used for IUSS. Metal and nonporous items are processed at: 270°F for 3 minutes. Complex items with lumens or instrument tape (plastic, metal, rubber) or that are porous require 10 minutes. Lumens should be flushed with water and sterilized wet.

      Documentation includes: time, temperature, items processed, type of sterilizer, cycle, date, load number, patient's name, reason for IUSS, chemical and biologic indicators, operator of sterilizer, and person who accepted the sterilized items.

      For more information, visit the Association for the Advancement of Medical Instrumentation (AAMI) website (https://www.aami.org/). AORN (Association of periOperative Registered Nurses), AAMI, and CDC Guidelines for IUSS include (immediate-use statement: https://www.aami.org/publications/standards/ST79:2017):

    1) Only use IUSS if necessary, not for convenience or shortage of instruments. Frequent use of IUSS is an indicator of the need for additional stock instruments.

    2) IUSS should never be used for implants according to the CDC, AAMI, and AORN.

    3) Leave instruments unwrapped, open, and disassembled.

    4) Rigid containers must be IUSS approved, and contents used immediately. There is no storage of IUSS items.

    5) A biologic (*G. stearothermophilus*) and chemical indicator must be used.

    6) IUSS for gravity and prevacuum sterilizers are time specific:
      a) 270°F for 10 minutes for gravity
      b) 270°F for 4 minutes for prevacuum

  d. **Dry heat** sterilization is used for items that are heat stable but cannot be exposed to moisture. Dry heat requires a longer period to let the hot air circulate, which coagulates protein and destroys microorganisms. Delicate instruments, sharp items such as burrs, small amounts of oil, talc, items packed in glass, test tubes, and small jars (lids can be used) can be sterilized by dry heat. The sterilizer should be loaded according to the IFU. Process time is determined by items and packaging. Dry heat is used in many dental offices.

    1) Peel pouches and woven packaging can be used if the temperature is not above 400°F. Packaging IFU should indicate if safe for use in dry heat sterilizer. Some packaging could ignite if exposed to high temperatures. Foil packaging, metal, or glass containers are commonly used.

    2) Biologic indicator with *B. atrophaeus* is used.

    3) Items should cool before removal from the sterilizer; burns are a hazard of dry heat.

Additional Methods of Sterilization

1. **Ozone** is a low-temperature sterilization process that works by oxidation. Ozone uses oxygen and water. Ozone is commonly used by manufacturers for metal, plastic, and heat-sensitive items.
  a. The process works in four phases, takes about 4.5 hours, only one setting, and requires no aeration.
  b. Can use nonwoven wrapping material or pouches (no paper) and aluminum containers.
  c. *G. stearothermophilus* biologic indicator is used.

2. **Ionizing radiation** is a very effective form of commercial sterilization. Cobalt-60 is the radioactive isotope converted to thermal and chemical rays, which kill microorganisms. The radiation passes through most materials. Effectiveness depends on the density and thickness of the item. The process is monitored and documented.
  a. Ionizing radiation is used on heat- and moisture-sensitive items.
  b. Items are packaged in FDA-approved containers and nonwoven pouches.
  c. A chemical indicator should be placed on the outside of the item, and a biologic indicator is used inside.
  d. Sterilization can take 10 to 20 hours. Ionizing radiation is done off-site at a commercial facility.

Additional Considerations for Sterilization

All items must be processed with an internal biologic and an outside chemical indictor. Terminal sterilization permits the item to be stored in a clean storage area. Sterilization equipment must be routinely checked with a biological indicator (process challenge device [PCD]) performed. The results are documented per facility policy.

1. **Loaner instruments:** Borrowed items that are sterilized outside of the facility must be taken out of their container, decontaminated, cleaned, and sterilized in-house before use.

2. **Instrument sets:** Wrapped wire trays and closed container systems are sterilized flat without obstruction for steam to pass through the entire set. Instrument trays should not weigh more than 25 pounds. Trays may have a count sheet enclosed, but it must be medical-grade paper. Printer toner material should not be permitted to contact the instruments during processing. Do not put count sheet in a peel pouch.

3. **Metal basin sets:** Wrapped metal basin sets should not weigh more than 7 pounds and are sterilized on the side with a slight forward lean so the steam can contact all surfaces. Basin sets should be separated by wicking material so they sterilize and dry completely.

4. Hot items should cool on designated wire racks after heat sterilization. Do not set hot trays on a cold surface, because condensation will cause strike-through, creating contamination.

5. Some complex packaged trays such as orthopedic trays may need additional processing time per IFU. They are usually steam sterilized by prevacuum for 15 minutes at 270°F.

6. Eye instrumentation should be cleaned and sterilized separately from other instrumentation. Improper processing can cause toxic anterior segment (TASS) syndrome.

Special Circumstances

1. **Emergency implant sterilization.** Implant sterilization is not a preferred activity.
   a. If an implant must be sterilized in an emergency, follow facility guidelines and manufacturer's written instructions.
   b. An internal biological indicator and an external chemical indicator must be used.
   c. Implants should be quarantined until the biologic indicator is negative. If the implant is used before the biologic indictor results are known, detailed documentation is needed in the patient's medical record and the facility implant log.

2. **Prions and Creutzfeldt-Jakob disease (CJD).** Prions are not living microorganisms. They are proteins that attach to the surface of instruments and are extremely difficult to remove. Despite processing, a prion can be transferred to another patient, causing cross-contamination if the instrumentation is incorrectly processed.
   a. If CJD is suspected before the surgical procedure, use all disposable items if possible. It is preferable to use disposable instruments and remove any nonessential equipment from the room. Cover everything else with disposable drapes.
   b. If CJD is suspected during the surgical procedure, but not yet confirmed by biopsy, these steps can be taken:
      1) Keep the instrument set moist during the surgical procedure. Dried material is hard to remove.
      2) Soak in sodium hypochlorite solution 1:10 H_2O (bleach) or sodium hydroxide solution 40 g:1 L H_2O (lye) for 1 hour.

      3) Rinse the tray of instruments well and place it in a steam autoclave for terminal steam sterilization.
         Gravity displacement at 270°F for 1 hour.
         Prevacuum at 274°F for 18 minutes.
      4) When the tray of instruments is cool, it is sent to the processing department. Notify the processing department that the tray of instruments has been pretreated and should be run through the automated washing system without other instrument sets.
      5) When the automated washing cycle is complete, the tray of instruments should be isolated from other sets until the patient's biopsy results are reported.
      6) If the patient's biopsy is negative, the set can be returned to service. If the biopsy is positive, the facility policy and procedure should be followed concerning disposition of the set.

Processing Flexible Endoscopes

Endoscopes should be cleaned according to the IFU. Processing should begin within an hour of use. Endoscopes and instrumentation that enter a cavity through a mucous membrane should be sterile according to the modified 2018 Spaulding Classification system found in the AORN *Guidelines for Perioperative Practice.*

1. Endoscopes should be precleaned at the point of use with an HLD or enzymatic solution.
2. Transport to the processing area in a closed biohazard container. The endoscope should be damp and placed horizontal.
3. Endoscopes should be processed in an area with necessary equipment, instrument air, single-use brushes, PPE, and emergency eyewash stations.
4. Before processing, flexible endoscopes are leak tested, manually cleaned, or ultrasonic cleaned; all channels are purged with air and inspected, with dry exterior. Some scope channels are rinsed with 70% to 90% isopropyl alcohol to hasten drying.
5. Wipe clean with a soft lint-free cloth. Suction with enzymatic solution followed by water. Alternate cleaning with compressed air and enzymatic solution flushing all lumens and channels during the process.
6. Flexible endoscopes are hung vertically with valves open in a closed drying cabinet equipped with a HEPA (high-efficiency particulate air) filter.

What Does the Perioperative Nurse Need to Know About Sterilization Packaging, Indicators, and Integrators?

Perioperative nurses must be familiar with the different packaging materials, containers, and sterility indicators. Each processed item must be inspected for integrity (moisture, holes, or tears) and whether the item has completed the sterilization process. All sterilized items should have an external chemical indicator and an internal chemical/biologic indicator.

1. **Wrapping materials** may be woven (fabric) or nonwoven (paper).
   a. The wrapping material should be correct for the method of sterilization and size appropriate (no gaps).
   b. Nonwoven materials are cellulose and rayon. They are disposable, lightweight, lint free, and can be layered. Nonwoven materials are also used for drapes. These drapes must not be cut to size at the sterile field because they will shed cellulose fibers into the surgical site that can cause granulomas or inflammation. Inflamed tissue is subject to frequent infections.
2. **Peel pouches** or packs have a transparent plastic side and paper on the other side; they are heat sealed or self-sealing. The paper side contains a chemical indicator. They are not used for heavy items.
   a. Labels, if used, should be placed on the clear plastic side so the sterilization process can penetrate the paper side without obstruction. This also prevents bleed-through of ink.
   b. Peel pouches are processed on their side so the sterilant can completely penetrate the paper side of the package. The steam will not penetrate the plastic side of the pouch if placed flat or inside a tray.
   c. If double pouching is permitted by the manufacturer, the inner pouch should be placed with the plastic facing in the same direction and fit inside without folding. The pouch must be sterilized on its side.
   d. Sterilized peel pouches must be stored on their sides to minimize the risk for puncture.
3. **Rigid sterilization containers** are constructed of metal, hard plastic polymer, or aluminum with a fitted, locking top. Each type contains a fitted mesh basket inside to hold instruments.
   The lid and the base unit contain filters that are changed between uses. The filter allows the sterilant to enter the container. The circulating nurse checks these for any signs of moisture. A damp filter means that the set is not considered sterile. The circulating nurse should remove and discard the filters after the sterile scrub person removes the wire mesh instrument tray. Removing the filters prevents accidently reusing them.
   a. Each style of closed container has a breakaway, tamper-proof, plastic locking system with an external chemical sterilization indicator.
   b. Identification information tag includes contents, lot number, assembler, and date.
   c. The inner basket contains the instruments and a chemical/biologic indicator or integrator.
   d. The sterile scrub person touches only the sterile handles of the inner basket and lifts it straight up without touching the outer container.
   e. When opening the sets, no additional sterile items are opened into the container because the outer surface is not considered sterile.

Six Classes of Chemical Sterilization Indicators/Integrators are Available for Specific Uses (Table 10.2)

1. **Class 1:** External: used to identify processed items from unprocessed items. First visible sign is the form of color changing tape or labels outside.
2. **Class 2:** Bowie-Dick chemical indicator is used to test dynamic air (prevacuum) sterilizer for recommended air removal. Should be run daily, with test load. If the sterilizer is new, relocated, or malfunctions, the machine is run three consecutive times to validate proper function.
3. **Class 3:** Measures one single parameter such as time or temperature placed inside.
4. **Class 4:** Multiparameter, two or more variables and time and temperature are placed inside; is commonly used for dry heat.
5. **Class 5:** Designed to display all variables such as time, temperature, and steam. Recommended for placement in all trays. Is placed inside tray.
6. **Class 6:** Responds to all variables; provides cycle verification. Placed inside. Chemical indicators are used along with biologic indicators.

Biological Indicators: Process Challenge Device (PCD)

1. The sterilization process is tested by placing a contained living endospore vial, strip, or ampule through the sterilization process. The processed sample is incubated along with an unprocessed sample or control. The processed sample will not grow if the sterilization process was complete Table 10.2.
2. Biologic indicators are required at least weekly, but most facilities use them daily. Chemical sterilizers routinely use biologic process challenge device (PCD) every load.
3. Biologic indicators are required in every load that contains an implantable device. The implant should not be used until the results from the biologic test are available and are negative.
4. The indicator should be specific for the sterilization method and placed according to IFU.

Sterilization Monitoring Systems

All processing methods have a monitoring program in place with detailed documentation. Items can be tracked by a scanning system.

Physical monitoring documentation includes method of sterilization, gauges, computer readouts, cycle times, temperatures, contents of the load, load identification number, results of chemical and biological monitors, and operator name.

1. Documentation is kept on file for tracking in case of a sterilization failure or recall of defective devices.
2. Each load has a lot number.

TABLE 10.2 Guidelines for Use of Chemical and Biologic Indicators

AAMI	AHA	AORN	CDC	TJC
Chemical				
Purpose: To indicate items exposed to the sterilization process; to monitor one or more sterilization parameters; to detect failures in packaging, loading, or sterilizer function. Indicators do not verify sterility.				
Placement				
External: On all packages except if internal indicator is visible	With each package; can be used inside or on outside	External: Visible on every package	External: Attached to each package	With each package, no designation to inside or outside
Internal: In center or area least accessible to sterilant within each package		Internal: Inside each package	Internal: Inside large pack	
Biologic				
Purpose: To document efficacy of sterilization process by killing resistant spores; to ensure that all process parameters are met; to detect nonsterilizing conditions in sterilizer.				
Steam				
Frequency: At least weekly, preferably daily	Frequency: Once a day	Frequency: At least once a week, preferably daily, and with each load of implants	Frequency: At least once a week, and with each load of implants	Frequency: At least weekly (daily is recommended), or with each load if sterilization activities are performed less frequently or if load contains implantable or intravascular material
Placement: Positioned in cold point in process challenge test pack, normally bottom front of sterilizer				
Ethylene Oxide				
Frequency: Every load	Frequency: Every load	Frequency: Every load	Frequency: At least once a week, and with each load of implants	Frequency: At least weekly (daily is recommended), or with each load if sterilization activities are performed less frequently or if load contains implantable or intravascular material
Placement: Inside pack in geometric center of load				

All organizations require that indicators and integrators be used routinely.
AAMI, Association for the Advancement of Medical Instrumentation; *AHA, American Hospital Association*; *AORN*, Association of periOperative Registered Nurses; *CDC*, Centers for Disease Control and Prevention; *TJC*, The Joint Commission.
From Phillips, N. (2017). *Berry and Kohn's operating room technique* (13th ed.). St. Louis, MO: Elsevier.

Reprocessing Single-Use Items

The FDA sets requirements for the reprocessing of single-use items. Reprocessing is highly regulated. Single-use critical items should not be reprocessed. Patients have the right to know if single-use reprocessed items were used. The facility is liable for purchasing or processing single-use items. The facility must be registered and list all items that are reprocessed following IFU.

1. Items must be labeled as "Reprocessed" with the manufacturer's name and lot number. The number of times the item has been reprocessed should be indicated on the packaging.
2. Items reprocessed are in two categories:
   a. Opened items but not used
   b. Opened used items

Storage of Packaged Sterile Items

1. Packaged sterile items shipped into a facility must be removed from the shipping containers. Cardboard boxes can contain vermin or other contaminants.
2. Packaged sterile items from distributors should be transported to the sterile storage area in covered carts with a solid bottom.
3. Packaged sterile items should be stored in a semi-restricted area with open shelving or cabinets, free from moisture and dust.

   a. Environmental control of storage
      1) Temperature is controlled between 60°F and 70°F
      2) Humidity 20% to 60%
      3) Heating, ventilation, and air conditioning (HVAC): four air exchanges (ACH) per hour with two outdoor exchanges
   b. Shelving must be more than 18 inches from the ceiling, 8 to 10 inches from the floor (bottom shelf should be covered, no wire), and 2 inches from an outside wall.
4. **Sterility is event related.**
   a. All items should be checked for expiration dates. Packages with unstable contents (i.e., custom packs: prep solution, suture, medication) will have an expiration date.
   b. Items are considered sterile as long as the packaging is not damaged and an unstable element is not inside.

The perioperative nurse must have knowledge of the different sterilization processes and be able to recognize the indicators for sterilization, both chemical and biologic. This knowledge and skill are essential when delivering instrumentation to the sterile field and maintaining aseptic technique throughout the surgical procedure.

LEARNING ACTIVITIES

MATCHING

INSTRUCTIONS: Match the term to the appropriate definition.

a. daily
b. decontamination
c. cavitation
d. radiation
e. vermin
f. point of use
g. 15
h. event
i. *Geobacillus stearothermophilus*
j. prion
k. immediate-use steam sterilization (IUSS)
l. 3
m. noncritical
n. steam
o. condensation
p. ozone
q. 4
r. parameters
s. endoscopes
t. Bacillus atrophaeus
u. Bowie-Dick
v. 10
w. critical
x. on side
y. reprocessed

_____ 1. The name for ultrasonic cleaning
_____ 2. At what point should instruments be cleaned during and after a procedure?
_____ 3. Which items are considered sterile according to Spaulding's Level of Care?
_____ 4. This process renders items safe for handling
_____ 5. How often should a biological indicator be run in sterilizer with *Geobacillus stearothermophilus*?
_____ 6. Which test is done to confirm the functioning of the air removal pump in a prevacuum sterilizer?
_____ 7. Which form of sterilization should be used only in emergency situations?
_____ 8. This form of sterilization is cost-effective, reliable, and destroys endospores and microorganisms
_____ 9. This method of sterilization uses low temperature with oxygen and water
_____ 10. The commercial method of cobalt-60 uses this form of sterilization
_____ 11. Hot items should not be placed on a cold surface because formation of this can cause contamination
_____ 12. A nonliving protein that is difficult to remove even after processing
_____ 13. The 2018 Spaulding Classification changed the guidelines for which instrumentation?
_____ 14. In which position should peel packs be sterilized and stored?
_____ 15. Sterility is _____ related

_____ 16. Packaged items shipped to a facility must be removed from containers because they can contain _____
_____ 17. Patients have the right to know whether these items have been used during a procedure
_____ 18. In a prevacuum sterilizer, wrapped instruments should be processed at 270°F for how many minutes?
_____ 19. Wrapped or packaged instruments sterilized by gravity displacement at 270°F should be processed for how many minutes?
_____ 20. Porous or complex items with lumens or tape should be sterilized at 270°F for how many minutes if IUSS gravity displacement autoclave is used?
_____ 21. Metal and nonporous items processed by IUSS in a gravity displacement sterilizer at 270°F should be processed for how many minutes?
_____ 22. Chemical indicators are used to show that _____ for sterilization have been met
_____ 23. The biologic indicator for steam sterilization contains which microorganism?
_____ 24. The biologic indicator used for dry heat contains which microorganism?
_____ 25. Blood pressure cuffs, tourniquets, or stethoscopes are considered what type of item according to Spaulding's Classification?

LEARNING ACTIVITIES ANSWERS

1. c
2. f
3. w
4. b
5. a
6. u
7. k
8. n
9. p
10. d
11. o
12. j
13. s
14. x
15. h
16. e
17. y
18. q
19. g
20. v
21. l
22. r
23. i
24. t
25. m

CHAPTER 11

Postoperative Patient Care

Postoperative patient care and teaching is another phase of the surgical process. The surgical procedure, intraoperative activities, and patient condition will determine which area of postoperative care will be necessary. Patients in critical condition may be sent to the intensive care unit (ICU) for specialized care. Other patients will be sent to the postanesthesia care unit (PACU) until they are stable enough to be transferred to another area for observation or continuation of care. Patients who have same-day surgery will recover from anesthesia in the PACU and return home.

Before the patient leaves the operating room (OR), the patient is prepared for the hand over to a perianesthesia nurse. The perioperative nurse, anesthesia provider, and surgeon should complete the final steps of a standardized surgical checklist. Examples of Universal Protocol and standardized checklists are the WHO (World Health Organization) Surgical Safety Checklist and AORN (Association of periOperative Registered Nurses) Comprehensive Surgical Checklist. The completed checklist becomes part of the patient's permanent medical record. For additional information about Universal Protocol, see Chapter 1.

Responsibilities of the Perioperative Nurse, Anesthesia Provider, and Surgeon Before the Patient Is Transferred to the ICU or PACU

Patients are usually extubated, semi-awake, and stable before going to the PACU. The patient will be received by a perianesthesia nurse, who will monitor the patient and provide the necessary information and teaching for discharge from the PACU.

1. What information should the perioperative nurse confirm and document before the patient goes to the PACU or ICU?
   a. The perioperative nurse affirms with the team that all counts are correct.
   b. The perioperative nurse confirms the name of the patient, specimen(s), and special handling, if necessary, with the surgeon.
   c. The perioperative nurse clarifies the surgical procedure with the surgeon and assigns the wound classification.
   d. The perioperative nurse clarifies any special instructions for the PACU with the surgeon and anesthesia provider.

1) Physiologic monitors: ventilator, oxygen, cardiac monitoring, and follow-up laboratory work
2) Continuity of care: X-ray, pain management, positioning devices, and ice pack
   e. The perioperative nurse completes the intraoperative portion of the universal surgical checklist to include blood loss or other complications.

2. In the OR, the anesthesia provider may need to use the **stir-up regimen** if the patient's respiratory rate is slow or the patient is too sleepy. This is done after the airway is removed and the patient's pain is being assessed. The stir-up is used to prevent venous stasis and atelectasis. It includes five steps:
   a. The patient is stimulated and asked to take deep breaths. Oxygen may be given.
   b. Position the patient so the head is slightly elevated or placed in a lateral position to prevent aspiration of secretions.
   c. Coughing is the best way for the patient to clear secretions. Suction should be available.
   d. Encourage the patient to wiggle the toes or flex the legs to keep the circulation moving.
   e. Assess the patient's pain and administer medication as appropriate. If the patient is shivering, a warm blanket is applied. Shivering can be a response to anesthesia.

3. **Hand-over to postoperative nurse (perianesthesia nurse).** Before the patient leaves the surgical suite, the perioperative nurse calls the ICU or PACU to give a preliminary report of the surgical procedure, patient's status, and when the patient will be brought over to the PACU. The phone call is important so that the postoperative nurse can have any special needed equipment ready, such as a ventilator. For information concerning the hand-over report, refer to Chapter 7 for additional information.

The perioperative nurse and anesthesia provider accompany the patient to the designated postoperative area, where the postoperative nurse (perianesthesia nurse) assumes direct care of the patient. According to Standard III-3 of the American Society of Anesthesiologists's (ASA's) Standards for Postanesthesia Care, an anesthesia provider must remain in the PACU until a nurse assumes the care of the patient. Nurses in the ICU and PACU are trained to use specialized equipment and recognize postoperative emergencies, and are trained in Advanced Cardiac Life Support or Pediatric Advanced Life Support. This is when the postoperative phase of patient care begins.

4. **Perianesthesia nursing care.** Activities of the perianesthesia nurse include having the necessary monitoring equipment ready for the patient. The perianesthesia nurse starts with an initial head-to-toe or body system assessment. The nurse observes the patient from the minute he or she arrives and may do a surgery-specific assessment first. The assessment includes (Box 11.1):

   a. The anesthesia provider will provide additional information such as the type of anesthesia and the patient's reactions, last dose of pain medication, intravenous (IV) lines or catheters, estimated blood loss (EBL), any surgical complications, and ongoing PACU orders. The nurse should identify the patient by checking the identification band and patient number against the paperwork or the electronic record.

   b. While information is being exchanged, the perianesthesia nurse will be plugging in monitoring devices for vital signs and connecting oxygen as appropriate. The immediate postoperative period focuses on basic physiologic needs of the patient.

      1) Assessment observations by the perianesthesia nurse include the following:

         a) Is the patient alert or sleeping? Does the patient respond and follow commands when his or her name is called? Can the patient hear? Does the patient have hearing aids that need to be applied?

         b) Does the patient's breathing look labored or shallow? Is there a risk for airway obstruction? Does the skin color look normal? Is the pulse oximeter reading within normal limits?

         c) Is the patient shivering and needs to be warmed? Is the shivering the result of anesthesia?

         d) Is the patient moaning or complaining of pain?

         e) Is the patient exhibiting any unusual behavior or complaints? Does the laparoscopic patient have gas pains or belching from (CO_2) gas insufflation?

         f) If the patient is a child: Is the child crying? Are the side rails up on the crib to prevent falls? Is a crib netting available? Is the child's bed or crib away from electrical equipment or sockets?

      2) Physical examination by the perianesthesia nurse includes the following:

         a) Respiratory status is assessed by auscultation of breath sounds, rate, depth, rhythm, and oxygen level. Patients under anesthesia for a long period may have excess mucous. Is the patient on a ventilator? Are the settings adequate? Is the alarm audible?

BOX 11.1 Suggestions for Hand-Over From Anesthesia Provider and Perioperative Nurse to PACU

Anesthesia Provider May Report:
- Patient name, allergies, surgical procedures performed
- Pertinent medical and/or surgical histories
- Current medications
- Anesthetic delivered
- Medications administered
- Regional anesthetic used
- Intraoperative course (anesthesia related)
- Lines, fluids, losses: The anesthesia provider may include estimated blood loss (EBL) in the handoff report to the PACU nurse. In some institutions a surgical Apgar score is calculated at the end of the surgical procedure from the EBL, lowest mean arterial pressure (expressed in mm Hg), and lowest heart rate rhythm recorded on the anesthesia record during the procedure. The score may be used to identify patients with a higher likelihood of development of complications after surgery (Wuertz et al., 2011).
- Anesthesia complications
- Pain and comfort management
- PACU orders
- Questions and answers

Perioperative Nurse May Report:
- Identity of patient
- Preoperative diagnosis
- Procedure performed
- Location of incision(s), dressings, drains, catheters, tubes, packing, stomas
- Surgical complications
- Allergies and reactions
- Medications, fluids, irrigations delivered by surgeon or RN
- Positioning during surgery
- Communication of other pertinent issues:
  - Location/presence of family or significant others
  - Special requests verbalized by the patient preoperatively
  - Special devices
  - Patient deficits
  - Questions and answers

Modified from American Society of PeriAnesthesia Nurses. (2016). *2017-2018 Perianesthesia nursing standards, practice recommendations and interpretive statements.* Cherry Hill, NJ: ASPAN; Chard, R. (2016). Care of postoperative patients. In D. D. Ignatavicius & M. L. Workman (eds.), *Medical-surgical nursing: patient-centered collaborative care* (8th ed.). St Louis, MO: Elsevier; and Odom-Forren, J. (2017). *Drain's perianesthesia nursing: a critical care approach* (7th ed.). St Louis, MO: Elsevier.

b) Assessment of vital signs includes blood pressure (BP), heart rate, pulse, temperature, and pulse oximetry. Any abnormal values are immediately reported to the anesthesia provider.

c) Is the patient moving all extremities? Are the peripheral pulses within normal limits?

d) Surgery-specific items are checked, such as IV sites or lines, surgical site, catheters, dressings, drains, peripads, casts, and splints.

e) All drains and catheters are monitored for patency, output, and color. Is the urinary output adequate?

f) Dressings and peripads are assessed for bleeding and color. Casted and splinted limbs are checked for temperature, color, peripheral pulses, and swelling.

g) The patient's pain will be assessed and treated.

h) Postoperative nausea and vomiting may need to be treated.

i) Abnormal findings are immediately reported to the surgeon or anesthesia provider if they are anesthesia related.

5. **Nursing process in the PACU.** The perianesthesia nurse formulates the appropriate nursing diagnoses as defined by the Perioperative Nursing Data Set (PNDS). For more information about the PNDS, see Table 1.2 and NANDA-I (North American Nursing Diagnosis Association International, Inc.). Refer also to Chapter 6 (see Box 6.2).

a. **Nursing diagnosis.** Common postoperative diagnoses include:
   1) Acute pain
   2) Ineffective breathing pattern
   3) Ineffective thermoregulation

b. **Outcomes.** Common desired postoperative outcomes: Identify the outcome according to PNDS.
   1) The patient will state a five or less on the pain scale.
   2) The patient will show an oxygenation level of 93% or higher.
   3) The patient is free from shivering and will have a normal body temperature on discharge.

c. **Planning and implementation.** The perianesthesia nurse continues the care plan based on the postoperative assessment. The nurse carries out patient-specific interventions recognized by NANDA-I. Some common interventions include:
   1) Assess the respiratory status and administer oxygen if needed.
   2) Monitor body temperature and observe for shivering.
   3) Assess patient's pain level and give pain medication if necessary.

d. **Evaluation.** Patients are constantly monitored in the ICU and PACU. The nurse evaluates the interventions, and the patient will not be discharged until outcomes are met. Some common postoperative outcomes may include:
   1) The patient is comfortable and has verbalized he or she is pain free.
   2) The patient is no longer shivering and is normothermic at discharge.
   3) The patient demonstrated deep breathing and adequate oxygenation at discharge.

6. **The perianesthesia nurse has tools available to help determine when it is safe to discharge a patient from the PACU.** Outcomes are measured by the **Aldrete scoring system** and **pain scales**. The Aldrete scoring system is used to determine whether patients can be safely discharged from the PACU based on his or her assessment numbers. The patient is assessed on admission to the PACU and at 15-minute intervals (15, 30, 45, and 60 minutes) (Table 11.1). The patient is assigned a number 0, 1, or 2 on admission to PACU. A patient must have a score of 8 to 10 for discharge; the maximum score is 10. There are five different assessment categories.

a. **Activity.** Can the patient move his or her extremities on command? If there is no movement, the score is 0. If the patient can move all four extremities on command, the score is 2.

b. **Respiration.** How is the patient breathing? If the patient presents with apnea or an obstructed airway, the score is 0. Limited breathing is given a score of 1. If the patient can cough, cry, or breathe without difficulty, the score is 2.

c. **Circulation.** BP is measured and compared with preanesthesia BP. If the patient's BP is below the preanesthesia number, the score is 0. A score of 2 is given if the BP is plus or minus 20 mm Hg based on the preanesthesia values.

d. **Consciousness.** The patient is scored based on whether he or she is awake. A score of 0 is assigned when the patient does not answer commands or does not move on command. A score of 2 is given if the patient is awake and can follow commands.

e. **Oxygen saturation.** If the patient's oxygen level is below 90%, the score is 0. If the level is between 90% and 92%, the score is 1. A patient is given a score of 2 if the oxygen level is above 92% on room air.

7. **Postoperative pain management.** Several pain scales can be used based on the age of the patient or communication level. Postoperative pain can be assessed using a pain scale with numbers, faces, or asked verbally if the pain is minimum to severe. Pain should also be assessed by observation and behavior. The nurse should remember that pain is whatever the patient says it is. If pain medication

TABLE 11.1   Aldrete Postanesthesia Scoring System

			Admission	15 Minutes	30 Minutes	45 Minutes	60 Minutes
Activity	Able to move voluntarily on command	4 Extremities	2	2	2	2	2
		2 Extremities	1	1	1	1	1
		0 Extremities	0	0	0	0	0
Respiration	Able to breathe deeply, cough freely		2	2	2	2	2
	Dyspnea or limited breathing		1	1	1	1	1
	Apnea		0	0	0	0	0
Circulation	BP + 20 of preanesthesia level		2	2	2	2	2
	BP + 20–50 of preanesthesia level		1	1	1	1	1
	BP + 50 of preanesthesia level		0	0	0	0	0
Consciousness	Fully awake		2	2	2	2	2
	Arousable on calling		1	1	1	1	1
	Not responding		0	0	0	0	0
O_2 saturation	Able to maintain O_2 saturation >92% on room air		2	2	2	2	2
	Needs O_2 inhalation to maintain O_2 saturation >90%		1	1	1	1	1
	O_2 saturation <90% even with O_2 supplementation		0	0	0	0	0

BP, Blood pressure.

Modified from Aldrete, A., & Wright, A. (1992). Revised Aldrete score for discharge. *Anesthesiology News, 18*, 17.

is administered in the PACU, the patient is reassessed and monitored.

a. **Adult pain assessment**
   1) For patients who can verbalize his or her pain, a numbered scale from 0 to 10, a visual analogue scale, or an intensity scale (Fig. 11.1) may be used.
   2) Signs of pain may be physiologic and psychological.
      a) Physiologic signs include increased BP, increased respiratory rate, chest pain, dizziness, headache, shortness of breath, splinting, increased heart rate, increase in urination, delayed bowel sounds, increased perspiration, dilation of the pupils, and decreased mobility.
      b) Psychological signs include anxiety, fear, confusion, stress, mental unstableness, and certain emotions. These can lead to chest pain, dizziness, numbness, shortness of breath, and headache.
b. **Pediatric pain assessment**
   1) **FLACC** (Face, Legs, Activity, Cry, and Consolability) scale is used for patients

2 months to 7 years old. This scale was created for children because the child may not talk or be able to express that he or she is in pain. Some behavioral signs of pain may include excessive crying, restlessness, kicking, quivering, moaning, or legs drawn up (Table 11.2).
   2) The **Wong-Baker FACES Pain Rating Scale** is a series of faces from happy to crying. This scale can be used for children and adults. This scale is easy to use because the patient just has to point to the face based on how he or she may feel. This is good for patients who have difficulty communicating (Fig. 11.2).

Home-Going Patients and Time in the Postanesthesia Care Unit

Most home-going patients do not spend a long time in the PACU. Preparing the patient for discharge from the PACU is the perianesthesia nurse's responsibility, but an anesthesia provider gives the final approval for discharge. This is based on the final assessment,

Pain Intensity Scales

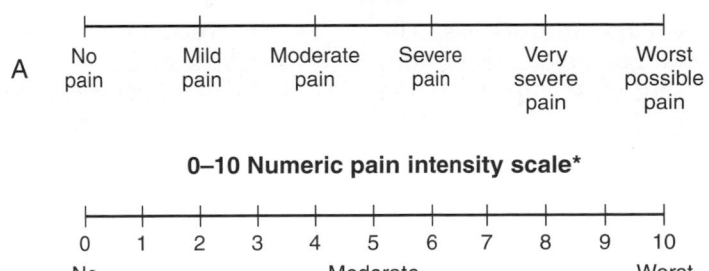

Simple descriptive pain intensity scale*

A | No pain | Mild pain | Moderate pain | Severe pain | Very severe pain | Worst possible pain

0–10 Numeric pain intensity scale*

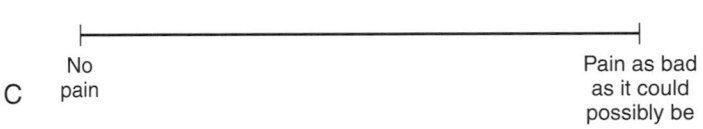

B | 0 1 2 3 4 5 6 7 8 9 10 | No pain | Moderate pain | Worst possible pain

Visual analogue scale (VAS)†

C | No pain | Pain as bad as it could possibly be

* If used as a graphic rating scale, a 10-cm baseline is recommended.
† A 10-cm baseline is recommended for VAS scales.

Figure 11.1 Examples of pain intensity and pain distress scales. *If used as a graphic rating scale, a 10-cm baseline is recommended. †A 10-cm baseline is recommended for visual analogue scales (VAS). (From Acute Pain Management Guideline Panel. [1992]. *Acute pain management in adults; operative procedures: quick reference guide for clinicians* [AHCPR Pub No. 92-0019]. Rockville, MD: Agency for Health Care Policy and Research [now Agency for Healthcare Research and Quality]. Available at https://www.ncbi.nlm.nih.gov/books/NBK52131/figure/A33641/?report=objectonly. Reprinted with permission of the U.S. Agency for Healthcare Research and Quality, successor to the Agency for Health Care Policy and Research.)

TABLE **11.2 FLACC Pain Assessment**

Categories[a]	Scoring		
	0	**1**	**2**
Face	No particular expression or smile	Occasional grimace or frown, withdrawn, disinterested	Frequent to constant quivering chin, clenched jaw
Legs	Normal position or relaxed	Uneasy, restless, tense	Kicking, or legs drawn up
Activity	Lying quietly, normal position, moves easily	Squirming, shifting back and forth, tense	Arched, rigid, or jerking
Cry	No cry (awake or asleep)	Moans or whimpers; occasional complaint	Crying steadily, screams or sobs, frequent complaints
Consolability	Content, relaxed	Reassured by occasional touching, hugging, or being talked to, distractible	Difficult to console or comfort

The FLACC scale was developed by Sandra Merkel, MS, RN, Terri Voepel-Lewis, MS, RN, and Shobha Malviya, MD, at C.S. Mott Children's Hospital, University of Michigan Health System, Ann Arbor, MI. Copyright © 2002, The Regents of the University of Michigan.
[a]Each of the five categories is scored from 0 to 2, resulting in a total score between 0 and 10.

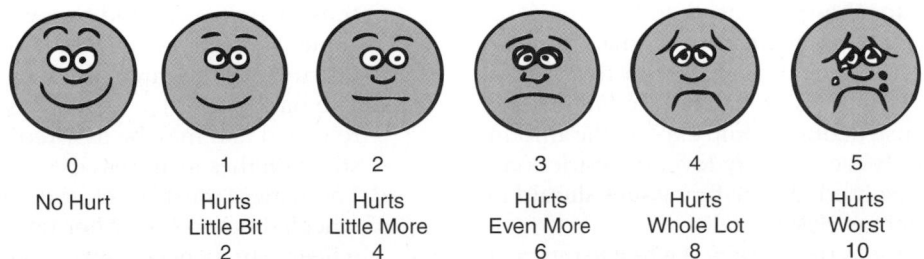

0	1	2	3	4	5
No Hurt	Hurts Little Bit	Hurts Little More	Hurts Even More	Hurts Whole Lot	Hurts Worst
	2	4	6	8	10

Figure 11.2 Wong-Baker FACES Pain Rating Scale. (From Hockenberry, M. J., Wilson, D., & Rodgers, C. C. [2017]. *Wong's essentials of pediatric nursing* [10th ed.]. St. Louis, MO: Elsevier. Used with permission.)

expected outcomes, and discharge instructions. The perianesthesia nurse must have good assessment skills and observe the patient closely so the needs of the patient going home will be met.

1. Criteria to consider before discharging a patient include the following:
   a. Did the patient understand the surgical procedure? Was family or a significant other present for preoperative teaching? Is there a language barrier or learning disability?
   b. Does the patient have family or someone to drive him or her home?
   c. Was a prescription for pain or other medication given to the patient? Does the patient understand the instructions for taking the prescribed medication? Can the patient afford medication and food? Can the facility social services department assist the patient with obtaining needed items?
   d. Will the patient be home alone? Is a home healthcare nurse needed?
   e. Is there a risk for falling? Does the patient have to walk up or down stairs to enter the home?
   f. Does the patient have all of his or her belongings before leaving? Are personal hearing aids inserted or spectacles worn to read written instructions?
   g. Does the patient understand the postoperative instructions? Does he or she know when to call the healthcare provider for help or advice? Does the patient have a ride to the follow-up appointment?

2. Postoperative instructions should be in writing and include the following:
   a. The patient is advised about the side effects of anesthesia: drowsiness, nausea, vomiting, or sore throat. The patient should not drive, drink alcohol, or operate heavy equipment for at least 24 hours. The patient should not make any important decisions or sign important papers. It may be recommended that the patient should not be left alone for a certain period.
   b. The patient is given information specific to the surgical procedure and site. Postoperative teaching should involve the patient and caregiver. The information should be explained in easy to understand terms or with hands-on demonstration. The learners should have time to ask questions and receive answers. The patient or caregiver may repeat the hands-on demonstration.

      Some surgical procedures may require preoperative teaching or classes to help reinforce learning. Examples may include stoma care, how to care for a dressing, and when/how to change it if necessary. If ice and elevation of a limb is needed, the instruction should explain the amount of time to apply ice. Activity level or restrictions should be explained. Any safety issues should be addressed such as risk for falls.
   c. The patient should be instructed when to return to a normal diet or be given written dietary materials if a special diet is needed. The patient may be instructed to increase dietary fiber, water, or take a stool softener if constipation-causing medications are prescribed. The patient should be instructed not to drink alcohol with prescription pain medications.
   d. The patient should have clear instructions with a phone number of when to call the healthcare provider. Examples may include increased bleeding through the dressing, fever, nausea and vomiting, severe pain or swelling, urinary retention, constipation, or redness at the surgical site.
   e. If new medications are prescribed, instructions on how to obtain the medication should be explained. Was the medication prescription electronically sent to the pharmacy? The instructions should include when the next dose of medication should be taken, correct dose, and how it is taken. Pain medications are given with caution, and the provider may order a limited amount to prevent addiction or patients seeking excessive amounts.

3. **Discharging the patient.** The patient may be discharged after he or she meets the criteria from the ASA, The Joint Commission, or the Accreditation Association for Ambulatory Health Care. These organizations have standards for discharge that reduce the risk for patient complications and returning to the healthcare facility for treatment. Discharge from the facility should include the following:
   a. The patient has stable vital signs according to the preoperative baseline and meets the standard on the Aldrete scoring system. The anesthesia provider must sign the patient out.
   b. The patient has written discharge instructions with phone numbers to call if questions arise when at home. The patient is informed of the next time the postoperative appointments with the surgeon are scheduled. The patient or caregiver signs the discharge papers acknowledging that the written material was given and understood.
   c. If the patient is going to an extended care or rehabilitation facility, a hand-over report is given to the registered nurse receiving the patient. The report should include the type of surgical procedure and the surgeon's name, vital signs, current medications, allergies and sensitivities, comorbidities, current laboratory values, mobility status, and any special instructions for care.
   d. The patient will have any personnel belongings returned and may be assisted with dressing into street clothes as necessary.
   e. The patient must have a ride home and may be wheeled out to his or her transportation in a wheelchair as necessary. If transferring to a different facility, the transport may be by ambulance.

4. **Follow-up.** Follow-up telephone calls are a common practice for outpatient surgery, same-day surgery, and ambulatory surgery centers. The calls are usually made 24 to 48 hours after discharge. Most surgical complications happen in the first 48 hours. The call uses open-ended questions extracted from information in the surgeon's discharge summary. The patient or caregiver is asked a series of questions about how the patient is feeling, managing pain and medications, eating and drinking, and activity level. The patient's personal concerns and any surgery specific questions are answered.

Patients who received follow-up calls were less likely to be readmitted to the healthcare facility because potential problems were addressed and patient compliance was reinforced. Fewer readmissions meets Centers for Medicare and Medicaid Services guidelines for reimbursement.

Postoperative care is a team effort by the perioperative nurse, anesthesia provider, surgeon, and perianesthesia nurse to help the patient return to a safe conscious level after anesthesia and surgery. Through communication, safe and efficient hand over, observation skills, and nursing interventions, the healthcare team can meet the needs of the patient with positive outcomes.

LEARNING ACTIVITIES

INSTRUCTIONS: Complete the crossword puzzle. Use the clues to help identify the words.

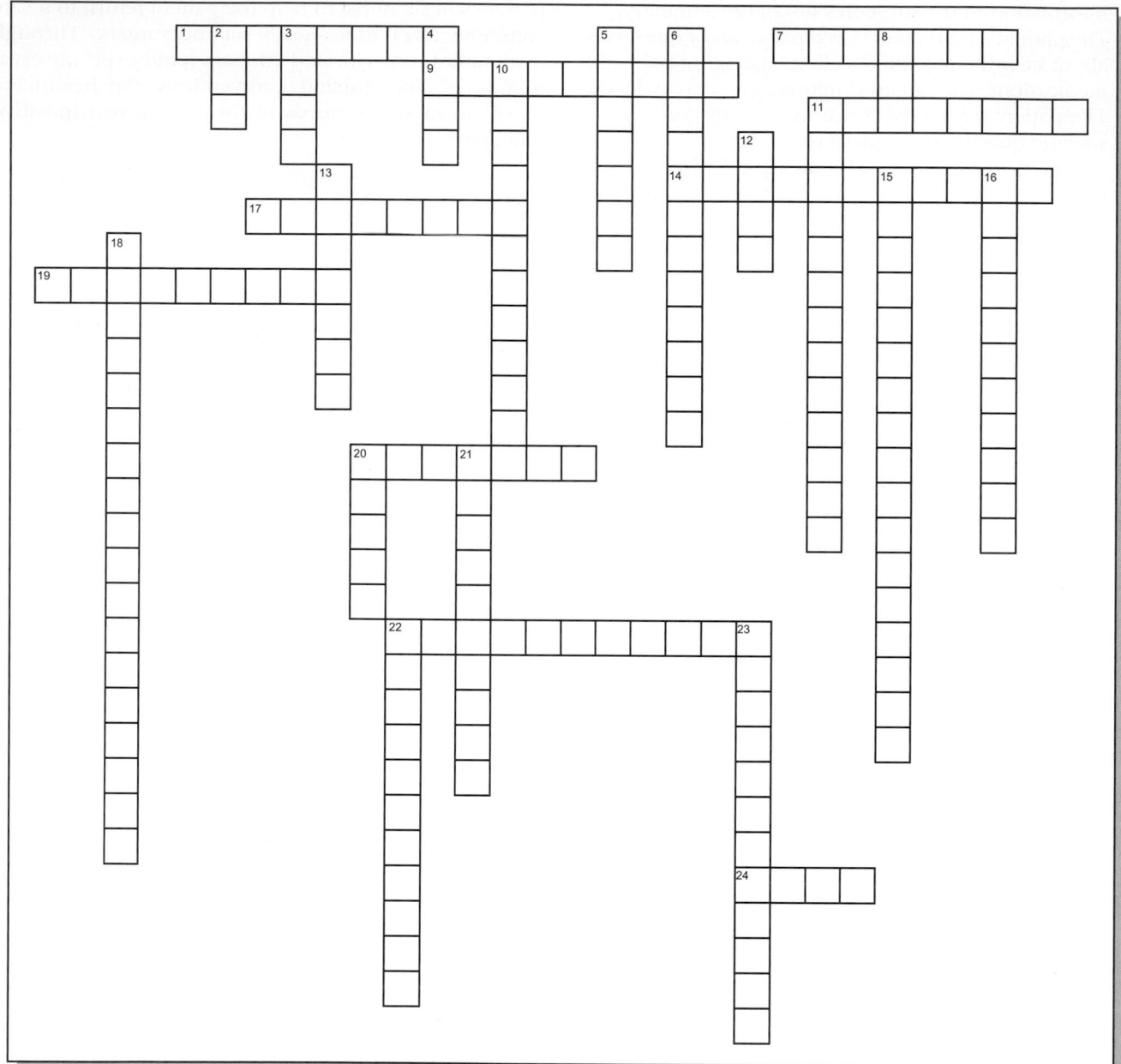

ACROSS

1. The perioperative nurse gives this verbal report to the perianesthesia nurse
7. Postoperative pain is decided by this person
9. Postoperative patients should avoid making these kinds of decisions and signing papers
11. This is the most effective way for a patient to clear secretions
14. Follow-up calls address problems and prevent _____ to the healthcare facility
17. This telephone call is made 24 to 48 hours after discharge from the PACU
19. This pain scale uses a series of faces ranging from happy to crying
20. Aldrete scoring is done starting with how many minutes?
22. The immediate postoperative period focuses on this basic need of the patient
24. Nurses who work in the ICU and PACU may have this training (use abbreviation)

DOWN

2. Which organization sets guidelines for discharge? (use abbreviation)
3. If a prescription is given, instructions should include the next time and exact _____
4. Before a patient is discharged, he or she must have a _____ home
5. The anesthesia provider may use this technique after the patient has been extubated if respiratory rate is slow due to sleepiness
6. These should be given to the patient in writing when discharged
8. Critical patients may be sent directly to this area (use abbreviation)
10. Some surgical procedures require this kind of teaching or classes to reinforce learning
11. These surgical problems usually happen within the first 48 hours
12. Patients should have clear instructions, a telephone number, and examples of when to _____
the healthcare provider
13. The scoring system that determines when a patient can safely be discharged according to measured outcomes
15. The WHO and AORN use this standardized tool, which becomes part of the patient's permanent record
16. The perioperative nurse uses this skill, as well as physical assessment
18. Who has the final say and responsibility for discharge of the patient from the PACU?
20. Pain scale used for children 2 months to 7 years old based on activity
21. Patients who have undergone anesthesia are advised to avoid driving, drinking alcohol, and operating heavy equipment for how many hours?
22. Pain can be physiologic, as well as _____
23. If pain medication is prescribed, a stool softener or increase in dietary fiber might be recommended to prevent this

LEARNING ACTIVITIES ANSWERS

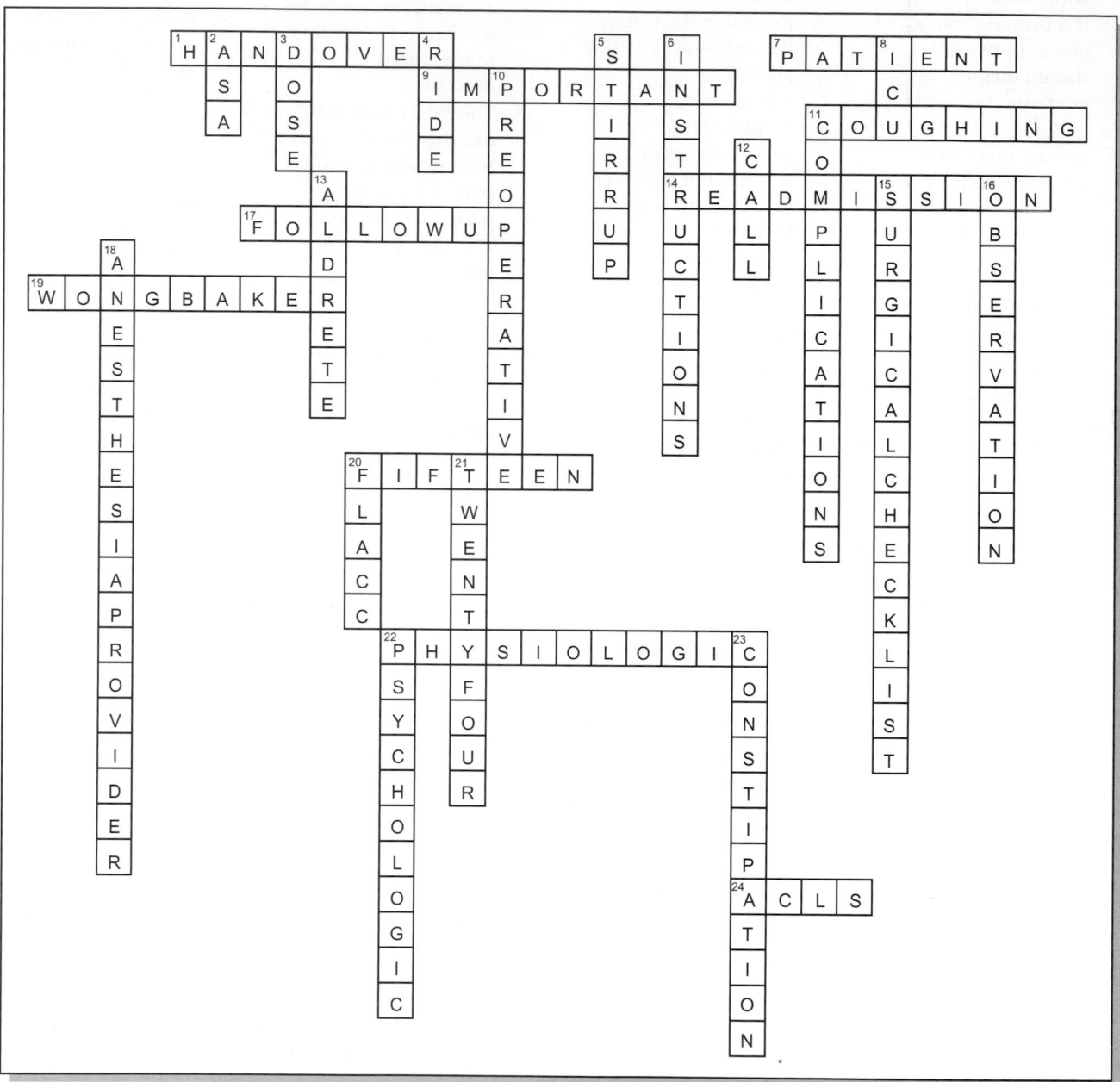

Special Topics

Energy-Powered Devices

Energy-powered devices used in surgical procedures are powered by electricity or an external gas source. The perioperative nurse must be educated and competent in the use and safety associated with each type of energy-powered device (see also Chapter 5).

Electrosurgical Unit

The type of electrosurgical unit (ESU) generator used during a surgical procedure is determined by the surgeon. Although the perioperative nurse prepares the ESU for use, the surgeon is the only person who should operate the device in the surgical field.

Each ESU is assigned an identification number for use tracking purposes. The perioperative nurse records the identification number in the patient's records. An ESU that malfunctions during the surgical procedure is removed from service and tagged with a description of the malfunction and the device identification number.

Important similarities in ESUs include the use of an active electrode and an inactive electrode. The path of ESU electrical current through the patient's tissues between the active and inactive electrode differentiates the particular machine's function during surgery.

Safety factors for all types of ESUs incorporate the use of audible alarms that must remain on at all times during use and adjustable power settings that are set to operate at the lowest setting possible as the surgical procedure progresses. ESU plume is a biologic contaminant and is evacuated into a suction evacuator. Solution bottles or basins must never be placed on top of the machine, to prevent an electric short within the device.

1. **Monopolar electrosurgery (ESU).** The monopolar ESU current flows from the generator to the active electrode (i.e., handpiece) and continues through the patient to the inactive electrode (also known as return electrode) and returned back to the generator (Fig. 12.1).
   a. **Inactive electrode.** The inactive electrode sends the electric current back to the ESU generator through an attached copper cable after it passes through the patient's tissues. Two types of inactive electrodes are used in monopolar procedures.
      1) **Return electrode pad.** An adhesive pad with a coated copper cable is positioned on the patient's body as close to the surgical site as possible when the patient is in the final position for the surgical procedure. The pad is placed over a large muscle mass that is clean, dry, and free from previous surgical scars, tattoos, and bony prominences. The cord is plugged into the generator (Fig. 12.2).
         a) The pad must never be cut to size or removed and replaced. If the patient must be repositioned, a new pad is applied. The patient's skin is assessed and documented before and after return electrode application.
         b) If an alarm sounds during ESU use, the first action is to check the return electrode attached to the patient.
         c) Some facilities require documentation of the lot number and expiration date of the pad used.
      2) **Capacitance return electrode.** A large 2 × 3 foot capacitance return electrode pad (i.e., Megadyne pad) is placed on the operating room (OR) bed mattress under the patient. The capacitance pad works in the same manner as the return electrode pad and returns the current to the generator.
         a) It is used for adults and children.
         b) No adhesive pad is attached to the patient. This is useful for patients who are sensitive to adhesives.
   b. **Monopolar active electrode tip.** The handpiece can be fitted with several types of tips, either Teflon coated or noncoated (i.e., loop, needle, ball, or blade).
      1) Clean coated nonstick tips with a moist sponge.
      2) Clean noncoated tips with a cleaning pad. Do not scrape eschar off with a knife.
   c. **Monopolar ESU settings.**
      1) *Coagulating:* seals small to medium vessels
      2) *Cutting:* constant current cuts tissue
      3) *Blended:* vessels are sealed as the tissue is cut
2. **Bipolar electrosurgery.** Bipolar ESU current flows from the generator to the active tip of the forceps, through the patient's localized tissue, and to the opposing inactive tip. The current does not pass through the patient's body. Bipolar ESU is used in

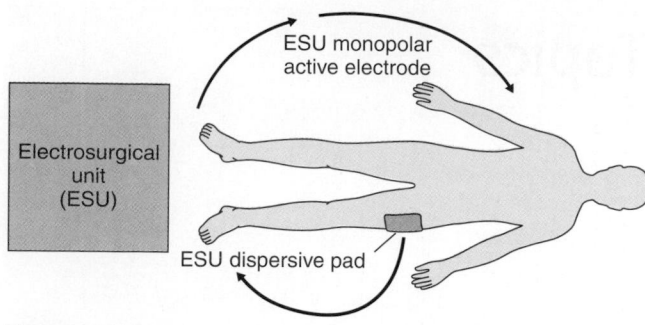

Figure 12.1 Monopolar current path. (From Phillips, N. [2017]. *Berry and Kohn's operating room technique* [13th ed.]. St. Louis, MO: Elsevier.)

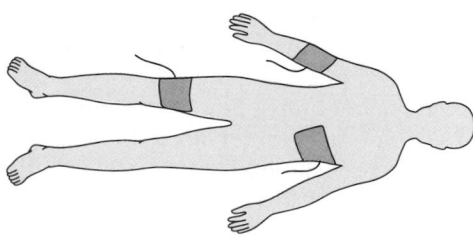

Figure 12.2 Placement of electrosurgical unit patient return electrode. (From Phillips, N. [2017]. *Berry and Kohn's operating room technique* [13th ed.]. St. Louis, MO: Elsevier.)

procedures that require lower voltage, such as pacemaker placement (Fig. 12.3).

a. No return electrode is used.

b. The handpiece looks like forceps (pick up), and the copper connecting cord has two prongs.

c. LigaSure is a form of bipolar electrosurgery that has its own generator, handpieces, and settings.

3. **Argon beam coagulator (ABC).** ABC is a form of a gas-enhanced monopolar ESU and uses a patient return electrode to return the current to the generator. It is commonly used for trauma of the spleen, liver, and kidneys.

a. Argon gas is nonflammable and used to create a current that causes a stream of gas to spray over a large area of tissue to disperse the electrical

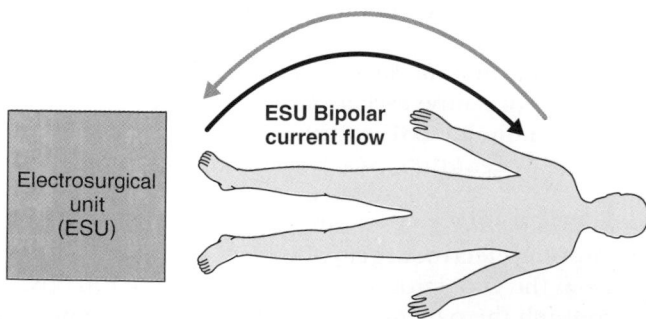

Figure 12.3 Bipolar current path. No patient return electrode is used. (From Phillips, N. [2017]. *Berry and Kohn's operating room technique* [13th ed.]. St. Louis, MO: Elsevier.)

current. The gas enhances the effects of the ESU by covering a broader area.

b. When using ABC during laparoscopic surgery, care must be taken to not overinsufflate the abdomen. A gas embolism could form.

Harmonic Ultrasonic Scalpel

A harmonic scalpel is an ultrasonic device with its own generator, settings, and special handpieces. The generator makes a humming sound during activation of the handpiece. There is less tissue damage and surgical plume.

1. The harmonic scalpel uses ultrasonic vibrations (high-frequency sound waves) turned into mechanical energy to cut and cauterize tissue.

2. The harmonic scalpel can be more precise in the dissection of tissue because it coagulates the vessels. It is available in a blade, hook, and shear grasper. It is commonly used in laparoscopic surgery.

Lasers

LASER is an acronym for light amplification by stimulated emission of radiation. Many types of lasers are available and process light into electromagnetic energy. Lasers are used in many surgical procedures to coagulate small blood vessels, ablation of tissue, vaporization of tissue, and cutting tissue. Lasers are regulated by the US Food and Drug Administration (FDA) (see Chapter 5 for specific laser safety discussion) (Table 12.1).

1. Wavelengths determine whether the color is visible; the energy of the beam is measured in watts. These two together can react on tissue by reflection, absorption, scatter, or transmission.

2. Lasers are class III medical devices, classified by numbers. Each laser has a standby button that is activated by the laser operator if the risk for injury is imminent.

3. The American National Standard for Safe Use of Lasers sets guidelines for the industry. Follow the manufacturer's instructions for training, proper eyewear, machine use, fire safety, and documentation. Laser credentialing is mandatory for surgeons (Box 12.1).

Rigid Endoscopes and Laparoscopy

Personnel should be trained on endoscopic and video equipment for proper use and safety. Minimally invasive surgery instrumentation is specialized and delicate. Robotics is an integral part of the endoscopic environment that uses rigid endoscopes.

1. **Laparoscopy.** Rigid endoscopes can be diagnostic (observation) or operative (used with instrumentation). Small openings are created in the body for laparoscopy with a trocar system (blunt or sharp) to view internal structures and use instrumentation during the surgical procedure. The openings are closed at the end of the procedure.

a. Laparoscopic procedures may use multiple trocars for the camera/telescope combination and instrumentation ports.

TABLE 12.1 Description of Common Lasers Used

Active Medium	Wavelength	Delivery System	Penetration	Characteristics
CO₂ laser (gas laser)	10,600 nm, infrared	Articulated arm, waveguide, scanner, microscope via microslad (micromanipulater)	Shallow penetration (0.1–0.2 mm), photothermal effect	Highly absorbed by water. Not color selective. Helium-neon aiming beam. Sometimes the handpiece has a tubing to conduct compressed air to keep plume from coating the lens. CO₂ energy can be delivered in a continuous wave or pulsed mode. When delivery system is attached, the laser must be test fired to ensure the aiming beam is aligned with CO₂ beam. Used on soft tissue, ablations, cutting, coagulation, vaporization.
Erbium : YAG laser (solid crystal laser)	2940 nm, infrared	Fiber (handpiece, microscope)	Shallow penetration, photothermal effect	Highly absorbed by water. Delivered in pulsed mode. Helium-neon aiming beam. Frequently used in dermatology for skin resurfacing and ablation. Also used in dentistry.
Holmium : YAG laser (solid crystal laser)	2140 nm, infrared	Fiber (handpiece, microscope)	Shallow penetration (0.4–0.6 mm), photothermal effect	Absorbed by water but can be delivered in a fluid environment within a vapor bubble if fiber is within 55 mm of target site. Helium-neon aiming beam. Pulse mode. Used for sculpting and ablating soft tissue. Has also been used on cartilage. Also used to fragment urinary or biliary stones with photo-acoustical effect.
Neodymium: YAG laser (Nd : YAG) (solid crystal laser)	1064 nm, infrared	Contact and noncontact fibers, contact tips, handpiece for dermatology, slit lamp for ophthalmology, microscope	Scatters in tissue (3–5 mm) for noncontact fiber. Shallow penetration (<1 mm) for contact delivery	Transmitted through clear solutions. Highly absorbed by pigmented tissue. Helium-neon aiming beam usually used. Used in continuous or pulsed modes. Ophthalmology Nd : YAG lasers (class 3B lasers) use special pulsed mode delivery (Q-switched) to provide photo-acoustical effect within the eye to rupture the secondary membrane.
KTP (potassium titanyl phosphate) laser (solid crystal laser)	532 nm, visible (frequency doubled YAG)	Fiber (handpiece, microscope)	1–2 mm depth of penetration	An Nd: YAG incident beam (1064 nm) is passed through a KTP crystal which doubles the frequency and halves the wavelength (532 nm). Aiming beam can be a low power KTP beam or helium-neon beam. Highly color selective. Transmitted through clear solutions. Often used in dermatology, urology, general surgery, gynecology.
Argon laser (gas laser)	Blue-green light of 488 and 514.5 nm (or 457 and 528 nm), visible	Fiber (handpiece, microscope, slit lamp)	1–2 mm depth of penetration	Intense visible blue-green laser light. Aiming beam can be a low power argon beam or a helium-neon beam. Highly color selective. Transmitted through clear solutions. Often used in ophthalmology, dermatology, and soft tissue procedures.

(Continued)

TABLE 12.1   Description of Common Lasers Used—cont'd

Active Medium	Wavelength	Delivery System	Penetration	Characteristics
Tunable dye laser (liquid laser)	Range of 400–900 nm visible	Fiber (handpiece, microscope, slit lamp)	Depends on wavelength	Can dial in desired wavelength within limited range of visible light. By changing dyes and other parameters, the wavelength can be altered. Laser energy formed by exposing a liquid dye to an intense light source, such as an argon beam. The dye absorbs the laser light and fluoresces over a broad spectrum of colors and with special prisms, diffraction gratings or filters, a specific wavelength is produced. Some wavelengths are highly absorbed by pigmented tissues. Can be delivered in continuous or pulsed modes. Often used in dermatology, ophthalmology, urology (fragment stones).
Diode laser (semiconductor crystal laser)	Varies (i.e., 532–910 nm), visible	Fiber (handpiece, microscope, slit lamp)	Depends on wavelength	Compact, reliable laser system. Often used for ophthalmology and dermatology.
Excimer laser (gas laser)	Ultraviolet (wavelength depends on chemical composition of active medium)	Fiber (handpiece, microscope, slit lamp)	Depends on wavelength (mostly <1 mm). Acts by disassociating cellular molecular bonds	"Excited dimer" laser. Most popular excimer lasers are argon fluoride (ArF) at 193 nm, krypton fluoride (KrF) at 248 nm, xenon chloride (XeCl) at 308 nm, and xenon fluoride (XeF) at 351 nm. Appropriate protective housing for laser needed because gases are extremely toxic. Extremely effective ablative capabilities. Used for corneal sculpting. Also used for other ablative procedures. Used experimentally to treat psoriasis and vitiligo.

From Rothrock, J. (2019). *Alexander's care of the patient in surgery* (16th ed.). St. Louis, MO: Elsevier.

BOX 12.1 Medical Device Regulations

FDA Classification of Medical Devices
Medical devices were classified in 1976 by the FDA according to their safety factors.

Class I: Subject to general controls

Class II: Devices for which general controls are not enough

Class III: Implants and life support devices

Classification of Lasers
Lasers are classified according to potential hazard of exposure.

Class 1: Enclosed system, considered safe based on current medical knowledge; no light emission escapes the enclosure.

Class 2: Limited to visible light (400–780 nm). Output power is 1 mW or less. Momentary viewing (0.25-second maximum permissible exposure) is not considered hazardous. Staring into the beam is not recommended. Protective eyewear of the correct optical density should be worn.

Class 3A: Emitted laser viewed directly through collecting optics would cause permanent eye damage. Output power is 0.5 mW or less. Protective eyewear of the correct optical density should be worn.

Class 3B: Continuous laser light with 0.5-watt or less output can cause permanent eye damage. Exposure to the beam should be avoided. Protective eyewear of the correct optical density should be worn.

Class 4: Laser light produced is hazardous to skin and eyes. Strict control measures are enforced. Protective eyewear of the correct optical density should be worn.

FDA, US Food and Drug Administration.
From Phillips, N. [2017]. *Berry and Kohn's operating room technique* (13th ed.). St. Louis, MO: Elsevier.

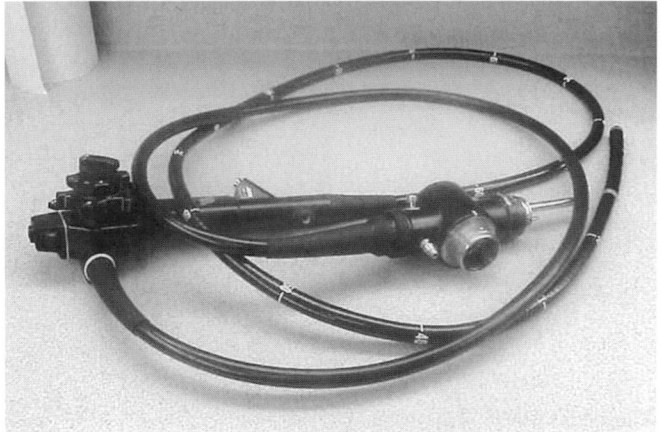
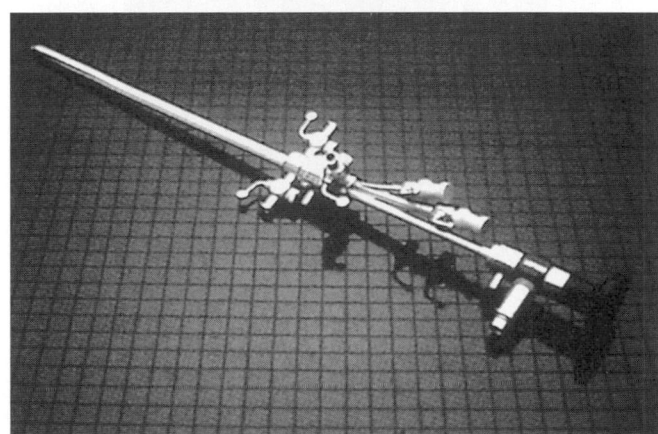
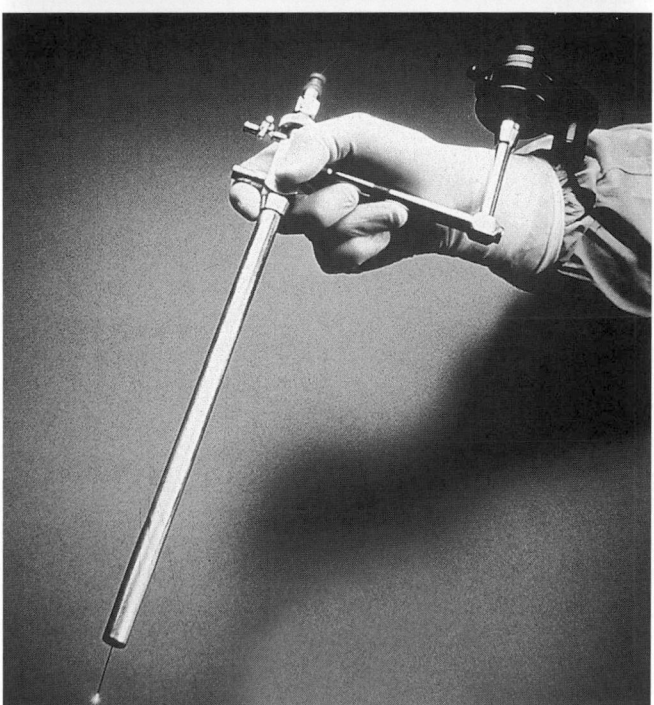

Figure 12.4 (A) Flexible endoscope. (B) Rigid endoscope. (C) Operative laparoscope. (B and C, From Ball, K.A. [1997]. *Endoscopic surgery*. St. Louis, MO: Mosby.)

b. Single-port laparoscopic trocar devices are used for select procedures. All devices and the telescope are passed through the same opening.

c. Hand-assisted laparoscopic procedures use trocar port devices, but also have a small 7-cm skin incision to remove larger organs.

2. Rigid endoscopes for laparoscopy and cystoscopy are available with different angled lenses (0, 30, 70, 120 degrees) for observing internal structures at different angles. Rigid scopes are available in varying diameters and lengths for different areas of the body (Fig. 12.4).

3. Rigid endoscopes are illuminated with a fiberoptic light cable for visualization on a video monitor. Fiberoptic light cables must not be dropped off the end of the sterile field or bent, because the tiny tubes that carry the light may break. See Chapter 5 for discussion about fire safety and the use of fiberoptic cables (Fig. 12.5).

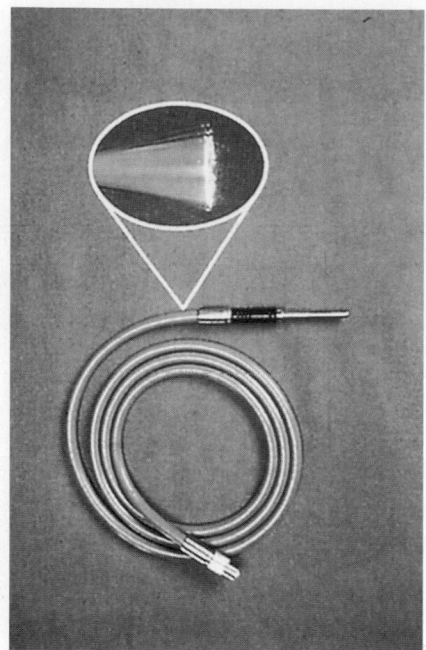

Figure 12.5 Inside the light cable are hundreds of glass fibers that transmit light. (From Ball, K.A. [1997]. *Endoscopic surgery.* St. Louis, MO: Mosby.)

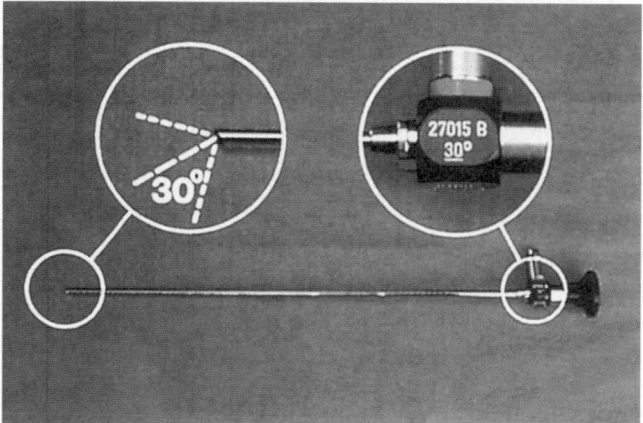

Figure 12.6 Lenses inside the endoscope determine the angle of view. (From Ball, K.A. [1997]. *Endoscopic surgery.* St. Louis, MO: Mosby.)

4. Rigid endoscopes can have a camera attached that is "white balanced" before the start of a procedure to clarify color and sharpness of the image (Fig. 12.6).
5. **Insufflation.** Carbon dioxide gas (CO_2) is used to expand the peritoneal cavity to create a working space for laparoscopy (pneumoperitoneum).
   a. Insufflation pressure should be between 12 and 18 mm Hg, based on body size and weight (12–15 mm Hg is the CO_2 pressure used for the average adult).
   b. CO_2 gas is cold when delivered to the patient. Care is taken to monitor the patient's body temperature and prevent hypothermia.
   c. When the case is completed, the CO_2 gas should be evacuated into the suction and not the room air.

The CO_2 gas from the patient's abdomen is a biologic contaminant.
6. Fluids are used to expand a working space in hollow organs (i.e., uterus, bladder, joint spaces). The perioperative nurse monitors and documents the amount of fluid administered and the amount returned.

Robotic Surgery

Robotic surgery is specialized and requires training to drape and operate the equipment. All robotic instrumentation should be cared for according to the manufacturer's instructions. A robotic surgical procedure employs the same principles as laparoscopy. Insufflation and trocars are used.
1. The surgeon controls the operating arms from a remote console area in the room. A sterile team is at the surgical field to assist.
2. Robotic instrumentation and the camera should be checked before use and placed back in containers when the case is over to prevent damage during transport for processing.
3. The robotic instrumentation is reusable for a prescribed number of times (usually 10) and is then discarded.

Powered Drills and Saws

Drills and saws can be powered by electricity, nitrogen gas, or reusable batteries.
1. Nitrogen gas is commonly used to power high-speed drills used in orthopedics, neurosurgery, and spine. A pressurized hose is plugged into a nitrogen tank or a piped-in wall delivery system. When activated, the hose is under pressure from the gas. The hose is not disconnected from the source until the gas is purged or an injury can occur.
2. All drills or saws with cords should be checked for cuts, devices should be powered off until use, and cords/hoses should be secured so they are not accidently severed. The safety lever on the handpiece should be on when not in use.
3. Drill tips and saw blades may be disposable or reprocessed. If a reprocessed item is used, check to make sure no debris has been left on the surface. Drill tip, saw blades, and burrs are counted items.
4. Battery-powered devices may require special handling if the batteries are sterile or unsterile. Processing batteries for sterile use must be done according to the instructions for use; the batteries are charged before sterile processing. Charged unsterile batteries are dropped into devices by the circulating nurse with a sterile guard to protect the device.

The perioperative nurse must be competent in the operation of energy-powered equipment, patient and personnel safety, and corresponding instrumentation.

Tourniquets

A tourniquet is used on a limb intraoperatively to establish a bloodless field during the surgical procedure.

Pneumatic tourniquets are the most common type of tourniquet used for hemostasis in an upper or lower extremity. When the Surgical Care Improvement Project (SCIP) protocol is used, the antibiotic should be administered intravenously (IV) at least 20 minutes before tourniquet inflation to allow for arterial circulation of the drug to the surgical site.

Anatomy and Physiology Review

Why is anatomy and physiology important to the perioperative nurse? The extremities where a tourniquet may be applied have distinct anatomic areas that are potentially injured when a tourniquet is used. The primary extremity anatomy is described here.

1. **Upper extremity:** The tourniquet is placed over the upper arm.
   a. Bones: humerus
   b. Musculature: primarily the biceps and the triceps brachii in linear form encased by fascial sheets
   c. Innervation is from the myocutaneous nerve arising from C5-C6
   d. Vascularity: arterial supply primarily from the brachial artery; venous drainage is via the basilic vein; lymphatics follow the vessels and drain into the axillary nodes
2. **Lower extremity:** The tourniquet can be placed over the thigh or occasionally the calf.
   a. **Thigh**
      1) Bones: femur
      2) Musculature is divided into two compartments separated by layers of the fascia lata
         a) Anterior compartment: sartorius and quadriceps femoris (rectus femoris, vastus lateralis, vastus intermedius, and vastus medialis)
         b) Posterior compartment: hamstring and adductor, three layers (gracilis, longus, and brevis)
      3) Innervation: arises from the lumbar plexus
         a) Anterior compartment: femoral and genitofemoral (medial)
         b) Posterior compartment: obturator and sciatic
      4) Vascularity
         a) Arterial supply: femoral arising from the external iliac and the obturator arising from the internal iliac
         b) Venous drainage: greater saphenous (superficial) and femoral (deep); the superficial and deep veins are connected by perforator veins; the lymphatic vessels follow the major veins and drain into the inguinal nodes
   b. **Calf**
      1) Bones: tibia and fibula
      2) Musculature is divided into three compartments covered by two layers of fascia that is continuous with the thigh fascia, both superficial and deep

a) **Anterior crural:** tibialis anterior, extensor digitorum longus, extensor hallucis longus, peroneus tertius muscles
b) **Lateral crural:** peroneus longus; peroneus brevis muscles
c) **Posterior compartment:** triceps surae (three superficial muscles—gastrocnemius, plantaris, and soleus; four deep muscles—popliteus, flexor hallucis longus, flexor digitorum longus, and tibialis posterior)
      3) Innervation is in three planes:
         a) **Anterior compartment:** deep common peroneal nerve
         b) **Lateral compartment:** superficial common peroneal nerve
         c) **Posterior compartment:** saphenous, peroneal, and sural nerves
      4) Vascularity in three planes:
         a) **Anterior compartment:** anterior tibial artery arising from the popliteal artery
         b) **Lateral compartment:** fibular and posterior tibial arteries
         c) **Posterior compartment:** posterior tibial artery arising from the popliteal artery
         d) Venous drainage is through the anterior and posterior tibial, fibular and popliteal veins; the lymphatics follow the vessels to the inguinal nodes

Nursing Assessment

1. **Physiologic assessment of patient.** For detailed physical assessment information, see Chapter 6.
   a. Identify the patient and confirm the correct surgical site marking.
   b. Observe limb size and preoperative mobility/ flexibility of joints and digits.
   c. Examine the skin of the planned site of the tourniquet application. Check the pulses in the limb.
   d. Note any history of previous or current contraindication for tourniquet use.
2. **Contraindications for pneumatic tourniquet use.**
   a. Peripheral vascular disease and diminished pulses
   b. Vascular access port or shunt, PICC line, other IV
   c. History of deep vein thrombosis
   d. Malignancy or tumor in limb
   e. Open fracture or history of healing fracture
   f. Rheumatoid arthritis
   g. Skin or other tissue grafting
   h. Hemoglobinopathy (e.g., sickle cell disease)
   i. Infection in the limb

Pneumatic Tourniquet Equipment

A powered control box with a pressure readout and alarm system uses compressed gas or ambient air to inflate a circumferential cuff around a limb to obstruct blood flow.

1. **Pressure delivery unit.** Alarms and settings must always be audible and visual during use as a safety measure for the patient. The machine should be

calibrated and checked as part of the facility policy and procedure. If the pressure changes during use, the alarm should sound and the readout will indicate the current pressure. The duration of inflation is part of the readout.

Unexpected decrease in pressure could cause the systemic release of local medication in a harmful bolus. Average tourniquet pressures are based on the patient's systolic blood pressure. The surgeon may make pressure adjustments according to the patient's limb size.

  a. **Upper extremity** pressure should be calculated at 30 to 70 mm Hg higher than the patient's systolic blood pressure. The average pressure usually ranges between 200 and 250 mm Hg. The widest cuff possible should be used with a 3- to 6-inch overlap with a secure Velcro closure.

  b. **Lower extremity** pressure is calculated at half value higher than the patient's systolic blood pressure. The average pressure for a **thigh** tourniquet usually ranges between 250 and 300 mm Hg, but in larger patients the pressure could be 400 mm Hg. A tourniquet for the **calf/ankle** uses pressure similar to use on an arm. Larger patients may need higher pressures. The widest cuff possible should be used with a 3- to 6-inch overlap with a secure Velcro closure.

2. A **single cuff** can be curved or straight with an inflatable bladder inside. Curved cuffs are used on the contour of a limb and may use slightly less pressure.

3. A **double cuff** is straight because each cuff segment is smaller than a single cuff and may need the higher ranges of pressure. The widest cuff possible should be used with a 3- to 6-inch overlap with a secure Velcro closure.

A double cuff is used in **Bier block regional anesthesia**. The double cuff is placed over the upper arm. An IV cannula is placed in the dorsum of the hand by the anesthesia provider and secured. The proximal cuff segment is inflated and local anesthetic is injected. The distal cuff segment is inflated when the local anesthetic takes effect. The proximal cuff segment is deflated and the surgical procedure can begin.

Procedure for Using Pneumatic Tourniquet

1. **Application to limb and prep.** The tourniquet location is wrapped in a lint-free padding. The tourniquet is applied. The inflation ports should be directed away from the surgical site. A plastic adhesive drape is wrapped around the tourniquet to prevent prep solution from running over the area and saturating the padding.

2. **Elevation and exsanguination.** The limb is elevated to facilitate venous drainage. During elevation, the limb is prepped. A sterile Esmarch or ACE is used to circumferentially wrap the limb

from the distal aspect of the digits to the proximal portion at the level of the tourniquet. The extremity is exsanguinated. This process minimizes the risk for thrombosis and embolus associated with stasis of blood.

3. **Inflation.** The tourniquet cuff is inflated and the sterile wrap is removed, rerolled, and kept on the instrument table in case it is needed again. The local anesthetic is injected. The result is a bloodless surgical field.

Precautions and Safety

1. **Medications**

  a. Antibiotics and SCIP protocol require the antibiotic to be circulating 20 minutes before tourniquet inflation.

  b. Local anesthesia is administered after the tourniquet is inflated. Larger amounts may be used. For additional information about regional anesthesia, see Chapter 8.

  c. Care is taken to prevent the prep solution from contacting or running under the tourniquet cuff. It can cause tissue damage.

2. **Timing.** The readout indicates the level of pressure and the duration of inflation. Inflation time should be limited to 1 hour, and the alarm system should be set to sound at that time with a reminder sound for each 15-minute interval.

Some surgeons will request reperfusion periods of 10 to 15 minutes followed by exsanguination and reinflation of the tourniquet.

Potential Complications

1. **Localized in limb.** Muscle, nerve, or other tissue damage can be caused by use of a tourniquet. Skin injury can be caused by wrinkles in the padding under the cuff. Pressure from the inflated cuff can cause a crush injury to muscles and nerves that can cause motor or sensory deficit.

  a. Extreme nerve injury can affect the local vessel's ability to vasodilate or constrict. A shifting tourniquet cuff can cause underlying tissue damage by shearing force.

  b. **Compartment syndrome** can happen when the muscles are damaged by swelling within the fascial sheath(s). The muscles degrade, causing rhabdomyolysis. Myoglobin is released into the circulation, causing organ damage. The swelling cannot be resolved by circulatory resorption. The only relief is surgical, by performing a fasciotomy (e.g., surgical linear cuts in the fascia to release the pressure).

2. **Systemic effects.** Deflation of the tourniquet can cause the release of a bolus of local anesthetic with toxic effects. Other effects of prolonged anaerobic tissue metabolism include the release of lactic acid and the potential for hyperkalemia, causing metabolic acidosis, myocardial depression, and cardiac arrest.

Documentation After Tourniquet Use

1. **Patient-oriented observation and assessment.**
   Assess the tourniquet site location. Did the patient offer any verbal complaints? Can the patient move all extremities and digits equally? Are the patient's vital signs at baseline? Are the distal pulses equal, strong, and regular bilaterally? Is the patient's skin intact and within normal limits where the tourniquet was placed? Any systemic or metabolic effects noted?
2. **Equipment documentation.**
   a. Pneumatic inflation device identifying serial number; tourniquet cuff type, padding, and size
   b. Who applied and removed the tourniquet cuff?
   c. Pressure settings and duration of inflation
      1) Were any reperfusion periods used? How long was the tourniquet cuff inflated before deflation? How long was the reperfusion period?
      2) What actions were performed before reinflation of the tourniquet cuff.

Perioperative nurses should have the knowledge and skill to apply tourniquets and monitor patients where tourniquets are used during surgical procedures. Recognition of potential complications is important for safe and effective use of the device.

Chest Tubes

Chest tubes are necessary to reestablish a closed vacuum within the thoracic cavity when the integrity of the chest wall has been penetrated intentionally or unintentionally. Several surgical procedures will require chest tubes postoperatively. Perioperative nurses should have the knowledge and skill to facilitate the insertion and maintenance of chest tubes.

Anatomy and Physiology Review

The thoracic cavity contains the lungs and is protected by the rib cage. The lungs are dependent on the diaphragm, innervated by the phrenic nerve, to function and are surrounded by two membranes: the visceral and parietal pleurae. The visceral pleura covers the surface area of the lungs, and the parietal pleura lines the chest wall and diaphragm. There is a space between the two membranes that contains about 25 to 50 mL of serous fluid that lubricates and allows the lungs to move easily under negative pressure when breathing.

Indications for a Chest Tube

A chest tube is necessary when a penetration of the visceral and parietal pleurae occurs after trauma, surgical procedure, or iatrogenic injury through the membranes. The penetration can cause air, blood, fluid, or pus to collapse the underlying lung (atelectasis).

Atelectasis can cause respiratory insufficiency, leading to cardiovascular collapse and death if not treated by restoring the negative pressure with chest tubes. The perioperative nurse must know the indications for chest tubes, placement, objectives, and proper care. One or two tubes may be used depending on the desired treatment function of the tube(s).

1. **Pneumothorax:** The chest tube is placed in the superior margin of the second or third intercostal space (depends on body size). The tube is positioned with the tip directed superiorly in the anterior plane in the midclavicular line between the pleural membranes. It may be used in combination with a second chest tube inferiorly for drainage.
   a. Trapped air in the pleural space must be removed.
   b. Restore negative pressure between the pleural space.
2. **Drain fluids from the intrapleural space:** The chest tube is placed in the superior margin of the fifth or sixth intercostal space in the midaxillary line. It may be placed lower in taller individuals. The tube is directed in a lateral direction with the tip directed inferiorly between the pleural membranes. It may be used in combination with a second chest tube superiorly for pneumothorax.
   a. **Pleural effusion**
      1) Transudate is most common in pathology such as cirrhosis in hypoproteinemia and accumulates in the base of the lungs/pleura.
      2) Exudate is most common in acute inflammation or impaired lymphatic absorption as in malignancy.
   b. **Hemothorax** drains blood from the pleural space.
   c. **Empyema** drains pus from the pleural space.
   d. **Chylothorax** drains lymph from the pleural space.
3. **Mediastinal chest tubes:** The chest tube is positioned in the mediastinum to evacuate air and fluids after cardiac or other mediastinal surgical procedure. The mediastinum forms a flexible separation between the bilateral lungs/pleurae and contains the esophagus, pericardial sac, and thymus.
   a. Can prevent cardiac tamponade and the resultant decrease in cardiac output caused by impaired venous return to the heart.
   b. Commonly used in postoperative cardiac surgery.
4. **Therapeutic chest tube** for chemotherapy or pleurodesis (poudrage). Can be used to sclerose the pleural surfaces together to prevent or minimize fluid transudate buildup.
5. **Thoracentesis** is inserting a needle to drain air or fluid from the pleural space above the ninth intercostal space. No chest tube remains in place.

Chest Tube Apparatus

1. **Tubing** is inserted through the chest wall in the necessary intercostal space. A stab incision is made in the chest and the tube is inserted with long forceps. The average adult size chest tube is 26 to 30 Fr. The tube is semirigid silicone or polyvinylchloride approximately 20 inches long with perforations along the insertion point. The perforations are completely inserted into the patient's chest. The tubing is ineffective if any of the perforations exit the chest wall. A negative pressure cannot be maintained.

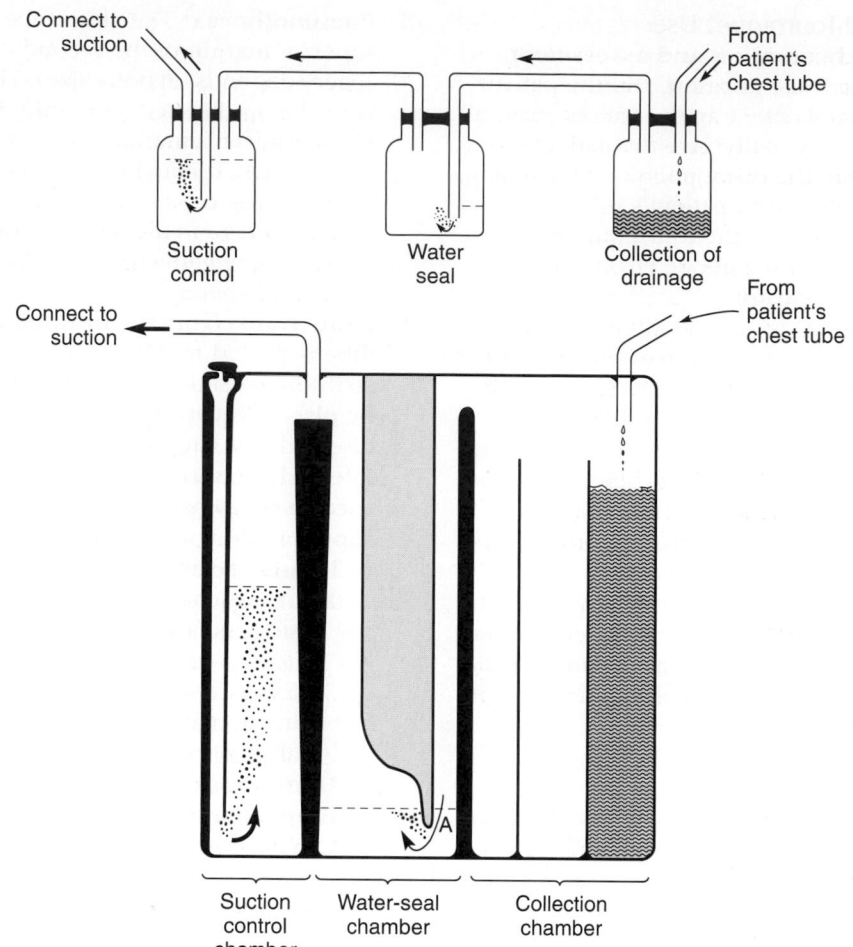

Connect to suction

From patient's chest tube

Suction control

Water seal

Collection of drainage

From patient's chest tube

Connect to suction

Suction control chamber

Water-seal chamber

Collection chamber

Figure 12.7 Comparison of a commercially available chest tube drainage system with a three-bottle system. (From Urden, L.D., Stacy, K.M., & Lough, M.E. [2006]. *Thelan's critical care nursing: diagnosis and management* [5th ed.]. St. Louis, MO: Mosby.)

The tubing can be secured with monofilament nonabsorbable suture and tape. Pediatric chest tube sizes range between 8 and 12 Fr. Placement can be confirmed by ultrasound or x-ray (Fig. 12.7).

2. **Receptacles** have three chambers that are used to re-create the vacuum for removing air from the chest. Single-chamber units are available. Contemporary types are commercially packaged sterile for assembly on the sterile field. Instructions include the volume of sterile water or saline to add to the water seal chamber fill line. When gravity water seal drainage is used, only two chambers of the receptacle are used. If mechanical suction is used, the third chamber is used to maintain pressure at 10 cm H_2O to approximate normal intrathoracic pressure.

The receptacle unit must remain below the level of the patient's lungs at all times for proper function. As air leaves the chest the fluid in the chamber will bubble demonstrating proper function.

3. **Precautions:** Do not clamp or kink the tubing. This could cause mediastinal shift. If ordered to clamp the tubing, use only a specified tube clamp. Reasons for clamping the chest tube include a full collection

chamber or if the collection unit must be raised above the patient's affected lung. Always have extra tubing and chest tube kits available. A thoracotomy tray should be in the room.

In the event of an unintentional tubing disconnection or malfunction of the receptacle, the chest tube can be submerged in a few inches of sterile water until a new water seal can be established.

Perioperative Patient Assessment

Checking the chest tubes and the effectiveness of the negative pressure is critical for the safety of the patient. Although placement of the chest tube is checked with x-ray, some anterior-posterior views can miss misplacement. The surgeon may order a chest computed tomography scan when in doubt. Observing the physiologic parameters of the patient with chest tubes can help troubleshoot potential complications.

1. Breathing assessment and breath sounds: Arterial blood gases may be ordered and drawn to ascertain the effectiveness of the oxygen exchange within the body. Observe respiratory effort. Pulse oximeter is used to evaluate O_2 saturation. The desired O_2 level

should be greater than 93%. In the postoperative area the head of the bed should be slightly elevated to 30 degrees to facilitate breathing and drainage.

2. Observe for drainage in the lower tube or mediastinal tube. The average capacity of chest tube drainage receptacle is less than 2 L. Prevent kinks in the tubing.
3. Observe for tracheal shift from midline. This may indicate mediastinal shift.
4. Assess the skin around the insertion point. Check for bleeding, puffiness, or crepitus (crackling air under the skin). The dressing should be clean and dry.
5. The drainage system is functioning when bubbling is present in the sterile water chamber. Encourage deep breathing and coughing to expand the lung within the pleural space. Elevating the head of the bed 30 degrees can provide some comfort. The drainage system must be below the level of the lung.
6. Pain management: Administer analgesics as ordered. Monitor respiratory rate for depression.

Complications of Chest Tubes

1. **Tension pneumothorax** occurs when the mediastinum moves lateral and compresses the unaffected side. The great vessels shift and compromise the cardiovascular system.
2. **Subcutaneous emphysema** can occur when air escapes into the tissues and causes the surrounding area under the skin to expand. When the tissue is compressed, it makes a crackling sound referred to as crepitus.
3. **Malpositioning** can occur at any time. The tube could press into the lung parenchyma and occlude the flow. The presence of fresh blood may indicate transection

of an artery by the tube. Careful observation of tube function can help detect malpositioning.
4. **Infection** is possible at any time. One of the first signs when observing the tubing is the presence of empyema.

Postoperative hand-over report to the receiving postanesthesia care unit nurse should include the reason for the chest tube(s), the size and type of tubes used, and any other pertinent information for the continuity care of care.

Pediatric Patients

The perioperative nurse should be knowledgeable about the physical and psychological differences to meet the needs of the pediatric patient and caregivers. Observation is an important part of the pediatric assessment to determine the appropriate way to interact with the patient. The pediatric physical assessment is focused on patient weight and age, emotional stage, nutrition requirements, heat and blood loss potential, and safety measures. The reason why the pediatric patient is having a surgical procedure can help guide the nursing assessment. The chronologic age may or may not match physical size and behaviors.

Pediatric Physical Assessment

Correct identification of the patient is critical for safe care. The parent or guardian must confirm the patient's name and birth date. An identification bracelet can be placed on an older child's wrist, but an infant may need the bracelet to be placed on an ankle.

Pediatric heart rate, respirations, and blood pressure differ according to weight, size, and age. Older adolescent vital signs closely match adult vital signs (Table 12.2).

TABLE 12.2 Pediatric Vital Sign Ranges

Age[a]	Heart Rate/Minute Awake	Heart Rate/Minute Asleep/At Rest	Respirations/Minute Asleep/At Rest	Blood Pressure Systolic[b] (mm Hg)
Newborn (2–3 kg)	100–180	80–160	30–60	60 ± 10
Infant				
1 month (4 kg)	110–150	70–120	26–34	80 ± 16
6 months (7 kg)	115–130	80–180	24–50	89 ± 29
1 year (10 kg)	100–150	70–120	22–30	96 ± 30
Toddler 18–30 months (12–14 kg)	110–130	70–100	22–28	99 ± 25
Preschool 4 years (16–18 kg)	80–120	60–90	20–30	99 ± 20
School Age				
6–9 years (20–32 kg)	70–115	60–90	20–30	100 ± 20
10 years (33 kg)	60–100	60–90	18–22	112 ± 20
Adolescent 14 years (50 kg)	60–100	60–90	16–20	120 ± 20

[a]Weights from the National Institutes of Health represent a combined estimate of weight for girls and boys.
[b]Blood pressure data are from Rodriguez-Cruz, E. (2017). *Pediatric hypertension*. Retrieved from Medscape website: http://emedicine.medscape.com/article/889877-overview.
Data from Novak, C. (2018). *Pediatric vital signs reference chart*. Retrieved from PedsCases website: www.pedscases.com/pediatric-vital-signs-reference-chart.

1. Is the child's weight appropriate for the age? Size may not always correlate to age. For infants, the rule of "10s" can be used: 10 lb, 10 weeks, and 10 g of hemoglobin. Underweight or overweight pediatric patients may indicate a nutrition deficit.
2. Assess the skin for birthmarks, rashes, cuts, or scars. Any suspected signs of abuse, such as burn marks, bruising, genital injuries, history of multiple broken bones, broken vessels in the eyes, or abrasions, must be reported to appropriate authorities per facility policy and procedure. Pictures may be taken as evidence.
3. Check the surgical site. Is it obvious, such as a defect, broken bone, or an infection? Is it marked correctly according to facility policy and procedure?
4. Is the patient verbal? Is the patient able to move all extremities equally?
5. Older children may be uncomfortable about removing undergarments. They can be removed in the OR after the induction of anesthesia.

Psychologic Assessment

Psychologic development depends on the child's age, home environment, culture, ethnicity, and socioeconomic status (Table 12.3).
1. The developmental stage and chronologic age can determine how the child will interact with the perioperative nurse. Some facilities offer a tour for parents and children before the day of surgery.
2. A parent or caregiver may help a child cooperate and understand what will happen. Avoid upsetting a child; crying can cause the pharyngeal membranes to swell, making intubation difficult. A child may bring a favorite toy in the OR for security.

Preparing the Child for Surgery

Preparing the child for surgery includes NPO status, transporting the child to the OR, maintaining normothermia, safety, blood loss, and pain control.
1. **NPO status** is determined by the age of the child. Children should be scheduled early in the day for surgery if possible. This way the child can return to normal feeding and caloric intake sooner. Special considerations for NPO status are based on age and individual health conditions.
   a. Breast milk may be given up to 4 hours before surgery.
   b. Formula may be given up to 6 hours before surgery, then clear liquids up to 2 hours preoperatively.
   c. Toddlers may have clear liquids 2 to 4 hours before surgery.
   d. Children 5 years and older may have clear liquids up to 6 hours before surgery.
   e. Bright-colored fluids, Jell-O, or popsicles should be avoided in case of vomiting; they could be mistaken for blood.
   f. Fluid intake and urine output are closely monitored. Infants can easily become dehydrated

because they have a large body surface area to body mass ratio.
2. **Transporting the child to the OR** requires planning and can be done in many ways depending on the child's age and maturity level. The anesthesia provider can give the child an anesthesia mask to play with. The mask can be scented with flavored lip balm. This can make the anesthesia delivery process less frightening. Avoid using words that can scare a child, such as "you will be put to sleep." This could relate to a pet that never returned. Instead, use gentler words, such as "you will breathe a funny smell and it might make you sleepy."
   a. Infants and small children may be transported in an enclosed crib to prevent falls. Some facilities use a wagon with sides for transport. At no time is the child left unattended.
   b. Older children may be taken to the OR on a transport cart. Give the child the choice of sitting up or lying down. Reassure the child that the parent or caregiver will be waiting for them after the surgical procedure.
   c. Some facilities permit a caregiver to accompany the child to the OR. The caregiver should be informed of the anesthetic process and what to expect. The perioperative nurse should stay close by, because it can be emotional when the child falls asleep after inhaling anesthetic gas. When the child is asleep, the caregiver should be escorted to the waiting area by assistive personnel.

Maintaining Normothermia

Maintaining normothermia in children is very important. Normal body temperature can range from 97°F to 100°F. The anesthesia provider monitors the child's vital signs including body temperature. Early signs of hypothermia include a change in heart rate, respirations, or temperature fluctuation. The body temperature is closely monitored to avoid overheating and sweating. Sweating causes fluid loss. Considerations for maintaining normothermia include:
1. Room temperature should be turned up before the procedure to 85°F.
2. Irrigation and IV fluids should be warm.
3. Use adjunct warming devices such as fluid warming pads and heating blankets, covering the child's head, or a radiant heat lamp.
4. Infants have physiologic differences in temperature regulation.
   a. Infants younger than 3 months do not have the mechanism to shiver because the neurologic system is not fully developed.
   b. Infants older than 3 months can shiver to create body heat. Shivering can increase the need for oxygen 200% to 500%.
5. **Heat loss.** Heat loss can occur from different sources. Heat can be lost by evaporation, convection, radiation, and conduction.

TABLE 12.3 Psychological Developmental Stage Theories

Chronologic Age Ranges (Approximate)	Developmental Stage by Theorist			Characteristics of Psychological Development
	Erikson	**Piaget**	**Loevinger**	
Birth–18 months	Trust vs. mistrust	Sensorimotor	Presocial	Learns to view self as being separate from the environment; begins to develop the concept of hope; learns to develop attachments to others; is dependent on caregiver for warmth, security, nourishment, nurturing, and stimulation; begins to use sounds and short words to communicate ideas; may view hospitalization as abandonment
19 months–3 years	Autonomy vs. shame/doubt	Preoperational	Symbiotic	Develops a two-way relationship with primary caregiver; suffers separation anxiety when isolated from established relationships; has short trials of independence; personality becomes introverted or extroverted; establishes a sense of will; uses sentences for communication; has fear of immediate threats; does not project thoughts beyond the present situation
4–6 years	Initiative vs. guilt	Preoperational	Impulsive	Asserts a separate identity; begins to have fear of real and imagined situations; senses peer acceptance or rejection; is concerned about disfigurement; may act out feelings; believes that every action has a purpose, either reward or punishment; learns to be self-protective; fears death or nonexistence; death is not always understood as being permanent; develops short-term self-control; uses compound sentences to communicate; mimics terminology used by fantasy characters
7–11 years	Industry vs. inferiority	Concrete operational	Conformist	Imitates actions and attitudes of peers and heroes; is aware of the differences of others and identifies with a particular social group; fears loss of self-control; understands the world in moderate detail; prefers honest explanations and reassurance of safety; does not want to be treated like a baby; strives for competency in daily tasks; can distinguish between fact and fantasy; has a greater understanding of death and its permanence; wants to be accepted as an individual; communicates well verbally and with basic writing skill
12–16 years	Identity vs. role confusion	Formal, operational	Self-aware, conscientious	May change opinion in response to stereotypes; develops close relationships; understands values, rules, and ideals; begins to feel more important as an individual; fears alienation; body image is extremely important; is capable of abstract thought and reasoning; has a sense of aesthetic beauty; can merge sensory information and logic to derive a conclusion; prefers privacy and confidentiality; may question authority; is aware of opposite sex; may explore sexual activity; dreams about future lifestyle; wants to prove self-worth; globally communicates verbally and in writing
17 years–adulthood	Intimacy vs. isolation	Formal, operational	Individualistic	Becomes aware of and accepts the interdependence of mankind; may feel some hostility toward authority; sometimes torn between the desire to be totally independent and dependent; seeks companionship of opposite sex; may be sexually active; refines interpersonal skills; demands privacy and confidentiality; plans for independent lifestyle as approach; refines verbal and written communication skill

From Phillips, N. (2017). *Berry and Kohn's operating room technique* (13th ed.). St. Louis, MO: Elsevier.

a. **Evaporation.** Evaporation can occur if the patient is wet or overheated. Sweat can evaporate and cause a drop in temperature.

b. **Convection.** Air currents cause the warm air to rise, and the cool air sinks and causes transfer of heat. It can come from anything wet or cold.

c. **Radiation.** Radiation occurs from the transfer of body heat into the air. Open body cavities radiate heat.

d. **Conduction.** Placing a patient on a cold bed can cause the warm body temperature to transfer to the cold bed.

Child Safety

Child safety is a priority. Ways to keep children safe can include the following:

1. Never leave a child unattended at any time. A parent or caregiver can stay with the child preoperatively and postoperatively.
2. Cribs with a top can be used to avoid falls.
3. Do not place cribs or beds near electrical sockets, IV poles, monitors, or any item that is within reach. IVs should be covered so they cannot be pulled out, and an arm board may be used.
4. Use appropriate size instrumentation, drapes, safety straps, and positioning aids. Do not cut large nonwoven drapes to size; cellulose fibers can fall into the surgical site creating inflammation followed by infection.
5. After a surgical procedure, place the child in a left lateral position or sitting up to prevent aspiration.
6. The ESU return electrode should be weight specific and placed on an area without gaps. Pediatric return electrodes are for patients less than 30 pounds.
7. The number of medication errors is much higher in children than in adults because of the variation of weight. Medications are dosed according to weight in kilograms. Double-check all medication doses and allergies.
8. Uncuffed endotracheal (ET) tubes are used for children younger than 8 years.

Blood Loss in Children

Measurement of blood loss is critical in children. A measurement commonly used is 1 g of blood weight equals 1 mL of blood. Weighing sponges is one method of calculation of blood loss.

1. **Calibrate (Tare) the digital scale and set a baseline in grams.** Place a small basin on the scale and set the readout to zero. Weigh 10 slightly moistened Raytec sponges in the basin and record the total in grams. Remove the Raytec sponges; then place five slightly moistened laparotomy tapes in the same basin and record the total in grams. Remove the laparotomy tapes and leave the empty basin on the scale. This method allows for the calculation of baseline materials and moisture before weighing for blood loss.
2. **Weighing bloody sponges.** Place 10 bloody Raytec sponges in the basin and record the weight in grams.

Subtract the baseline weight in grams from the bloody sponge weight in grams. The total will be the amount of blood loss in grams minus the baseline material weight. The same method is used for weighing laparotomy tapes.

Pain Management in Children

Children display signs of pain differently than an adult. For additional information concerning pain management, see Chapter 11.

1. Observe the child for signs of pain that can include crying, moaning, facial expressions, verbal expression, kicking, body movement, rocking, or restlessness.
2. The **Wong-Baker FACES Pain Rating Scale** can used for children 3 years and older (see Fig. 11.2).
3. For children 2 months to 7 years old, the **FLACC behavioral scale** can be used for pain assessment (see Table 11.2).

Caring for pediatric patients is a very specific role in nursing. The perioperative nurse should have the knowledge of child development, vital signs, childhood illnesses, and surgical procedures. Pediatric perioperative nurses need to be nurturing, calm, patient, and compassionate toward the children and caregivers.

The Geriatric Patient

Geriatric patients are considered 65 years and older. Caring for a geriatric patient can be complicated because many surgical procedures are done in emergency situations. Older adults may have multiple comorbidities and take numerous medications that can lead to slower surgical recovery times. Anesthesia drugs may take longer to clear the patient's system because of decreased renal and liver function.

Physical and psychologic assessment should be completed to determine the patient's level of function, formulate critical nursing diagnosis, and identify special needs for postoperative care.

1. **Physical assessment.** The physical assessment may be extensive depending on the patient's health. Evaluating body systems may be a good way to assess the patient. With observation, smell, and listening, the perioperative nurse can learn a great deal about the patient. Some important points of the physical assessment include the following (Table 12.4):

   a. **Vital signs.** Are the vital signs within normal range? Checking blood glucose is common. Is the patient taking medications (e.g., cardiac medications, diuretics, anticoagulants, or diabetic medications [insulin or hyperglycemics]) that affect vital signs such as blood pressure?

      1) **Cardiovascular assessment.** Does the patient have a pacemaker, implantable defibrillator, or history of heart surgery? Cardiac testing is usually required to clear a geriatric patient for surgery. Assess the peripheral pulses and observe the color of the nails, hair pattern, and whether edema is present.

TABLE 12.4 Physiologic Changes Associated With Normal Aging Processes in the Geriatric Patient

Age-Related Factors	Assessment Factors
Integumentary System	
Decreased subcutaneous fat, decreased turgor (elasticity)	Thin dry skin, wrinkles
Diminished sweat glands, dulled tactile sensation Thickened connective tissue	Poor thermoregulation, heat and cold sensitivity Keratosis (patchy overgrowths of dermis), warts, skin tags (especially on face and neck)
Increased fat deposits over abdomen and hips	Poor excretion of fat-soluble drugs
Diminished capillary blood flow, reduced vascularity, capillary fragility	Pressure sores, delayed wound healing, purpura or lentigo (liver spots), bruises
Dry mucous membranes, decreased salivation and secretions	Dry mouth and vagina
Musculoskeletal System	
Diminished protein synthesis in muscle cells, decreased muscle mass and tone	Muscle weakness, reduced strength, muscle wasting
Erosion of cartilage, thickened synovial fluid, fibrosed synovial membranes	Joint pain, swelling, stiffness, diminished range of motion
Diminished mobility, flexibility, and balance	Poor gait, poor posture, risk of falling
Increased porosity and demineralization of bone, thinning of intervertebral discs, decreased height	Ankylosing spondylosis, kyphosis, osteoporosis
Respiratory System	
Atrophied respiratory muscles, kyphosis or other postural changes, rib cage rigidity	Chest wall limitations
Reduced vital capacity	Dyspnea
Risk of pneumonia	Ineffective cough
Cardiovascular System	
Decreased cardiac output and stroke volume	Chronic fatigue and dyspnea, orthostatic hypotension
Myocardial irritability and stiffness, decreased size of sinoatrial and atrioventricular nodes	Slow heart rate and circulation, dysrhythmias and murmurs
Increased vascular resistance, rigidity in arteries	Hypertension
Thickening and dilation of veins	Venous insufficiency, varicosities
Decline in renal blood flow	Edema in tissues
Gastrointestinal System	
Decreased esophageal peristalsis, slowed emptying of stomach	Indigestion, frequent antacid use
Diminished saliva production, which slows breakdown of carbohydrates; reduced gastric secretion of hydrochloric acid, which impairs absorption of vitamins and minerals; hepatic insufficiency, which affects absorption of fats	Malnutrition Diarrhea, fecal incontinence Constipation, frequent laxative use
Loss of perineal and anal sphincter tone	
Decreased intestinal peristalsis, loss of abdominal muscle turgor, reduced mucosal secretions in intestines	
Endocrine System	
Reduced hormonal activity, decreased physical activity	Slowed basal metabolic rate, subnormal temperature
Slowed release of insulin from pancreas	Impaired glucose metabolism
Reduced thyroid hormone production	Dry skin, temperature intolerance, poor appetite, lethargy, memory lapse
Disturbed fluid and electrolyte balance	Hydration status
Genitourinary System	
Decreased renal blood flow, reduced number of glomeruli, reduced glomerular filtration rate, decreased excretory ability	Diminished renal function, risk of acid-base imbalance and drug toxicity
Loss of elasticity and muscle tone in ureters, bladder, and urethra	Urinary frequency, urgency, and nocturia

(Continued)

TABLE 12.4   Physiologic Changes Associated With Normal Aging Processes in the Geriatric Patient—cont'd

Age-Related Factors	Assessment Factors
Decreased bladder muscle and sphincter tone, estrogen deficiency in female	Stress incontinence
Enlarged prostate in male	Urinary retention
Reduced testosterone levels, hypertrophied prostate, sclerosis of penile arteries and veins	Male: slow erection and ejaculation
Reduced estrogen levels; atrophied vulva, clitoris, and vagina	Female: sagging breasts, painful intercourse
Nervous System	
Decreased number of brain cells, reduced cerebral blood flow, reduced oxygen supply to brain	Cognitive deficits: delirium, temporary state of confusion, forgetfulness, disorientation, irritability, and insomnia; dementia, a permanent state of cognitive impairment
Decreased neurons	Paresthesia, akinesia, diminished pain perception
Diminished neurotransmitters, decreased neurons	Tremors, head nodding, and other repetitive movements
Degeneration of myelin sheath, which lessens motor neuron conduction	Slowed reflexes and reaction time
Reduced sound transmission as eardrum thickens, decreased hair cells and neurons, reduced blood supply to cochlea	Auditory impairment
Weakened lens muscles; hardening of lens; flattening of cornea; reduced blood supply, which leads to macular deterioration; increased rigidity of iris; reduced pupil size	Visual impairment: decreased acuity, poor perception of light and color, poor peripheral vision

From Phillips, N. (2017). *Berry and Kohn's operating room technique* (13th ed.). St. Louis, MO: Elsevier.

2) **Respiratory assessment.** Are the lungs clear to auscultation? Does the patient have any respiratory conditions such as chronic obstructive pulmonary disease, chronic cough, or asthma? Does the patient smoke? Did the surgeon order a preoperative chest x-ray?

b. **Skin assessment.** Observe the skin for color, temperature, and turgor. Is the skin in good condition? Is it dry or moist? Does the patient have sores or bruising? Are there any signs that could indicate abuse (Box 12.2)?

c. **Musculoskeletal assessment.** Can the patient walk and move all extremities? Is there a history of musculoskeletal disease such as arthritis, broken bones or total joint replacement? Does the patient seem frail or a fall risk? A wristband indicting a fall risk should be placed on the patient.

Can the patient perform the activities of daily living? Activities include self-care, from feeding to grooming, preparing meals, housework, and socializing.

d. **Neurologic assessment.** Can the patient answer questions coherently? Is the speech slurred? Does the patient have tremors? Does the patient have spectacles, hearing devices, or dentures? Allow the patient to wear spectacles and hearing devices before surgery. Hearing devices may be worn in the OR to hear the anesthesia provider or the surgeon. Spectacles and dentures should be removed and properly secured with the patient's name and kept with the belongings.

BOX 12.2   Signs of Elder Abuse

The older person demonstrates *excessive* agreement or compliance with the caregiver.

- The older person shows signs of poor hygiene, such as body odor, uncleanliness, or soiled clothing or underpants.
- The older person has malnutrition or dehydration.
- The older person has burns or pressure sores.
- The older person has bruises in various stages of healing that may indicate repeated injury.
- The older person lacks adequate clothing or footwear.
- The older person has not received adequate medical attention.
- The older person verbalizes lack of food, medication, or care.
- The older person verbalizes being left alone or isolated in some way.
- The older person verbalizes fear of the caregiver.
- The older person verbalizes his or her lack of control in personal activities or finances.

Modified from Williams, P. (2016). *Basic geriatric nursing* (6th ed.). St. Louis, MO: Elsevier.

e. **Nutrition assessment.** Does the patient's weight and nutrition status seem adequate for age and height? Are there any gastrointestinal issues? If obese, a weight-appropriate OR bed is necessary. Does the patient wear dentures? Missing teeth or poor oral health can lead to low nutrition intake. Does the patient lack resources to purchase food?

2. **Psychological assessment.** The psychological assessment can help the perioperative nurse plan for postoperative care. The patient's views and attitude can help decide whether a patient will need additional or continued care after a surgical procedure. Psychological issues may include the following:
   a. Is the patient participating in his or her own care? Did the patient sign the surgical consent and demonstrate understanding of the surgical procedure? Is the patient accompanied by family or a significant other?
   b. Culture can influence how well a patient recovers from surgery. Positive attitude, family, and socializing will give the patient encouragement to recover.
   c. Depressed patients who feel helpless, alone, or have no self-worth may decline in health. Many older patients admitted to the intensive care unit suffer from delirium.
   d. Cognitive ability should be assessed because impairment can lead to confusion or disorientation. Any change in mental status should be evaluated because there can be an underlying cause.

Nursing Process for the Geriatric Patient

1. **Examples of perioperative nursing diagnoses**
   a. Ineffective tissue perfusion
   b. Ineffective thermoregulation
   c. Risk for perioperative positioning injury
2. **Examples of perioperative nursing interventions**
   a. Use sequential compression devices if possible to prevent thrombus formation and emboli caused by slow circulation or hypotension
   b. Use warm blankets or a forced warm air device, head cover, and booties. Irrigation and IV solutions should be warm. Hypothermia occurs when the core body temperature decreases to less than 96.8°F (36°C).
   c. Use patient lifting devices if the patient cannot move over to the OR bed. When positioning, do not force limbs into a position. It could cause fracture or dislocation of a joint. Extra gel padding may be necessary for bony prominences to avoid pressure injuries.

The geriatric patient requires a comprehensive nursing assessment before surgery to meet individual needs for safe care. A complete history and physical with cognitive assessment can identify risk factors. Accurate nursing diagnosis and planning can provide a safe and caring environment with positive outcomes for geriatric patients.

Disaster Preparedness

Disaster training should be a part of every facility. Disasters can happen inside the facility, such as a fire, or outside the facility. The Joint Commission requires healthcare facilities to have practice drills twice a year for emergency situations.

Types of Disasters

The types of disasters for which healthcare providers should be prepared include:
1. **Internal disasters**
   a. Fire
   b. Explosion
   c. Intruder or person with criminal intent
2. **External disasters**
   a. Natural disasters: tornadoes, floods, volcanoes, hurricanes
   b. Train, plane, or auto accidents
   c. Explosion
   d. Biologic or pandemic
   e. Chemical
   f. Gun fire
   g. Mass casualty

Role of Perioperative Nurses During Disasters

Perioperative nurses should know what to do in different types of disasters. They should also make sure they have safety equipment (personal protective equipment) available if necessary. Internal and external disaster victims may have multiple injuries requiring surgical intervention that include contamination exposure. The patients of external disasters are triaged before coming to the OR and have likely been decontaminated if exposed to chemicals or biologic agents. What information should the perioperative nurse consider during an internal disaster?

1. **Fire and/or explosion in the facility**
   a. Follow RACE (Rescue anyone in immediate danger. Activate the fire alarm. Contain the fire if possible [close the door]. Extinguish the fire [some facilities use Evacuate].) and PASS (Pull the ring from the handle. Aim the nozzle at the base of the fire. Squeeze the handle. Sweep the spray over the base of the fire.) training. Know the location of fire extinguishers and fire alarms. For information concerning RACE and PASS, see Chapter 5.
   b. Close all doors to contain the fire and prevent spread.
   c. If the source of explosion is gas or oxygen, can it be turned off? The perioperative nurse should know where the shutoff valves are located.
   d. Do patients need to be evacuated to another wing or area?
2. **A natural disaster affecting the facility, such as a hurricane, tornado, or flood**
   a. Do patients need to be moved to a safe place away from windows?
   b. Do patients need to be moved to a higher floor in the case of flooding?
   c. Do patients need to be evacuated from the facility?
3. **Internal facility crisis with intruder or person with criminal intent**
   a. Shelter self and patients in place as possible. Lock door, turn off lights. Remain silent.

b. Summon help (silence cell phone, use texting).
c. Assist injured individuals as much as possible until danger has passed and help arrives.

4. **External biologic or pandemic crisis. What is the microorganism?**
    a. Can the healthcare staff safely treat patients after triage and decontamination?
    b. Do patients need to be quarantined?
    c. Will any of the contaminated patients need a surgical procedure?

5. **Chemical or toxic exposure after an external disaster. What chemicals or toxins are involved?**
    a. Is there an antidote for the chemical or toxin?
    b. Does the perioperative nurse know how to access the material safety data sheet or government agency for information?
    c. Will any of the contaminated patients need a surgical procedure?

6. **Mass casualty.** Healthcare providers will be triaging patients in the healthcare facility and at the disaster site. All personnel report to a command post within the facility and will be assigned a specific roll according to need. The emergency internal and external disaster policy and procedure should be known throughout the facility.
    a. Patients can have multiple injuries and/or exposures.
    b. Patients can be any age or condition. Multiple injuries can be present that are not immediately apparent.

Triage of Patients During a Disaster

Experienced perioperative nurses may be in a situation where they are assisting in the triage of disaster patients. Personal safety measures must be used when trying to help patients. Nurses in a triage situation face difficult ethical decisions if they have to pass over critically ill or seriously injured patients. A physician will make the final triage decision concerning patient categories and care. There are two primary triage systems in use for mass casualty:

1. **START system:** Simple Triage and Rapid Treatment. It has four categories:
    a. Deceased or beyond help
    b. Injured, in need of immediate help to survive
    c. Injured but less severe
    d. Minor injuries, not requiring urgent help

2. **TAG system.** Patients are triaged by the physician and assigned a color tag or wristband to indicate level of immediate care. At the site of the disaster a colored tent may be present to house differing levels of triaged patients.
    a. *Black tag* (expectant): extensive injuries, will not survive
    b. *Red tag:* in need of immediate care or will not survive
    c. *Yellow tag* (observation): not in immediate danger of dying
    d. *Green tag* (wait): walking wounded, eventually need care
    e. *White tag* (dismiss): minor injuries, do not need doctor's care

Competencies

In 2009, the World Health Organization and the International Council of Nurses developed the Framework of Disaster Nursing Competencies. Competencies included communication, planning, decontamination, safety, command system, and ethics. These competencies are for all nurses worldwide to help them prepare for a disaster. The nurses are required to demonstrate their knowledge of disaster planning. This information was updated in 2017 to help nurses all over the world be better prepared for any disaster.

Volunteer Groups

Some nurses belong to volunteer groups that are deployed during disasters and may go to other states and countries to help. The American Nurses Association has a position statement on the rights and responsibilities related to work release during a disaster. The document defines what constitutes a disaster.

1. Nurses, who belong to state and federal teams, are trained and prepared for disaster relief. This includes select perioperative nurses.
2. The nurse must be preapproved and have permission to leave from his or her employer.
3. The statement defines the nurse's rights if he or she is away for a long period.
    Healthcare providers who care for patients in disasters or mass casualty situations risk their own lives to help others in need. They often struggle with the emotional burden of trying to save everyone in need. Through preparation drills and extensive training, nurses can be organized, calm, and mentally prepared to assist during internal and external disasters.

LEARNING ACTIVITIES

INSTRUCTIONS: Complete the word search puzzle. Use the clues to help identify the words.

```
E X G J I N K J C Z Z P V Q Y I I P F N P U T U P Z M K Y U
W M G S V P L V T A R V H T P L V O J C O B T E W Q L O W L
S K X U B I O A Y D P B I P O L A R B A O E L I E B L S B N
O E A B L C E J R T B A D W V N C B T V F E T H G Z T U M X
J T A H K A M N F G E Q C V P R L U K W N N G G V P V D P E
H R F L S O P K S O E P R I I K V T L U E T W Y E U U O Z G
S I H B S T I A H D B M P P T Z D G O T P G U U E U T N V B
E A A C M A I N R X Q C C O A A W H D U K G U B W C Y K J C
M G M Q Q O T N N O I H B H J T N Z D J R Y N W X T N T R U
C E L Q Y C O P S R S T E F E J I C X C H N V O E E Y R Q E
K R N V X U E S T U G C S S F S S E E F H I I F X K X A G C
D C F S Q T K A Y L F A O I N N T M N Z O I A Q J W H U F X
D Y B K C C I X X Z I F B P L B R T L T F S L J U D D M E B
Y E S W T D O Y H B P U L F Y E R E U H P C I D Q E T A N W
U M S H E X U U A X Y X R A R U P U P B Y F S A R N T I P X
B J B P R P E W W W P V O U T D Q C I P E H D X A E V O O L
E H V W C Q O Z X J R R S O E I O B O S K H B T H G N S S A
G Y S M T S D M F T H A O D Q L O X X W I R S H W M O F T S
M X N Z V G Z N T Q G V N X D L T N J U B N X Q Z C K T A E
N M S W C T T V T I S E C V I S Z P X H O D G I M J F J T R
D C E Y J I M A L Z L J O J H M J X V C W W F C J V J C U Q
B W F G Z B I W H B W U X G K H A G E R I A T R I C T I S W
O Y Y P T M R J W V Q M H P C O S L G I U F T X O J L I C Z
R P R D G U L T R A S O N I C R R H L R Y W J M M B Q J Z R
U G Y A V J A S R V W S T Q F C B O Y L R V B U G C V Y D H
E P W Q M J Y A Z Z G O N U C P G X F J S R J G S S W L M S
U G G O D M Y S F Q B I N A C T I V E E L E C T R O D E Z B
Q R K H T Y H K U O D Z W E J T X F Z M V Q E U B T A M Y
P Z J D O E Y I R V X A U D I B L E V F E X Y O H Z Z D Y Q
A X U B P H X R E F U P N A H E A T L O S S E D A G S U U F
```

CLUES

1. ESU units have _____ alarms that should be on at all times for safety.
2. A _____ ESU sends the current from the generator to the active tips of the forceps. No return pad is needed because the current does not pass through the patient's body.
3. Monopolar ESU setting that is _____ can seal vessels and cut tissue.
4. Assess the skin. If signs of abuse, such as _____ , cuts, burns, scars, broken blood vessels in the eyes, or abrasions, are suspected, they must be reported to the authorities per facility policy.
5. A _____ return electrode is placed on top of the OR mattress under the patient.

6. Indications for a _____ include trauma, surgical procedure, and injury. Penetration of the visceral and parietal pleurae can cause air, blood, fluid, or pus to collapse the lung. Tubing is inserted through the chest wall and attached to a receptacle with chambers to create a vacuum for normal intrathoracic pressure.

7. The Wong-Baker FACES Pain Rating Scale is used for ages 3 years and older, and the FLACC behavioral pain scale can be used for _____ 2 months to 7 years old.

8. The monopolar ESU setting that cuts has a _____ current.

9. A return electrode pad must never be _____.

10. The _____ patient is considered 65 years or older. A physical and psychological assessment should be completed to determine the patient's level of function and ability to perform the activities of daily living (ADL).

11. Shivering can increase the need for oxygen 200% to 500% in infants. _____ can come from different sources: evaporation, convection, radiation, and conduction.

12. The ESU sends the current back to the generator after it _____ through the patient's tissues.

13. The peritoneal cavity is expanded with carbon dioxide gas. _____ pressure should be between 12 and 18 mm Hg for the average adult.

14. Rigid endoscopes can be diagnostic or operative. Small openings are created in the body for _____ with the use of trocars.

15. A return electrode pad should be placed over a _____ muscle. Avoid bony prominences, scars, and tattoos.

16. Light Amplification by Stimulated Emission of Radiation (_____). Lasers are regulated by the FDA.

17. _____ is a form of bipolar electrosurgery with its own generator and hand pieces.

18. Children are usually scheduled for surgery earlier in the day so they can return to normal feeding as soon as possible. _____ is different depending on age, nutrition source, and surgical procedure.

19. Monopolar electrosurgery flows through the generator to the active electrode or hand piece through the _____ and back to the generator.

20. Assessment for pediatric patients may not correlate to age. The numbers for vital signs are not the same as adults. Psychological development depends on the child's age and home environment.

21. A Bier block uses a double tourniquet cuff. The _____ cuff is inflated first and the local anesthetic is injected. The distal cuff is inflated after the local takes effect. The proximal cuff is deflated. At the end of the procedure the tourniquet should be deflated slowly to prevent a bolus of anesthetic from causing toxicity.

22. _____ surgery requires special training and instrumentation. The surgeon controls the operating arms from a remote console.

23. Children have different _____ requirements, such as: Never leave them unattended, do not place cribs or beds near equipment or electrical sockets, ESU pads are weight specific (30 pounds and under), and uncuffed ET tubes are used for children younger than 8 years.

24. The monopolar ESU setting for coagulation _____ small to medium vessels.

25. A _____ creates a bloodless field. Antibiotics should be given at least 20 minutes before inflation. The average pressure for an upper extremity is between 200 and 250 mm Hg. The average pressure for a lower extremity is between 250 and 300 mm Hg (pressure could be higher than 400 mm Hg for larger patients).

26. The Argon beam coagulator uses gas to create the current. A return electrode pad is used to return the current to the generator. It is commonly used for _____ because it can cover a larger area with a stream of gas.

27. There are two main _____ systems: START system and the TAG system. Disaster drills should be held at all facilities.

28. Harmonic scalpel uses _____ vibrations as energy to cut and cauterize.

LEARNING ACTIVITIES ANSWERS

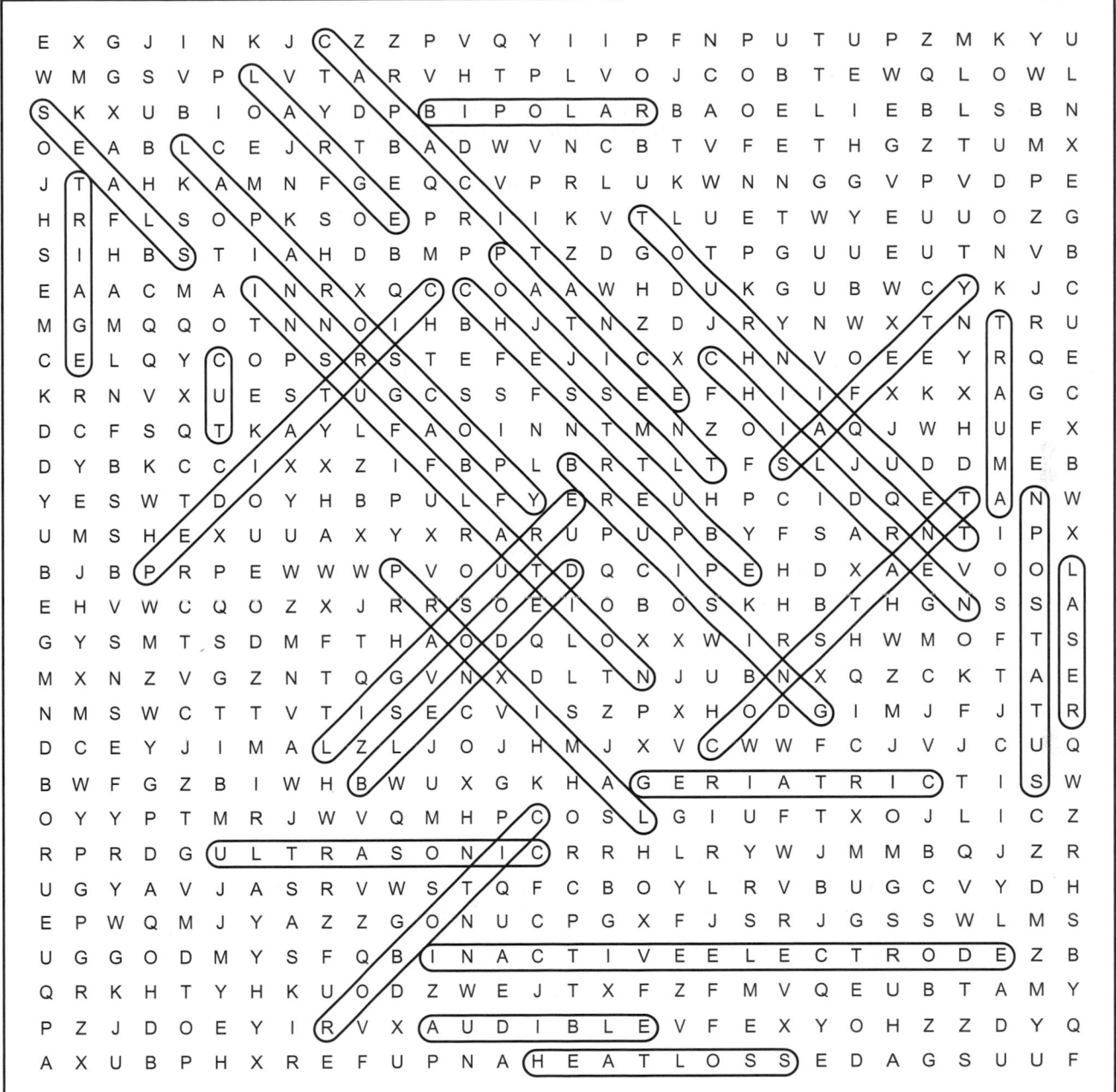

CLUES

1. ESU units have **audible** alarms that should be on at all times for safety.
2. A **bipolar** ESU sends the current from the generator to the active tips of the forceps. No return pad is needed because the current does not pass through the patient's body.
3. Monopolar ESU setting that is **blended** can seal vessels and cut tissue.
4. Assess the skin. If signs of abuse, such as **bruising**, cuts, burns, scars, broken blood vessels in the eyes, or abrasions, are suspected, they must be reported to the authorities per facility policy.
5. A **capacitance** return electrode is placed on top of the OR mattress under the patient.

6. Indications for a **chest tube** include trauma, surgical procedure, and injury. Penetration of the visceral and parietal pleurae can cause air, blood, fluid, or pus to collapse the lung. Tubing is inserted through the chest wall and attached to a receptacle with chambers to create a vacuum for normal intrathoracic pressure.

7. The Wong-Baker FACES Pain Rating Scale is used for ages 3 years and older, and the FLACC behavioral pain scale can be used for **children** 2 months to 7 years old.

8. The monopolar ESU setting that cuts has a **constant** current.

9. A return electrode pad must never be **cut**.

10. The **geriatric** patient is considered 65 years or older. A physical and psychological assessment should be completed to determine the patient's level of function and ability to perform the activities of daily living (ADL).

11. Shivering can increase the need for oxygen 200% to 500% in infants. **Heat loss** can come from different sources: evaporation, convection, radiation, and conduction.

12. The ESU sends the current back to the generator after it **passes** through the patient's tissues.

13. The peritoneal cavity is expanded with carbon dioxide gas. **Insufflation** pressure should be between 12 and 18 mm Hg for the average adult.

14. Rigid endoscopes can be diagnostic or operative. Small openings are created in the body for **laparoscopy** with the use of trocars.

15. A return electrode pad should be placed over a **large** muscle. Avoid bony prominences, scars, and tattoos.

16. Light Amplification by Stimulated Emission of Radiation (**LASER**). Lasers are regulated by the FDA.

17. **LigaSure** is a form of bipolar electrosurgery with its own generator and hand pieces.

18. Children are usually scheduled for surgery earlier in the day so they can return to normal feeding as soon as possible. **NPO status** is different depending on age, nutritional source and surgical procedure.

19. Monopolar electrosurgery flows through the generator to the active electrode or hand piece through the **patient** and back to the generator.

20. Assessment for pediatric patients may not correlate to age. The numbers for vital signs are not the same as adults. Psychological development depends on the child's age and home environment.

21. A Bier block uses a double tourniquet cuff. The **proximal** cuff is inflated first and the local anesthetic is injected. The distal cuff is inflated after the local takes effect. The proximal cuff is deflated. At the end of the procedure, the tourniquet should be deflated slowly to prevent a bolus of anesthetic from causing toxicity.

22. **Robotic** surgery requires special training and instrumentation. The surgeon controls the operating arms from a remote console.

23. Children have different **safety** requirements, such as: Never leave them unattended, do not place cribs or beds near equipment or electrical sockets, ESU pads are weight specific (30 pounds and under), and uncuffed ET tubes are used for children younger than 8 years.

24. The monopolar ESU setting for coagulation **seals** small to medium vessels.

25. A **tourniquet** creates a bloodless field. Antibiotics should be given at least 20 minutes before inflation. The average pressure for an upper extremity is between 200 and 250 mm Hg. The average pressure for a lower extremity is between 250 and 300 mm Hg (pressure could be higher than 400 mm Hg for larger patients).

26. The Argon beam coagulator uses gas to create the current. A return electrode pad is used to return the current to the generator. It is commonly used for **trauma** because it can cover a larger area with a stream of gas.

27. There are two main **triage** systems: START system and the TAG system. Disaster drills should be held at all facilities.

28. Harmonic scalpel uses **ultrasonic** vibrations as energy to cut and cauterize.

1. Why is it important to keep the doors of the operating room (OR) closed?
   A. Because the air pressure gradient is positive inside the room and negative in the hallway to minimize particulate transfer from the hall.
   B. Because the air pressure gradient is negative inside the room and negative in the hallway to keep the airflow equalized.
   C. Because the air pressure gradient is positive inside the room and positive in the hallway to keep the airflow equalized.
   D. Because dust and particulates are contained in the room when the door is closed.

2. What is an advantage of steam sterilization?
   A. All instrumentation can be cleaned in less than 4 minutes
   B. It is convenient, inexpensive
   C. Long processing time, expensive
   D. Nontoxic, expensive

3. Relative temperature and humidity of the OR should be maintained between which of the following levels?
   A. 58°F–65°F and 50%–75% humidity
   B. 70°F–85°F and 50%–70% humidity
   C. 60°F–70°F and 30%–70% humidity
   D. 68°F–75°F and 20%–60% humidity

4. Which of the following hemostatic agents is derived from beef (bovine) products?
   A. Thrombin
   B. Gelfoam
   C. Surgicel
   D. Oxycel

5. Which pathogen causes Creutzfeldt-Jakob disease (CJD)?
   A. Virus
   B. Bacteria
   C. Prion
   D. Dementia

6. Methods for affixing a burn dressing include all of the following except:
   A. Staples
   B. Tape
   C. Sutures
   D. Ties

7. Which form of cold high-level disinfection solution may be used for plastics, rubber, and some endoscopes?
   A. Bleach
   B. Isopropyl alcohol
   C. Glutaraldehyde
   D. Cobalt-60

8. How does Spaulding's classification identify the three levels of patient care items?
   A. Critical, semicritical, noncritical
   B. High, medium, low
   C. Clean, dirty, contaminated
   D. Sterile, clean, dirty

9. Which packaging material is best for processing small single instruments?
   A. Peel pack or pouch
   B. Rigid container
   C. Nonwoven blue wrapping material
   D. Custom pack

10. Which process is used to determine the total body surface area (TBSA) burned in an adult?
    A. Lund-Browder
    B. Multiply body weight by 9 and divide by 4
    C. Rule of nines
    D. Divide body weight (in kilograms) by height (in centimeters)

11. LASER plume is best managed by which of the following methods?
    A. Smoke evacuator
    B. Wall-mounted suction
    C. Canister suction with a gauze sponge over the tip
    D. Irrigation of the site to prevent plume accumulation

12. During a malignant hyperthermia crisis, dantrolene (Dantrium) is reconstituted with which of the following solutions?
    A. Sterile water for injection
    B. Sterile saline for injection
    C. Sterile Ringer's lactate for injection
    D. Sterile dextrose for injection

13. Epinephrine is commonly added to injectable local anesthetics for which of the following reasons?
    A. Prevents stinging and burning of the tissues
    B. Provides a palpable surgical landmark by plumping up the skin
    C. Dilutes the anesthetic to increase the safety margin of administration
    D. Hemostasis

14. Reprocessing of single-use items is regulated by which organization?
    A. US Food and Drug Administration (FDA)
    B. Centers for Disease Control and Prevention (CDC)
    C. Environmental Protection Agency (EPA)
    D. Association for the Advancement of Medical Instrumentation (AAMI)
15. Which organization oversees the safety of the workplace and has the authority to fine an institution for breaches of safety guidelines?
    A. The Joint Commission (TJC)
    B. Association for the Advancement of Medical Instrumentation (AAMI)
    C. Occupational Safety and Health Administration (OSHA)
    D. Association of periOperative Registered Nurses (AORN)
16. Which endospore is used in the biological indicator for dry heat processing?
    A. *Geobacillus stearothermophilus*
    B. *Bacillus atrophaeus*
    C. *Clostridium perfringens*
    D. *Proteus vulgaris*
17. Which of the following is an early sign of malignant hyperthermia (MH)?
    A. Unexplained tachycardia
    B. Trismus
    C. Elevated body temperature
    D. Convulsions
18. Bipolar electrosurgery does not require the use of an inactive dispersive electrode for which of the following reasons?
    A. The radiofrequency current passes through the active tip of the forceps to the patient's tissue and returns it to the generator through the inactive tip of the same forceps.
    B. The radiofrequency current passes through the bipolar forceps and disperses into the patient's tissues.
    C. The radiofrequency current is very weak and does not need to return to the generator.
    D. The radiofrequency current is applied to tissue only in short bursts and is of no risk for injury to the patient.
19. The Association for the Advancement of Medical Instrumentation (AAMI) recommends that sterile items be stored in a designated area with ventilation and air-conditioning under which conditions?
    A. Humidity >75%, temperature at 75°F
    B. Humidity between 25% and 45%, temperature at 65°F
    C. Humidity between 30% and 70%, temperature <75°F
    D. Humidity between 20% and 50%, temperature <50°F

20. Which of the following is a malignant hyperthermia trigger?
    A. Nitrous oxide
    B. Halothane
    C. Sodium pentothal
    D. Oxygen
21. Improper cleaning and processing of eye instrumentation can cause which of the following conditions?
    A. Glaucoma
    B. Cataracts
    C. Toxic anterior segment syndrome (TASS)
    D. Evisceration
22. The dispersive electrode pad placement during monopolar electrosurgery depends on which of the following for safety?
    A. The electrode is placed over a fleshy area close to the surgical site.
    B. The electrode is cut to fit the area if the patient is smaller than 60 pounds in body weight.
    C. The electrode is repositioned if it becomes lose or fails to stick completely.
    D. The electrode should be applied before the patient is positioned for the procedure.
23. Air exchange in the OR is controlled for atmospheric safety. How many total air exchanges take place per hour in the OR, and how many of these are fresh air from the outside?
    A. 15 total exchanges with 3 fresh air exchanges
    B. 20 total exchanges with 4 fresh air exchanges
    C. 25 total exchanges with 5 fresh air exchanges
    D. 15 total exchanges with 5 fresh air exchanges
24. When not in use, the safest place for the electrosurgical handpiece is in which of the following?
    A. In the handpiece holder attached to the Mayo stand
    B. In the dominant hand of the first assistant for immediate use
    C. In the small basin at the working end of the sterile instrument table
    D. In the fold of the drape at the edge of the incision
25. Why would intraluminal isopropyl alcohol be used during the processing of an endoscope?
    A. To decrease drying time
    B. To remove any residual bioburden
    C. For sterilization of the channels
    D. As a backup to sterilization
26. What is the purpose of the inactive dispersive electrode pad attached to the patient's skin during monopolar electrosurgery?
    A. Returns the radiofrequency current from the active electrode to the generator
    B. Grounds the patient
    C. Prevents electrical shock in team members
    D. Eliminates the risk for surgical burns in the patient

27. Which of the following attire is worn in the unrestricted area of the OR?
    A. Scrub suit and hair cover are required
    B. Cover gown or lab coat should be worn over scrub suit
    C. Scrub suit, mask, and hair cover are required
    D. Street clothes

28. Endoscopic use of electrosurgery is safest when which parameter is followed?
    A. The foot pedal is operated by the user of the cautery device.
    B. The foot pedal is operated by the first assistant.
    C. The metallic electrosurgical forceps are used with a mixed composition trocar and sleeve.
    D. The char on the end of the forceps is dipped in sterile saline.

29. What safety features should be near the disinfection and sterilization areas in case of exposure?
    A. Safety signs
    B. Eyewash and showers
    C. Extra gloves
    D. Lids for chemicals

30. Trendelenburg's position is used for which of the following purposes?
    A. To shift abdominal contents cephalad
    B. To provide a closer working space for general surgical instruments
    C. To provide clear access to the stomach for gastric procedures
    D. To shift the gallbladder into grasping range

31. Antiseptic solutions used for surgical skin cleansing of the face and ears should not contain which of the following chemicals?
    A. Saline
    B. Chlorhexidine (Hibiclens)
    C. Iodophor (Betadine)
    D. Parachlorometaxylenol (PCMX)

32. The patient is positioned for a craniotomy. The anesthesiologist indicates that a venous air embolus is suspected. What immediate actions are taken by the team to alleviate the problem?
    A. The surgery is stopped and the incision closed in rapid succession.
    B. The patient is positioned in reverse Trendelenburg's with the left side elevated.
    C. The patient is positioned in steep Trendelenburg's with the right side elevated.
    D. The surgeon packs the surgical site and calls for an x-ray because the air will look darker than the surrounding tissue.

33. Intestinal stomas are considered contaminated. Which of the following nursing actions is one method for containing and preventing stomal contamination during the surgical procedure for stomal closure?
    A. Cleanse and dry the stoma last and cover with a clear adherent adhesive dressing.
    B. Cleanse the stoma first and cover with a Betadine-saturated gauze sponge.

C. Prep the skin around the stoma without touching the contaminated intestinal tissue.
D. Prep the stoma immediately after the incision line and incorporate the surrounding skin of the abdomen.

34. What is the weight limit of instrument trays for sterilization?
    A. No more than 10 pounds
    B. No more than 15 pounds
    C. No more than 25 pounds
    D. No more than 50 pounds

35. Which endospore is used to test steam sterilization, and when is it used?
    A. *Geobacillus stearothermophilus*, every load
    B. *Geobacillus stearothermophilus*, required weekly, every load with implants
    C. *Bacillus atrophaeus*, weekly
    D. *Bacillus atrophaeus*, daily

36. The patient indicates that she uses herbal preparations for brain circulation and memory improvement. What should the perioperative nurse know about herbs used for this reason?
    A. Most herbs used for this reason can affect the patient's clotting mechanisms.
    B. Herbs such as this are purchased over the counter and have no impact on the surgical procedure.
    C. Many herbs are the cause of thrombosis if the patient is immobile for more than 2 hours.
    D. Herbs are essentially harmless if taken in small quantities.

37. Surgical dyes are used to stain tissue during surgery. Which of the following surgical dyes is also used for intraoperative renal diagnostics?
    A. Methylene blue
    B. Brilliant green
    C. Scarlet red
    D. Gentian violet

38. The anesthesia provider is intubating the patient and indicates that the patient is demonstrating gastric reflux. Which of the following actions is performed by the perioperative nurse to assist with the intubation?
    A. Durant procedure
    B. Valsalva maneuver
    C. Crede maneuver
    D. Cricoid pressure

39. Safe administration of local anesthetics from the sterile field includes which of the following actions of the scrub person?
    A. Labeling the medicine cup and the syringe before the drug is poured
    B. Drawing up the drug as the circulating nurse holds the vial in position for the label to be read by both team members
    C. Removing the needle as soon as the surgeon hands the syringe back
    D. Labeling the medicine cup and the syringe after the drug is poured

40. What is the purpose of a biologic indicator?
    A. To make sure no microorganisms are left in the sterilizer
    B. To make sure the set temperature was achieved
    C. To document that process parameters were met
    D. To determine the length of time to kill endospores

41. The patient is having a gynecologic procedure that will result in several individual specimens of endometrial tissue. What information is important to include on the pathology specimen requisition that will facilitate a correct diagnosis?
    A. Antibiotic use
    B. Last menstrual period date
    C. Marital status
    D. Sexual orientation

42. The patient has had four gallstones removed and the surgeon has ordered these sent to the pathologist for diagnostic testing. The perioperative nurse performs which of the following actions?
    A. The stones would be sent to pathology in a dry cup with a lid.
    B. The stones would be sent to pathology in a cup of 10% formalin with a lid.
    C. The stones would be placed in a cup of Bowen's solution with a lid.
    D. The stones would be placed in a cup of normal saline with a lid.

43. How should peel packs or pouches be sterilized and stored?
    A. Plastic side down
    B. Inside of a tray
    C. Paper side down
    D. On their side

44. Which of the following statements is true concerning patients who are having a surgical procedure while positioned in the prone position?
    A. The patient is positioned and prepped, then anesthetized.
    B. The patient is anesthetized in the lateral position and prepped, then rolled onto the abdomen.
    C. The patient is anesthetized on the operating bed, then turned by the team before they perform the prep.
    D. The patient is anesthetized on the transport cart in the supine position.

45. Reverse Trendelenburg's position is used for which of the following surgical procedures?
    A. Bariatric procedure
    B. LAHV (laparoscopic-assisted vaginal hysterectomy)
    C. Laparoscopic tubal ligation
    D. Spinal fusion

46. Which sterilization process would be utilized if instrumentation is possibly contaminated with prions from Creutzfeldt-Jakob disease?
    A. Soak in hypochlorite solution for 1 hour, steam sterilize for 1 hour at 270°F
    B. Soak in hydrogen peroxide for 30 minutes, steam sterilize for 30 minutes at 270°F
    C. Soak in sterile water for 1 hour, steam sterilize for 1 hour at 270°F
    D. Soak in ethylene oxide for 30 minutes, steam sterilize for 18 minutes at 270°F

47. Placing a supine patient's arms on the armboards can cause nerve damage under what conditions?
    A. Adduction of the arm greater than 10 degrees
    B. Abduction of the arm greater than 90 degrees
    C. Circumduction of the glenoid fossa in a 45-degree circumference
    D. Extension of the shoulder less than 10 degrees

48. The patient is in the operating room (OR) for x-ray contrast studies of the gallbladder. Which of the following is avoided to minimize error in diagnosis?
    A. Shaking the syringe containing the contrast media
    B. Mixing the contrast media with sterile normal saline for injection
    C. Placing the contrast media in a metallic medicine cup on the field
    D. Using room-temperature IV saline as a diluent

49. Which of the following drugs is given intraoperatively as a thrombolytic agent?
    A. Heparin
    B. Warfarin
    C. Protamine
    D. Streptokinase

50. The patient is having an excisional biopsy of her left breast. The surgeon indicates that the specimen needs to go to pathology for a frozen section. Which of the following can best facilitate the frozen diagnostic process?
    A. Sending the specimen in a cup of saline with a lid
    B. Sending the specimen fresh in a cup with a lid
    C. Sending the specimen fresh in a clamp
    D. Sending the specimen in a cup with a few drops of formalin and a lid

51. The patient will have a plaster splint applied to the right arm at the end of the case. Which of the following methods is the correct way to prepare a plaster splint?
    A. The plaster bandage is dipped in cool to tepid water immediately before use.
    B. The plaster is soaked in warm water for 10 minutes before use.
    C. The plaster roll is dipped in warm saline so the patient will not become chilled during the application process.
    D. The plaster bandage is allowed to partially dry before application.

52. Which heated solution provides high-level disinfection (HLD) and sterilization by passing through ultraviolet light and then rinsed with filtered tap water?
    A. Ozone
    B. Ionizing radiation
    C. Peracetic acid
    D. Ethylene oxide

53. A man aged 29 years is having a right inguinal herniorrhaphy. The surgeon has requested a 1-inch Penrose drain. What information should the circulating nurse know about the use of this drain?
    A. The drain is secured to the patient's skin with a 3-0 nylon suture at the end of the case.
    B. A safety pin is attached to the end of the drain during closure.
    C. A half-inch Penrose drain should be available in case the 1-inch drain is too long.
    D. The drain is used during the procedure only as a retractor and is discarded at the end of the case.

54. Which of the following statements best describes when wound class should be assigned for each surgical procedure according to the Centers for Disease Control and Prevention (CDC)?
    A. Wound class is the basis for the selection of a preoperative antibiotic preparation.
    B. Wound class is assigned at the end of the case as a predictor of the risk for postoperative infection.
    C. Wound class is assigned at the start of the case as a prevention of cross-contamination.
    D. Wound class is determined preoperatively to help the team prepare the correct instrumentation for the procedure.

55. A surgical procedure involving entrance into a natural body orifice is classified by the Centers for Disease Control and Prevention (CDC) as which of the following?
    A. Class I
    B. Class II
    C. Class III
    D. Class IV

56. Which of the following cultures renders inaccurate results when exposed to room air?
    A. Aerobic culture
    B. Tissue culture
    C. Anaerobic culture
    D. Bone marrow culture

57. Which recommendations should be followed when preparing items for sterilization and disinfection?
    A. Follow facility policy.
    B. Follow manufacturer's instructions for use (IFU).
    C. Follow Universal Protocol.
    D. Follow the Association for the Advancement of Medical Instrumentation (AAMI) guidelines.

58. The shelf life of sterile packages and instrumentation depends on which of the following?
    A. Time
    B. Process
    C. Date
    D. Related

59. The surgeon plans to do a cell block and washing of the peritoneal cavity. Which of the following statements is true concerning the performance of this procedure?
    A. The surgeon will instill sterile normal saline into the peritoneal cavity. The solution is aspirated and sent to the laboratory for cancer diagnosis.
    B. The surgeon will instill sterile water into the peritoneal cavity. The solution is aspirated and spun down for fibrin content.
    C. The surgeon will instill sterile normal saline into the peritoneal cavity. The solution is aspirated and sent to the radiology department for measurement of the radioactive assay.
    D. The surgeon will instill sterile normal saline into the peritoneal cavity to remove abscessed tissue. The solution is aspirated and discarded before the primary incision is created.

60. The patient is having a frozen section biopsy under local anesthesia. The surgeon indicates that the specimen is to go directly to the waiting pathologist, who will in turn immediately report the results. Which of the following patient care activities can the perioperative nurse implement to minimize the patient's stress in this circumstance?
    A. Provide a warm blanket.
    B. Prevent excess exposure of body parts during the skin prep.
    C. Place a sign on the door indicating that the patient is awake.
    D. Indicate on the pathology slip that the patient is awake.

61. A 62-year-old patient is scheduled for a bone marrow biopsy. Which of the following statements is correct concerning this procedure for this patient?
    A. The specimen will be taken from either the sternum or the iliac crest.
    B. The specimen will be taken from the distal end of the tibia or the femur.
    C. The specimen will be obtained after the administration of radio contrast.
    D. The specimen will be obtained under fluoroscopy to confirm needle placement.

62. The adult patient is scheduled for a tonsillectomy. Which of the following actions would be appropriate for care of the specimens?
    A. The specimens are combined in one cup and covered with saline.
    B. The specimens are sent for gross inspection and discarded.
    C. The specimens are sent in two separate cups labeled left and right.
    D. The specimens are cultured for beta strep.

63. Thrombin is used in the following manner for hemostasis over a large body surface?
    A. Thrombin is used as a topical hemostatic agent.

B. Thrombin is mixed with sterile injectable saline and injected slowly over a period of 3 minutes.

C. Thrombin is titrated by the anesthesia provider.

D. Thrombin is used as a component of intraperitoneal irrigation in the event of hemorrhage.

64. Which of the following is a contraindication for the use of a tourniquet?
    A. Infection in the limb
    B. Hypertension
    C. Geriatric
    D. Amputation

65. Which best describes the definition of sterile?
    A. Free from most microorganisms, but not endospores
    B. Free from endospores and all microorganisms
    C. Free from biofilm
    D. Reduction in microorganisms

66. During carbon dioxide (CO_2) laser use, which of the following safety precautions apply?
    A. Green-colored glasses with side shields, covered windows, and locked doors
    B. Clear plastic or glass eyewear with side shields, no shiny surfaces, and moist drapes around the surgical site
    C. Orange-yellow–colored glasses with side shields, covered windows, and a fiber splitter
    D. Specialized contact lenses and eye-caps on the telescope, covered windows, and a metallic handpiece

67. Which of the following is a porcine hemostatic agent?
    A. Avitene
    B. Surgicel
    C. Gelfoam
    D. Epinephrine

68. For what purpose is a Bowie-Dick test performed?
    A. Confirms the air vacuum is working
    B. Removes debris from the sterilizer
    C. Confirms sterility
    D. Measures internal air pressure

69. Which of the following methods is appropriate for prevention of wrong site surgery according to The Joint Commission?
    A. The site is initialed by the surgeon and validated by the perioperative nurse.
    B. The site is identified by the perioperative nurse and initialed by the patient.
    C. The site is identified by the patient and initialed by the perioperative nurse.
    D. The site is identified by the perioperative nurse and initialed by a second nurse as validation

70. Appropriate sterile attire consists of which of the following?
    A. Scrub suit, gloves, cap, and mask
    B. Gown, gloves, cap, mask, and eyewear
    C. Scrub suit, cap, and mask
    D. Cover gown, shoe covers, and mask

71. Venous pooling in the patient's pelvis is most pronounced in which of the following positions?
    A. Seated
    B. Prone
    C. Lateral
    D. Lithotomy

72. Which of the following is a necessary component of a fire or explosion?
    A. Nitrogen
    B. Oxygen
    C. Hydrogen
    D. Ether

73. What are the three most important factors to remember concerning the safety of the team in the presence of ionizing radiation?
    A. Age of the x-ray machine, shielding, time
    B. Time, shielding, age of the x-ray machine
    C. Time, shielding, distance
    D. Bone penetration, shielding, distance

74. Which chemical processing method produces a gas or vapor to sterilize sensitive items by low-temperature oxidation?
    A. Peracetic acid
    B. Isopropyl alcohol
    C. Hydrogen peroxide
    D. Ionizing radiation

75. Standard Precautions applies to which of the following?
    A. Blood
    B. All body fluids, secretions, and excretions except sweat, regardless of whether they contain visible blood
    C. Mucous membranes and nonintact skin
    D. All of the above

76. Critical items are processed to which degree for patient use according to the Spaulding's classification of the importance of patient care items?
    A. Disinfected
    B. Sterile
    C. Aseptic
    D. Decontaminated

77. Sterility of a packaged item is in question if:
    A. A peel pack was used for a metal object.
    B. The tape on the outer wrapper has more than three stripes.
    C. A stain is seen on the lower end of the wrapper.
    D. The item is sequentially wrapped.

78. Which of the following is not one of the four elements of malpractice?
    A. Abandonment
    B. Duty
    C. Causation
    D. Damages

79. The standard acronym RACE is used in the event of fire in the OR or other patient care areas. Which of the following represents what the acronym stands for?
   A. Remove patients. Activate alarm. Close doors. Extinguish the fire.
   B. Rescue patients. Activate alarm. Contain fire. Evacuate.
   C. Remove fuel source. Activate alarm. Cover burned areas. Exit the area.
   D. Recover patient belongings. Activate alarm. Call for help. Evacuate.

80. In which situation can immediate-use steam sterilization (IUSS) be applied?
   A. To flash a tray for faster turnover time
   B. To sterilize implants
   C. In emergency situations
   D. It should never be used

81. The process of sterilization can best be described as which of the following?
   A. A physical or chemical process rendering an item free from all microbial life and endospores
   B. Use of a steam sterilizer
   C. Decontamination rendering an item safe to handle with bare hands
   D. Chemical process rendering an item free from all microorganisms

82. Which of the following gloving methods is appropriate for inserting a Foley catheter?
   A. Closed gloving
   B. Open assisted gloving
   C. Closed assisted gloving
   D. Open gloving

83. When prepping a patient for a perineal and abdominal surgical approach, which of the following areas should be prepped first?
   A. Perineum
   B. Umbilicus
   C. Lower abdomen
   D. Midline abdomen

84. Which of the following retains its own blood supply?
   A. Allograft
   B. Xenograft
   C. Free flap
   D. Pedicle flap

85. Which of the following best describes the function of the argon beam coagulator?
   A. Monopolar coagulation
   B. Vasoconstriction caused by gas
   C. Mini flame thrower
   D. Bipolar coagulation

86. Heparin does which of the following?
   A. Promotes clots
   B. Prevents clots
   C. Dissolves clots
   D. Mobilizes clots

87. Which of the following is a passive drain?
   A. Hemovac
   B. Penrose
   C. Jackson-Pratt
   D. Sump

88. Sellick's maneuver is also known as which of the following?
   A. Cricoid pressure
   B. Intubation
   C. Extubation
   D. None of these

89. In an ileorectal anastomosis where the stapler is introduced through the rectum, how are the two round specimens labeled when removed from the internal circular stapler?
   A. Together with a suture around the distal specimen
   B. Separately as two specimens marked distal and proximal
   C. Together with a suture around the proximal specimen
   D. None of these

90. Where should used surgical instrumentation cleaning begin?
   A. After the case
   B. In the processing department
   C. At point of use
   D. Wiped before handing up to the sterile field

91. Which two organ systems are closely observed when the patient has low blood pressure?
   A. Cardiac and renal
   B. Neurologic and respiratory
   C. Endocrine and integument
   D. Musculoskeletal and digestive

92. A chemical trigger for malignant hyperthermia is which of the following?
   A. Intravenous narcotics
   B. Nitrous oxide
   C. Nondepolarizing muscle relaxants
   D. Depolarizing muscle relaxants

93. What is the drug of choice for reversal of hypnotic and sedative drugs?
   A. Epinephrine
   B. Atropine
   C. Heparin
   D. Narcan

94. Laparoscopic surgical cases require instrument, sponge, and sharps counts for which of the following reasons?
   A. The case can convert to open very quickly.
   B. The instruments can slip into the puncture site.
   C. The sets can easily get mixed together.
   D. Replacement parts are very expensive.

95. The timed cycle for wrapped instruments processed in a gravity displacement sterilizer should be?
   A. 240°F (115.6°C) exposure for 5 minutes
   B. 250°F (121°C) exposure for 10 minutes
   C. 270°F (132°C) exposure for 25 minutes
   D. 275°F (135°C) exposure for 10 minutes

96. Dry heat is a form of sterilization used for what type of items?
    A. Retractors
    B. Sponges
    C. Talc or glass
    D. Implants

97. Which of the following is true concerning carbon dioxide gas (CO_2) used during inflation for laparoscopy?
    A. Is sterile
    B. Is warm
    C. Contains particulate
    D. Is delivered as a fluid to the patient

98. Epinephrine has which effect on the patient's physiology?
    A. Increases heart rate
    B. Decreases heart rate
    C. Dilates blood vessels
    D. None of these apply

99. Compartment syndrome is treated by which of the following methods?
    A. ACE wrap
    B. Fascial incisions
    C. Plaster casting
    D. Amputation

100. Which of the following is included in the restricted area?
    A. Storage areas for sterile supplies used in the OR
    B. Preoperative holding area
    C. OR director's office
    D. Dressing rooms

101. Which stage of general anesthesia can lead to patient death?
    A. I
    B. II
    C. III
    D. IV

102. Fluid bottles may be recapped and reused under what conditions?
    A. If the fluid is to be warmed
    B. If the bottle is sterile
    C. If the pourer is wearing gloves
    D. Fluid bottles may not be recapped and reused

103. Contrast medium used during a surgical procedure:
    A. Is administered only by anesthesia personnel.
    B. Enhances visualization during diagnostic imaging procedures.
    C. Is tinted for easy identification.
    D. Is used only in full strength.

104. Skin that is taken from an unburned area of a patient and used as a transplant is referred to as which of the following?
    A. Autograft
    B. Homograft
    C. Heterograft
    D. Allograft

105. Which of the following general inhalation anesthetics is not a malignant hyperthermia trigger?
    A. Nitrous oxide
    B. Halothane
    C. Forane
    D. Enflurane

106. When sterilizing a wrapped instrument in a prevacuum sterilizer, what is the appropriate temperature setting and exposure time?
    A. 250°F (121°C) for 30 minutes
    B. 250°F (121°C) for 45 minutes
    C. 270°F (132°C) for 4 hours
    D. 270°F (132°C) for 4 minutes

107. Which is not true about endospores?
    A. They persist on a semicritical item.
    B. They persist on a sterile item.
    C. They persist after high-level disinfection.
    D. They persist after intermediate-level disinfection.

108. Tumescence is performed before which of the following surgical procedures?
    A. Blepharoplasty
    B. Mentoplasty
    C. Liposuction
    D. Rhytidoplasty

109. Bier block anesthesia uses which of the following techniques?
    A. Double tourniquet
    B. Single tourniquet
    C. Elevated head of the operating bed
    D. Cricoid pressure

110. Manufacturers commonly use which low-temperature sterilization process using oxygen and water for plastics, metal, and heat-sensitive items?
    A. Radiation
    B. Ozone
    C. Dry heat
    D. Glutaraldehyde

111. An abnormal filmy attachment of two surfaces or structures that are normally separate is which of the following?
    A. Hemorrhage
    B. Adhesion
    C. Herniation
    D. Fistula

112. The scrub nurse establishes the sterile field by first performing which of the following actions?
    A. Gowning and gloving with the open technique
    B. Gowning and gloving with the closed technique
    C. Gowning and gloving with the assisted open technique
    D. Gowning and gloving with the assisted closed technique

113. Semicritical items are processed to which degree for patient use?
    A. Decontaminated
    B. Sterile
    C. Disinfected
    D. Aseptic

114. Which statement(s) is/are true about sterile persons as they move about in the sterile field?
    A. Pass back to back
    B. Pass face to face
    C. Both of these
    D. None of these

115. Counting sponges, sharps, and instruments at the end of the surgical procedure should be performed in which order?
    A. Mayo stand, incision, table, and off-field sponge receptacle
    B. Off-field sponge receptacle, table, Mayo stand, and incision
    C. Table, Mayo stand, incision, and off-field sponge receptacle
    D. Incision, Mayo stand, table, and off-field sponge receptacle

116. Bier, spinal, and epidural blocks are common types of which form of anesthesia?
    A. Local infiltration
    B. MAC
    C. General anesthesia
    D. Regional anesthesia

117. Eyewear worn as protection during LASER use is determined by which of the following?
    A. Thickness
    B. Color
    C. Optical density
    D. Composition

118. Why should instrumentation taken from a steam sterilizer not be placed on a cold surface?
    A. It may cool to fast.
    B. It may create fog.
    C. Moisture may develop, causing contamination.
    D. It could melt the surface.

119. The toxic level of lidocaine used as a local anesthetic for an average adult is which of the following doses?
    A. 20 mg
    B. 200 mg
    C. 100 mg
    D. 125 mg

120. Which of the following is true regarding the actions of heparin?
    A. It is used to prevent clots.
    B. It is used to break down clots.
    C. It is used to encourage coagulation.
    D. None of these answers apply.

121. Which of the following is used as a topical solution for coagulation at the surgical site?
    A. Heparin
    B. Surgicel

122. Informed consent is obtained by which of the following surgical team members?
    A. Perioperative nurse
    B. Surgeon
    C. Nurse practitioner
    D. First assistant

123. Atropine is administered preoperatively to control which of the following physiologic properties?
    A. Lower blood pressure
    B. Decrease secretions
    C. Prevent vomiting
    D. None of these apply

124. "Balanced anesthesia" refers to the maintenance of which stage of anesthesia?
    A. Stage I
    B. Stage II
    C. Stage III
    D. Stage IV

125. Bacteria forms a protective mechanism known as an endospore that is best destroyed by which process?
    A. Precleaning
    B. Steam under pressure
    C. High-level disinfection
    D. Decontamination

126. Which chemical used for sterilization can be toxic and requires special personal protective equipment (PPE)?
    A. Ethylene oxide
    B. Peracetic acid
    C. Ozone
    D. Hydrogen peroxide

127. How should metal basin sets be sterilized?
    A. Individually
    B. Face down
    C. Face up
    D. On the side, slight lean forward

128. Saline solution should not be used to clean stainless-steel instruments because of which of the following reasons?
    A. Saline will bond with the instrument at a chemical level.
    B. The salt will pit the stainless-steel finish on the instruments.
    C. It may not be available.
    D. It is expensive.

129. What is the process that ensures that all microorganisms including endospores are killed?
    A. High-level disinfection
    B. Asepsis
    C. Enzymatic action
    D. Sterilization

130. A wound expected to heal by primary intention is considered to be which of the following?
    A. Packed wound
    B. Draining incision
    C. Sutured incision
    D. Complicated wound

C. Gelfoam
D. Thrombin

131. Chemical indicators can be placed on the outside and inside of packages. There are different classes. Where is a class 1 indictor placed?
    A. Inside a ridged container
    B. Inside a peel pack
    C. On the outside of all packaging and containers
    D. Inside drapes

132. The safety belt is not used in which of these positions?
    A. Kraske
    B. Supine
    C. Lithotomy
    D. Prone

133. Which person is responsible for the independent actions of the surgical technologist at the sterile field?
    A. Surgeon
    B. Circulator
    C. Surgical technologist
    D. Charge nurse

134. Reverse Trendelenburg's position requires which of the following OR bed attachments?
    A. Shoulder support and pads for the ear
    B. Footboard and thigh strap
    C. Two armboards and adhesive tape
    D. Allen stirrups and four towels

135. Which method of commercial sterilization uses a radioactive isotope?
    A. Cobalt-60
    B. Cobalt-49
    C. Cobalt blue
    D. Cobalt ion

136. Noncritical items should be processed in this manner according to Spaulding's theory of the importance of patient care items?
    A. Have been autoclaved for 3 minutes or more
    B. Have not been sterilized, but high-level disinfected
    C. Have only one wrapper instead of two
    D. Have no need to be sterile at any time

137. The lithotomy position is accomplished by which of the following?
    A. Holding both ankles up so the knees remain straight during the transition
    B. Frog-legging the patient to externally rotate the hip joints first so they will move freely
    C. Raising the legs into stirrups one at a time so the blood pressure remains stable
    D. Two people raising the legs up into stirrups at the same time

138. If adult response to drug therapy is considered the norm, pediatric patients are observed for which difference in response?
    A. There is no variance in response
    B. Unusual responses to some drugs
    C. None of these apply
    D. Decreased responses to some drugs

139. The presence of food or fluid in the stomach during surgery increases the danger to which body system?
    A. Surgical site
    B. Digestive system
    C. Respiratory system
    D. Urinary tract

140. The pediatric patient's mother accompanies him to the OR. She begins to cry as she sees her child go under anesthesia. Why is she having this reaction?
    A. The environment is strange.
    B. The sleep state resembles death.
    C. Her child looks very small and helpless.
    D. All of these apply.

141. The formation of which toxic product can be formed if the preparation and aeration is not done correctly when using ethylene oxide?
    A. Ethylene peroxide
    B. Ethylene glycol
    C. Ethylene dioxide
    D. Ethylene chloride

142. What is the purpose of chemical sterilization indicators?
    A. Verification that the item is sterile
    B. Indicates the parameters of sterilization were complete
    C. Placed in implant trays to verify sterilization
    D. Determines that the item was packaged correctly

143. The pediatric patient is being prepped for a femur fracture. You notice that there are several round, burnlike sores at the base of the patient's buttocks. What is your first action?
    A. Bring this to the attention of the surgeon.
    B. Observe that this may be an abuse situation and you should mind you own business.
    C. Rest assured that someone else will follow up on this finding and complete your sterile setup.
    D. It is probably caused by incontinence and not a concern at this time.

144. How many vials of dantrolene should be stocked to stabilize a patient during a malignant hyperthermia crisis?
    A. 10
    B. 12
    C. 22
    D. 36

145. Pediatric intubation requires which of the following considerations?
    A. Cuffed endotracheal tubes from birth
    B. Uncuffed endotracheal tubes after the age of 8 years
    C. Uncuffed endotracheal tubes before the age of 8 years
    D. No special considerations

146. The pathogenic material responsible for Spongiform encephalopathy is predominately found in which tissue?
    A. Neurologic
    B. Muscle
    C. Bone
    D. Blood

147. The surgeon wants to measure the urine produced by each kidney. Which of the following drainage devices would the nurse prepare?
    A. Foley catheter
    B. Urethral catheter
    C. Ureteral catheter
    D. None of these

148. When inspecting a rigid container before opening, the nurse notices the plastic breakaway locks are missing. What action should be taken?
    A. Open the lid slowly toward the body.
    B. If the lid is tight, use it.
    C. Consider the tray unsterile.
    D. Check the indicator inside.

149. In 2018, the Spaulding's classification regarding endoscopes and instrumentation processing changed. How did the processing recommendation change?
    A. An endoscope and instrumentation should be processed in a steam sterilizer.
    B. An endoscope and instrumentation should be processed with dry heat.
    C. An endoscope and instrumentation should be ozone processed.
    D. An endoscope and instrumentation should be sterile.

150. A pregnant patient is demonstrating hypotension when placed in the supine position. The surgical team positioning the patient can provide hemodynamic support by performing which of the following actions?
    A. Place the patient in reverse Trendelenburg's position.
    B. Place the patient in low Trendelenburg's position.
    C. Elevate the patient's left hip.
    D. Elevate the patient's right hip.

151. Which of the following drugs is used to counteract heparin?
    A. Thrombin
    B. Mannitol
    C. Protamine
    D. Atropine

152. Sterile saline is safe to use for irrigation at which of the following temperatures?
    A. 104°F
    B. 108°F
    C. 115°F
    D. 120°F

153. The circulating nurse records the lot number for implants when used in a patient for which of the following reasons?
    A. To ensure that the correct implant was used
    B. To track the implant in the event of a recall
    C. To record the implant use for inventory replacement
    D. To confirm the implant was safe for use

154. What is the purpose of the Surgical Care Improvement Project (SCIP)?
    A. To prevent positioning injuries
    B. To prevent wrong site surgery
    C. To prevent pressure injuries
    D. To prevent surgical site infection

155. Universal Protocol requires which of the following for every patient having a surgical procedure?
    A. Time out and the use of a checklist
    B. Patient's signature on the OR record
    C. Surgeon's signature on verbal orders
    D. None of the above

156. Which of the following is considered a "never event" by the Centers for Medicare and Medicaid Services (CMS) and is not reimbursable?
    A. Delayed arousal from anesthesia
    B. Retained surgical items (RSI)
    C. Wound class III
    D. Resolved incorrect count

157. Bacterial secretions that persist on infected surfaces and resist antibiotic therapy are referred to as which of the following?
    A. Primary secretions
    B. Differential exudate
    C. Transudate
    D. Biofilm

158. When should the processing of a flexible endoscope begin?
    A. At the point of use, within 4 hours
    B. At the point of use, within 1 hour
    C. At the point of use, within 3 hours
    D. At the point of use, when time permits

159. When a surgical count is incorrect, the first action by the circulating nurse should be which of the following?
    A. Call x-ray.
    B. Inform the surgeon.
    C. Check the trash bin.
    D. Notify the supervisor.

160. A patient experiencing local anesthetic systemic toxicity (LAST) will exhibit which of the following symptoms as a first indicator of a reaction?
    A. Numbness of the lips and tongue
    B. Bradycardia
    C. Sleepiness
    D. Hallucinations

161. A pressure injury assessment does not include which of the following?
    A. Age
    B. Use of handheld retractors
    C. Body mass index (BMI)
    D. Nutrition status

162. What is the purpose of documenting every load number and parameters after sterilization or processing?
    A. To make sure the correct instruments are in the tray
    B. To keep records in case there is a recall or sterilization failure
    C. To make sure all the instruments are returned
    D. To keep track of loaner trays

163. Noise and extraneous commotion should be avoided during which of the following activities?
    A. Phase III of anesthesia
    B. Patient positioning
    C. Emergence from anesthesia
    D. Patient prepping

164. Incapacitated patients need assistance to move from the transport cart to the operating bed. How many personnel are required to move this patient from one surface to another?
    A. 2
    B. 3
    C. 4
    D. 6

165. Which of the following organizations set the standard for reporting of sentinel events?
    A. AAMI (Association for the Advancement of Medical Instrumentation)
    B. NIOSH (National Institute for Occupational Safety and Health)
    C. TJC (The Joint Commission)
    D. APIC (Association for Professionals in Infection Control and Epidemiology)

166. When placing the patient in the supine position, where should the safety belt be secured?
    A. Over the thighs, 2 inches above the knees
    B. Over the abdomen at the level of the iliac crest
    C. Over the anterior tibia, 2 inches below the knees
    D. Over the chest, below the axillary line

167. The Perioperative Nursing Data Set (PNDS) is the standardized language that captures nursing care data in the perioperative environment. Which of the following defines data associated with the PNDS?
    A. Nursing process
    B. Domains that frame the nursing diagnosis
    C. Documentation of nursing intervention
    D. Identification of desired outcomes

168. National Patient Safety Goals (NPSG) are established by which professional organization to promote patient safety in the healthcare environment?
    A. ANA
    B. AORN
    C. CDC
    D. TJC

169. Patients who report a sensitivity to shellfish are likely allergic to which of the following substances?
    A. Iodine
    B. Fish protein
    C. Prep solution
    D. Chlorhexidine

170. Patients positioned in steep Trendelenburg's position are at risk for which of the following complications?
    A. Cerebral edema
    B. Intestinal ischemia
    C. Urinary retention
    D. Foot drop

171. Comorbidities associated with immediate postoperative complications include which of the following conditions?
    A. Allergies and sensitivities
    B. Previous surgical incisions
    C. Cardiorespiratory disease
    D. Urinary tract infection

172. Patient privacy is protected by laws enacted by the Department of Health and Human Services (HHS) branch of the federal government. Which of the following protects the patient's healthcare information?
    A. CDC
    B. FDA
    C. OSHA
    D. HIPAA

173. Implants should be sterilized with a biologic and which class chemical indicator?
    A. Class 2
    B. Class 3
    C. Class 4
    D. Class 5

174. Medication given by the anesthesia provider to decrease intraocular pressure during cataract surgery is which of the following?
    A. Mannitol
    B. Benzodiazepine
    C. Diazepam
    D. Fentanyl

175. Select the best method for transporting contaminated instruments to the processing area?
    A. Instruments soaking in saline in a red bin, inside a case cart
    B. Instruments soaking in sterile water, inside a case cart
    C. Back table covered with a drape
    D. Instruments sprayed with an enzymatic cleaner, sharps secured, placed in a closed cart

176. Which of the following communicable diseases is spread by direct contact?
    A. Mumps
    B. Measles
    C. Hepatitis C
    D. Tuberculosis

177. The patient with a DNR (do not resuscitate) order on file is coming to the OR for placement of a central line. The circulating nurse knows which of the following statements is false?
    A. The patient is having a palliative procedure.
    B. The DNR order is always suspended when a patient comes to the OR.
    C. The patient wants to have the central line inserted to prolong comfort.
    D. The patient wants to make autonomous end-of-life care decisions.

178. The female patient has body piercings. What is the best, understandable explanation the circulating nurse can give to the patient for removing the piercings before the surgical procedure?
    A. The piercings are unattractive.
    B. The piercings will reflect the OR lights, causing distortion of the field.
    C. The piercings could interfere with the electrosurgical device (ESU) used during the procedure.
    D. The piercing could be lost during the procedure.

179. After the lid of a rigid container is opened, what is the next step for validating correct processing parameters?
    A. Hold the container so the scrub nurse can reach the sterile handles.
    B. Place the lid under the opened tray.
    C. Inspect the filters in the lid.
    D. Take the count sheet out of the tray.

180. The patient has donated blood in advance of his scheduled surgical procedure. The circulating knows which of the following is true concerning the use of his blood?
    A. The blood is for autologous use only.
    B. The blood can be used for other patients.
    C. The blood has been typed and cross-matched.
    D. The blood has been frozen for storage.

181. A complication of overheating the patient during the procedure is which of the following?
    A. The surgical procedure will be extended in time.
    B. The patient can lose undetectable fluids through sweat.
    C. The instrumentation will become slippery.
    D. The monitoring devices will not record the vital signs accurately.

182. One feature of the SCIP (Surgical Care Improvement Project) is preoperative administration of antibiotics as appropriate. Which of the following best describes this aspect of the SCIP protocol?
    A. Routine antibiotic administration the night before surgery
    B. Vancomycin administration 2 hours before the incision
    C. Addition of an antibiotic to all irrigation solutions
    D. Administration of Benadryl before antibiotic use to minimize the risk for allergic reaction

183. The patient has signed a declination for the use of blood during surgery for religious reasons. The circulating nurse knows that hypovolemia can be treated by which of the following interventions without violating the patient's wishes?
    A. Plasma infusion
    B. Packed cell infusion
    C. Crystalloid infusion
    D. Vasoconstrictor infusion

184. Which is the proper way to mark an instrument for identification?
    A. Place a colored sticker on the handle before sterilization.
    B. Engrave a name on the handle.
    C. Have a number laser etched on the instrument.
    D. Carve the instrument name on it.

185. Select the correct statement regarding the handling of loaner trays.
    A. Loaner instruments should be delivered to the processing department, inspected, and sterilized.
    B. Loaner instruments can be used if they are unopened and sterile.
    C. Loaner instruments can be sterilized in the delivered containers.
    D. Loaner instruments can be brought in by a vendor and flashed.

186. Which of the following is acceptable for use as a prep in the vagina if the patient has a Betadine sensitivity?
    A. Chlorhexidine in saline
    B. Alcohol in saline
    C. Iodine in saline
    D. Baby shampoo in saline

187. The patient is having a cataract extraction under local anesthesia. During the procedure the patient will have a nasal cannula for oxygen. What risk is apparent to the circulating nurse as the patient is draped?
    A. The patient could suffocate.
    B. The nasal cannula can cause oxygen to accumulate under the drape, causing a fire.
    C. The surgical field could be obscured by the drape.
    D. The drape is too short to protect the surgical site.

188. The surgical procedure requires the use of lead protection because of ionizing radiation used during the procedure. The circulating nurse knows which of the following is true concerning the use and care of lead aprons?
    A. After use, the aprons are folded and stored in the closet.
    B. After use, the aprons are sent to the instrument processing area.
    C. After use, the aprons are hung on hooks to prevent creases and breaks in the lead lining.
    D. After use, the aprons are stored in the radiologist's locker.

189. The electrosurgical unit (ESU) is alarming intermittently. The circulating nurse's first action should be which of the following?
    A. Check the integrity of the dispersive return electrode.
    B. Call the biomed department.
    C. Turn off the power to the ESU.
    D. Turn up the power to increase the current.

190. Which of the following statements is the correct way to handle incoming supplies for storage?
    A. Check the inventory list and place the shipping carton in the designated spot in the sterile core.
    B. Label the shipping carton and stack it on the floor near the substerile room.
    C. Remove all items from the shipping carton and place them in the sterile core.
    D. Place the shipping carton under the sink in the substerile room.

191. The patient is having a total thyroidectomy and parathyroidectomy. What is the physiologic risk to the patient postoperatively when the thyroid and the parathyroid glands are removed?
    A. Unattractive scarring at the neckline
    B. Aversion to iodized salt
    C. Convulsions caused by calcium release
    D. Torticollis associated with adhesions

192. The surgeon is using a tourniquet for the surgical procedure. The circulating nurse should do which of the following actions as the procedure progresses?
    A. Decrease the inflation pressure every 15 minutes.
    B. Inform the surgeon when inflation time has reached 1 hour.
    C. Increase the inflation pressure every 15 minutes.
    D. Inform the surgeon when inflation time has reached 2 hours.

193. The patient is known to be HIV-positive. What precautions should the circulating nurse take to prevent transmission to the surgical team?
    A. Use only disposable supplies for the procedure.
    B. Request extra personnel for patient positioning.
    C. Wear double gloves for the prep.
    D. Proceed with the room preparation as with any other case.

194. The circulating nurse observes that the patient has a dry ulcer on the anterior surface of his right leg. The leg appears pale, white, and hairless. This observation indicates which of the following conditions exists in the patient's leg?
    A. The patient has impaired arterial circulation in the right leg.
    B. The patient has serious heart disease.
    C. The patient has a form of cancer in the leg.

    D. The patient has an injury to the ileo-inguinal canal on the right.

195. Which wound class will be assigned at the end of the surgical procedure when bile leaks into the abdomen during a cholecystectomy?
    A. Class I
    B. Class II
    C. Class III
    D. Class IV

196. Large, powered instruments such as drills and saws may contain which of the following that may not be sterile?
    A. Saw blade
    B. Drill bit
    C. Battery
    D. Reamer

197. The surgeon indicates that he or she will be seated for the surgical procedure. The circulating nurse prepares the room for which of the following scenarios?
    A. Seats for the surgeon and first assistant
    B. Seats for all the sterile team members
    C. Seat for the surgeon only
    D. Seat for the surgeon and the scrub person

198. The intended surgical procedure on the patient's arm will be performed on a hand table attached to the operating bed. How is the patient's arm positioned on the hand table?
    A. The arm is extended 45 degrees onto the hand table.
    B. The arm is circumducted to protect the glenoid fossa.
    C. The arm is abducted 90 degrees onto the table.
    D. The arm is pronated on the table.

199. The abdominal prep boundaries for an abdominal aortic aneurysm procedure are outlined as which of the following?
    A. Begin at the incision line and prep to the periphery.
    B. Begin at the nipple line and prep to the pubis.
    C. Begin with the umbilicus followed by the incision line to the periphery.
    D. Begin with the periphery moving toward the incision line.

200. The abdominal skin has been prepped with an alcohol-based prep. What steps minimize the hazard associated with using this type of prep?
    A. Allow the solution to dry completely before draping.
    B. Dry the surface with a sterile towel before applying drapes.
    C. Allow the solution to pool in the umbilicus to prevent infection.
    D. Cover the prepped area with a fenestrated drape to hasten drying.

201. If a single-use item is reprocessed, what information must be included on the package label?
    A. The reprocessed date and time
    B. The facility where it was reprocessed
    C. Manufacturer's name, lot number, number of times the item was reprocessed
    D. How the item was reprocessed, name of the person who processed it

202. The circulating nurse communicates with the postoperative care nurse at the conclusion of the surgical procedure. The communication during this phase of care is referred to as which of the following?
    A. Postoperative report
    B. Hand-over report
    C. Exchange of assessment
    D. Perioperative data exchange

203. Surgical site closure is defined by three methods employed to promote healing. The approach used for chronic wounds where the skin edges cannot approximate is referred to as which of the following?
    A. Packed wound
    B. Primary closure
    C. Secondary closure
    D. Tertiary closure

204. The abdominal surgical incision site is verified by the patient and the perioperative nurse during the preoperative assessment. Visual confirmation is denoted by which of the following indicators?
    A. The surgeon's initials on the site
    B. The X on the skin
    C. The patient points to the area
    D. The sticker placed over the organ

205. Dantrolene will be administered to a patient during a malignant hyperthermia crisis starting at which dose?
    A. 25 mg/hour
    B. 25 mg/L
    C. 2.5 mg/kg
    D. 25 mL/hour

206. A necessary retractor is accidently dropped on the floor. What action can the circulating nurse take?
    A. Wash the retractor in a designated sink, then flash the retractor in a prevacuum sterilizer for 3 minutes at 270°F.
    B. Clean the retractor in the scrub sink and flash it in the prevacuum sterilizer for 4 minutes at 270°F.
    C. Spray the retractor with enzymatic cleaner, then flash it in the prevacuum sterilizer for 3 minutes at 270°F.
    D. Wipe it with alcohol and return it to the sterile field.

207. Instrumentation placed in a washer-decontaminator goes through which phases?
    A. Rinsing, sterilization
    B. Prerinse, wash, rinse, steam, heat
    C. Prerinse, wash, sterilization
    D. Prerinse, wash, dry, sterilization

208. The boundaries of the surgical scrub include which areas of the hands and arms?
    A. Nails, hands, and arms to the mid-forearm
    B. Nails, hands, and arms to 2 inches above elbows
    C. Nails, hands, and arms to the antecubital fossae
    D. Nails, hands, and arms to the axilla

209. The first assistant is using sponges during electrosurgical use for hemostasis. What consideration for patient safety is the primary concern during this process?
    A. A sponge could be left in the patient
    B. The sponge could ignite if not moistened
    C. The sponge count could be incorrect
    D. The sponge could be too small to be effective

210. Minimizing the risk for particulate in the surgical site prevents adhesions. The use of sponges can generate lint that can enter the patient. How can the scrub nurse minimize the dispersal of lint in the patient?
    A. Moisten the sponges by dipping them into the irrigation basin.
    B. Moisten the sponges by placing them in the irrigation basin before the solution is poured.
    C. Moisten the sponges by using the Asepto syringe before handing to the field.
    D. Moisten the sponges by wringing them out over the irrigation basin before use.

211. The patient is scheduled for a surgical procedure of the right leg. The surgeon plans to use a tourniquet but declines at the last minute because of which of the following contraindications?
    A. History of deep vein thrombosis (DVT)
    B. Anticoagulation therapy
    C. Diabetes
    D. Obesity

212. The patient is having CO_2 laser excision of human papillomavirus (HPV) of the uterine cervix under local anesthesia. The circulating nurse protects the patient from the contaminated plume by which of the following methods?
    A. Placing drapes over the patient's face
    B. Placing a LASER mask over the patient's nose and mouth
    C. Placing extra drapes over the abdomen
    D. Placing an oxygen cannula in the patient's nose

213. The surgeon wants to visualize the patency of the patient's fallopian tubes during a laparoscopic procedure. The circulating nurse should prepare and instill which of the following as directed during the procedure?
    A. Contrast media mixed with sterile saline via a uterine cannula
    B. Monsel's solution mixed with sterile saline via a uterine cannula
    C. Methylene blue dye mixed with sterile saline via a uterine cannula
    D. Acetic acid solution mixed with sterile saline via a uterine cannula

214. The patient will have fluoroscopy for a closed reduction during the surgical procedure. The circulating nurse will provide which of the following for the patient's protection during the use of ionizing radiation?
    A. Lead shields for the gonads, thyroid, and abdomen
    B. Additional drapes as protection from contamination
    C. Radiolucent arm boards
    D. Dosimeter on the patient's gown

215. Which of the following bacteria form endospores that are resistant to sterilization?
    A. Staphylococcus
    B. Streptococcus
    C. Clostridia
    D. Spirochetes

216. The patient is in lithotomy in sling stirrups. Which nerve group is at risk from this position?
    A. Femoral
    B. Peroneal
    C. Inguinal
    D. Tibial

217. The patient has a swollen, red leg with a weeping, anterior tibial ulcer. This observation by the circulating nurse indicates which of the following conditions?
    A. Alcoholism
    B. Diabetes
    C. Crohn's disease
    D. Venous return complications

218. CNOR is the designated credential used when officially certified. What is the significance of these initials?
    A. It means certified operating room nurse.
    B. It means certified perioperative nurse.
    C. It is an acronym.
    D. It is a permanent credential.

219. Patient assessment by the circulating nurse begins with which of the following activities?
    A. Patient identification by name and date of birth
    B. Checking the patient's wristband
    C. Reading the charted notes
    D. Confirming the signature on the consent form

220. The scrub nurse needs to change a contaminated glove during the surgical procedure. The circulating nurse, wearing examination gloves, removes the contaminated glove for the scrub nurse. Which method is appropriate for the scrub nurse to don a new sterile glove?
    A. Closed gloving
    B. Open gloving
    C. Closed assisted gloving
    D. Double gloving

221. A sterile team member needs to change both the contaminated gown and gloves. Which of the following actions is the best approach to reestablish the sterile attire?
    A. Remove the gown before removing the gloves.
    B. Untie the gown and open new gloves on the back table.
    C. Remove gloves followed by the gown.
    D. Remove the gloves, then the gown, and rescrub.

222. The circulating nurse manages metallic forensic evidence using which of the following methods?
    A. The metallic specimen is taken to the laboratory in a metal basin.
    B. The metallic specimen is placed in a plastic cup with saline.
    C. The metallic specimen is placed in a dry plastic cup.
    D. The metallic specimen is given directly to the supervisor.

223. Autologous tissue is taken for reuse by the patient at a later date. The circulating nurse should consider the following best practice when storing the patient's tissue according to facility policy?
    A. The container is placed in a plastic bag.
    B. The container is labeled with the patient's name and date.
    C. The container is immersed in dry ice.
    D. The container is filled with sterile water.

224. The surgeon requests Gelfoam during an open spinal surgery. What property concerning this hemostatic agent should the circulating nurse understand for this type of procedure?
    A. Gelfoam should not be retained in confined spaces.
    B. Gelfoam is only used dry.
    C. Gelfoam is available only in a powdered form.
    D. Gelfoam should be left in place for hemostasis.

225. The patient is scheduled for a surgical procedure using magnetic resonance imaging (MRI). The preoperative nurse should assess the patient for which of following?
    A. Allergy to iodine
    B. Implanted metallic devices
    C. History of hiatal hernia
    D. Sensitivity to general anesthesia

226. An adolescent male is reluctant to remove his underwear and don a gown for surgery. The preoperative nurse should take which of the following actions?
    A. Instruct him to completely undress despite his protests.
    B. Call the main desk and have his parents brought to the preoperative area.
    C. Allow him to wear the gown over his underwear and inform the circulating nurse.
    D. Call the main desk and cancel the surgical procedure.

227. The fire marshal is inspecting the surgical suite. The resulting report indicates which of the following is a violation of safety?
    A. Shelving is 12 inches above the floor
    B. Shelving is 6 inches from the wall
    C. Shelving is layered 24 inches apart
    D. Shelving is 10 inches from the ceiling

228. Anesthesia personnel check the gas machine before each surgical procedure. The circulating nurse should understand which of the following concerning waste anesthetic gas?
    A. The gas is recirculated through the machine.
    B. The exhaled gas from the patient is evacuated via the scavenger capture hose.
    C. The machine does not lose gas into the room air.
    D. The need for excess gas capture has been eliminated by the use of a microprocessor.
229. Which of the following is true about prion contamination?
    A. Prions are transferred via droplets.
    B. Prions are killed via steam under pressure.
    C. Prions can multiply on inanimate surfaces.
    D. Prions are not living and cannot be killed.
230. A capacitative return electrode has which of the following characteristics?
    A. Is positioned under the patient's full body length
    B. Attaches to two limbs
    C. Is only used with bipolar electrosurgery
    D. Is only used with argon beam coagulators
231. What is the primary hazard associated with surgery of the head and neck?
    A. Retained surgical items
    B. Tissue damage from radiation can distort the surgical planes
    C. Fire is an extreme risk when electrosurgery (ESU) is used near or around the airway
    D. Loss of airway control
232. The surgeon requested biologic fibrin sealant. The circulating nurse knows the following about the prepacked delivery unit?
    A. The product is kept on ice until used.
    B. The product is supplied in two syringes.
    C. The product is mixed with 50-mL platelets.
    D. The product is preheated before use.
233. The patient received a packed cell transfusion in the emergency department before arriving in the OR. The circulating nurse assesses the patient and suspects a transfusion reaction. What signs have aroused the nurse's suspicion?
    A. The patient has an elevated body temperature greater than the admitting baseline
    B. The patient is unconscious
    C. The patient seems confused
    D. The patient is complaining of thirst
234. The patient is jaundiced and scheduled for a cholecystectomy. Which of the following conditions can present during the surgical procedure?
    A. Incontinence of the bladder
    B. Hypertension
    C. Hypoglycemia
    D. Impaired coagulation
235. The female patient is having an abdominal surgical procedure that is anticipated to last 4 or more hours. Which set of steps is appropriate for the surgical prep?
    A. Prep the abdomen, the perineum, then insert the Foley using a fresh prep setup.
    B. Prep the perineum, the abdomen, then insert the Foley using a fresh prep setup.
    C. Prep the perineum, insert the Foley, then prep the abdomen using a fresh prep setup.
    D. Prep the abdomen, insert the Foley, and then prep the perineum using one prep setup.
236. Vaccination for communicable diseases is recommended for all healthcare workers. Which of the following diseases is also known as rubella and is spread through droplet transmission?
    A. Chickenpox
    B. Mumps
    C. German measles
    D. Small pox
237. The patient is having a toe amputation for gangrene. The circulating nurse knows the following is true concerning gangrene?
    A. Gangrene is caused by a virus.
    B. Gangrene is caused by a form of clostridia.
    C. Gangrene is caused by ischemia.
    D. Gangrene is caused by cross-contamination.
238. The surgeon requests 1 ounce of a pharmacologic solution. The circulating nurse dispenses how much solution to the scrub nurse's medicine cup?
    A. 30 mL
    B. 20 mL
    C. 15 mL
    D. 10 mL
239. The patient has a fractured femur. Which of the following is a potential life-threatening complication?
    A. Air embolus
    B. Fat embolus
    C. Ileo-inguinal compression
    D. Foot drop
240. The patient is undergoing cataract removal surgery. The surgeon has requested medication to dilate the patient's pupils. The circulating nurse will provide which of the following eye drops for the surgeon's use?
    A. Miotic drops
    B. Mydriatic drops
    C. Fluorescein drops
    D. Viscoelastic drops
241. The surgeon injects the uterus with Pitressin during a hysterectomy. What is the purpose of this drug?
    A. Vasodilation
    B. Hormone suppression
    C. Hypertension control
    D. Vasoconstriction
242. Which of the following hemostatic agents is only used dry?
    A. Gelfoam
    B. Thrombin
    C. Avitene
    D. Silver nitrate

243. The surgeon has requested cultures of the patient's open wound before an incision and drainage (I&D) of an abscess. Which of the following is the best action of the circulating nurse?
    A. Culture the open wound before the site is prepped.
    B. Culture the wound after the site is prepped.
    C. Culture the wound after the abscess is opened.
    D. Culture the site before primary closure.

244. The patient has a deep laceration over the eyebrow. What does the circulating nurse know about preparing the patient's injury?
    A. The eyebrow is shaved.
    B. The eyelashes are trimmed.
    C. The eyebrow is not shaved.
    D. The eyelashes are coated with gel.

245. Which nerve is at risk during parotid gland surgery?
    A. Mastoid
    B. Facial
    C. Auricular
    D. Hypoglossal

246. The patient is having a split-thickness skin graft (STSG). The surgeon plans to expand the graft to cover more of the denuded area. Which process will the surgeon likely use to cover a large area with a small tissue sample?
    A. Free-hand graft
    B. Dermatome
    C. Mesher
    D. Braithwaite blade

247. The pediatric patient is having a cheiloplasty. The circulating nurse knows that this surgical procedure corrects which of the following congenital conditions?
    A. Cleft palate
    B. Baby bottle teeth
    C. Microtia
    D. Cleft lip

248. The patient is scheduled for a Bristow procedure. What position will be used for the patient's surgical procedure?
    A. Beach chair semi-Fowler's
    B. Supine with extra padding under the surgical site
    C. Lateral, with the surgical site elevated
    D. Prone, with the arms on armboards

249. The patient has a parathyroidectomy during a thyroidectomy. The parathyroid glands are saved for physiologic use by which of the following methods?
    A. Flash frozen for further studies
    B. Cut into small pieces and implanted in the patient's forearm
    C. Preserved in Bowen's solution
    D. Chilled in sterile saline for 2 hours after removal

250. The surgeon plans to use a postoperative suprapubic catheter. The circulating nurse knows which of the following is true about the use of this catheter?
    A. The patient will have a total cystectomy as part of the procedure.
    B. A urostomy will be created using the patient's ureters.
    C. Fluid is instilled into the bladder and the catheter is inserted in the lower abdomen.
    D. The catheter will be inserted using a nephroscope.

251. Which of the following drugs will be given by the anesthesia provider to reverse the effects of a nondepolarizing muscle relaxant?
    A. Neostigmine
    B. Narcan
    C. Tracrium
    D. Pavulon

252. During setup for the surgical procedure, when is the best time for the circulating nurse to open and dispense the dressings to the sterile field?
    A. After the initial count
    B. After the time out
    C. After the incision is made
    D. After the final closing count

253. The World Health Organization (WHO) is in place for which of the following purposes?
    A. To set health standards in the United States
    B. To promote universal health and wellness
    C. To enforce health standards in third world countries
    D. To globally monitor surgical practice

254. The surgeon requests a flat plate of the abdomen before the surgical procedure. What is a flat plate?
    A. A flat plate is an x-ray that uses nonionic contrast.
    B. A flat plate is an x-ray that uses ionic contrast.
    C. A flat plate is also known as a KUB (kidneys, ureters, and bladder) x-ray without contrast.
    D. A flat plate is also known as a KUB x-ray with contrast.

255. The circulating nurse is weighing sponges to estimate blood loss. The scale is balanced to account for extraneous weight of materials and irrigation. Which of the following is correct for estimating blood loss?
    A. 1 g = 1 mL
    B. 2 g = 1 mL
    C. 0.5 g = 1 mL
    D. 1.5 g = 1 mL

256. The circulating nurse adds a pack of hemostats to the sterile field at the request of the scrub nurse. Before delivering the instruments to the field, the circulating nurse does which of the following?
    A. Records the date and time of sterilization
    B. Asks the scrub nurse to count the number of hemostats currently present on the sterile field
    C. Inspects the package for integrity
    D. Records the number of hemostats being given to the scrub nurse

257. The circulating nurse prepares chest rolls for the patient's prone procedure. The placement is necessary for which reason?
    A. To elevate the spine for visualization of the surgical site
    B. To decrease pressure on the vena cava
    C. To protect the patient's genitalia
    D. To relieve the respiratory system

258. When should the patient's prep begin?
    A. Immediately after positioning
    B. After gowning and gloving
    C. After the anesthesia provider indicates the patient is stable
    D. As soon as the setup is completed by the scrub nurse

259. The patient is having a laminectomy. Where should the dispersive return electrode be positioned on the patient's body?
    A. On the patient's posterior thigh
    B. On the patient's biceps
    C. On the patient's gastrocnemius
    D. On the patient's chest

260. During the initial sponge count, the packaged number of the contents is wrong. What should the circulating nurse do to minimize error in the final count?
    A. Document the number and continue the count.
    B. Isolate the pack of sponges in a plastic bag and place it on the circulator's desk.
    C. Throw the pack of sponges in the clean trash bin for recycling.
    D. Add an additional sponge to make the count correct.

261. The patient is admitted directly from the emergency department. The emergency procedure begins as soon as the patient is placed on the OR bed. An initial count was not performed. At the conclusion of the surgical procedure, what should the circulating nurse do?
    A. Attempt to count as the procedure proceeds.
    B. Do not add any extra sponges to the sterile field.
    C. Add only 10 sponges at a time to the sterile field.
    D. Request an x-ray when the procedure is complete.

262. The pediatric patient is going to postanesthesia care unit (PACU) after a tonsillectomy. The best position for the child during transport is which of the following?
    A. In high Fowler's position
    B. Supine
    C. On the left side
    D. Seated

263. The C-arm will be used for the orthopedic extremity procedure. What can the circulating nurse do to protect the patient?
    A. Place lead shielding over the patient.
    B. Place lead shielding under the patient.
    C. Place lead shielding over the patient's thyroid.
    D. Place lead gonad shield over the patient's groin.

264. During an abdominal aortic aneurysm repair surgery, the surgeon may ask the circulating nurse to perform which action?
    A. Periodically check bilateral pedal pulses on the patient.
    B. Call the family to give updates every 15 minutes.
    C. Pour warm sterile saline into the surgical site.
    D. Inflate the tourniquet over the thighs.

265. The patient has been to x-ray for a needle localization biopsy. The circulating nurse performs the prep with the following in mind?
    A. The wire is removed immediately before the prep and discarded in the sharps box.
    B. The wire must remain in situ for accurate diagnosis.
    C. The wire can be bent to the medial side of the chest wall to facilitate the prep.
    D. The wire is not sterile and could contaminate the prepped area.

266. The patient is in lithotomy. The circulating nurse knows that hypotension can be minimized by which of the following actions?
    A. One leg at a time is removed from the stirrups and placed on the OR bed.
    B. Both legs are removed from the stirrups by two personnel and slowly lowered to the OR bed.
    C. The stirrups are lowered to the level of the OR bed before moving the legs to the OR bed.
    D. The patient is frog-legged before placing the legs on the OR bed.

267. Which type of local anesthesia is appropriate for a circumcision?
    A. 1% lidocaine plain
    B. 0.25% Marcaine with Wydase
    C. 1 % lidocaine with epinephrine
    D. 2 % Pontocaine plain

268. Which of the following measures should the circulating nurse follow when the patient is in the prone position?
    A. Ask the transporter to stand by for the specimen delivery.
    B. Position the crash cart near the door.
    C. A transport cart should be immediately available in case of the need to place the patient supine during an emergency.
    D. Provide a headlamp for the surgeon.

269. The patient is positioned supine with arms tucked in at the sides. Which of the following is the appropriate method of securing the arms with a drawsheet?
    A. The drawsheet extends over the elbows and is tucked under the mattress.
    B. The drawsheet encases the hands and forearms and is tucked under the mattress.
    C. The drawsheet cases the hands and forearms and is fan folded next to the patient.
    D. The drawsheet extends over the elbows and is tucked under the patient.

270. The patient will have a Foley inserted before the skin prep. The circulating nurse does which of the following before catheterizing the patient?
A. Asks the patient to void in the preoperative area
B. Pretests the Foley balloon
C. Positions the patient and prepares the Foley insertion supplies
D. Gowns and gloves using the closed gloving technique

271. The surgeon instructs the circulating nurse to label the specimen as a bezoar. What is this?
A. An ingested hairball
B. A staghorn stone
C. A tumor from the small intestine
D. A thyroglossal duct cyst

272. Which of the following practices decrease the risk for biologic exposure during a needlestick?
A. Rinsing the gloves with betadine
B. Double gloving
C. Using an alcohol-based hand hygiene product
D. Using a brush method scrub for the first scrub of the day

273. Which of the following is the most common cause of surgical site infection?
A. *Streptococcus*
B. *Escherichia coli*
C. *Staphylococcus aureus*
D. *Pseudomonas*

274. The patient has a wound infection scheduled for debridement. The defect cannot be sutured at the initial procedure but is planned for a few days later. What closure method will be used?
A. Primary closure
B. Secondary intention
C. Retention sutures
D. Delayed primary closure

275. The surgeon requests antibiotic irrigation in sterile saline. The circulating nurse prepares the medication in which manner?
A. Draws the medication into a syringe and expresses the drug into the irrigation basin through the needle
B. Draws the medication into a syringe and expresses the drug into the bottle of sterile saline before pouring to the sterile field
C. Pops the top of the vial and pours the drug into the sterile irrigation basin on the sterile field
D. Draws the medication into a syringe, removes the needle, and expresses the drug into the irrigation basin

276. The OR is equipped with laminar airflow. The circulating nurse knows that the purpose of this airflow is which of the following?
A. Provides ultra-clean filtered air for the sterile field
B. Removes particulate from the sterile field
C. Maintains the patient's body temperature
D. Sterilizes air before it reaches the sterile field

277. A potential complication associated with prone position is which of the following?
A. Epistaxis
B. Ocular ischemia
C. Deafness
D. Torticollis

278. The anesthesia provider uses capnography to monitor the patient. Which of the following parameters is observed using this method?
A. Carbon dioxide
B. Oxygen
C. Lactic acid
D. Acidosis

279. Which of the following methods is unsafe for delivering medications to the sterile field?
A. Pouring irrigation solution into a basin on the sterile field.
B. The circulating nurse draws the drug into a syringe before dispensing to the medicine cup.
C. The circulating nurse holds the vial while the scrub nurse pierces and withdraws the drug.
D. The circulating nurse dispenses the presterilized glass ampule to the sterile field.

280. When positioning a patient, which of the following does not provide a pressure reduction surface?
A. Gel pad
B. Towel roll
C. Egg crate foam
D. Memory foam mattress

281. Which of the following is correct for positioning the supine patient's legs?
A. Flex the knees 5–10 degrees on a pillow.
B. Place a safety strap over the tibia.
C. Maintain the heels in contact with the bed.
D. Flex the bed at the knee.

282. Which of the following is not a method of preventing hypothermia in the patient?
A. Place a forced air warming drape over the patient.
B. Place a blanket from the warming cabinet over the patient.
C. Place a warming blanket under the patient.
D. Pour warm irrigation into the scrub nurse's sterile basin.

283. The legs of a patient in a seated position should be arranged in which manner?
A. Frog-legged
B. Knees flexed 30 degrees
C. Straight
D. Abducted 10 degrees

284. Which of the following is a potential source of pressure injury during positioning?
A. Peripheral IV
B. Implanted pacemaker device
C. Dentures
D. Artificial nails

285. The patient is positioned laterally. Which of the following considerations is the best position for the legs?
    A. The upper leg is straight.
    B. The lower leg is straight.
    C. The upper leg is flexed.
    D. The lower leg is elevated.
286. When using kidney braces in the lateral position, which of the following is the correct placement?
    A. The shorter brace is placed anterior.
    B. The shorter brace is placed adjacent to the longer brace.
    C. The longer brace is placed anterior.
    D. The longer brace is placed posterior.
287. Which of the following best describes the padding under the patient in a lateral position?
    A. A chest roll under the thorax from axilla to iliac crest
    B. A blanket roll under the thorax above the diaphragm
    C. An axillary roll under the thorax at the level of the seventh to ninth rib
    D. A gel pad under the patient's neck above the clavicle
288. When the patient is prone, the arm boards should be in which position related to the patient's body?
    A. Even with the patient's chest
    B. Slightly lower than the patient's chest
    C. Even with the OR bed
    D. Angled greater than 45 degrees to the patient's body
289. The surgeon requests bilateral ureteral stent placement before performing an abdominal hysterectomy. What is the rationale for this additional procedure?
    A. Identification of the ureters during dissection
    B. Instillation of antibiotic irrigation
    C. Urinary measurement intraoperatively
    D. Injection of methylene blue
290. During an emergency in the OR, which of the following assessment notations facilitates prompt treatment of the patient's crisis?
    A. Notation of the chronologic age of the patient
    B. Notation of the location of the waiting family
    C. Notation of the patient's religion
    D. Notation of the patient's weight in kilograms (kg)
291. The patient has a penicillin allergy. Which of the following antibiotics is safe for use with this patient?
    A. Ampicillin
    B. Ciprofloxacin
    C. Amoxicillin
    D. Ticarcillin
292. When transporting a patient with chest tubes, which of the following is appropriate for managing the tubes during transport to the PACU?
    A. Clamp the tubes.
    B. Disconnect the tubing.

C. Keep the drainage receptacle below the chest.
    D. Drain the water from the collection unit.
293. Administration of large quantities of fluids during an emergency surgical procedure requires which of the following access lines?
    A. Central line
    B. Arterial line
    C. Additional peripheral line
    D. Arteriovenous shunt
294. The patient has thoracic outlet syndrome. Which of the following surgical procedures is performed to alleviate the patient's symptoms?
    A. Resection of the clavicle
    B. Resection of the first rib
    C. Resection of the anterior mediastinum
    D. Resection of the cervical nerve plexus
295. The patient is having a rhytidectomy. Which procedure is performed on the patient?
    A. Microdermabrasion
    B. Laser resurfacing
    C. Blepharoplasty
    D. Face lift
296. Precautions when using polymethylmethacrylate (PMMA) for the team include which of the following?
    A. Avoid wearing contact lenses.
    B. Avoid bright lights.
    C. Avoid moving about in the sterile field.
    D. Avoid glove changes.
297. The surgeon is performing an embolectomy. Which device will be requested for the completion of the surgical procedure?
    A. Guidewire
    B. A 20-cc syringe
    C. Fogarty catheter
    D. A swivel knife
298. The surgeon is performing a rhinoplasty. Which of the following drugs is drawn into the syringe for hemostasis?
    A. Thrombin
    B. Afrin
    C. Lidocaine with epinephrine
    D. Epinephrine
299. When obtaining a sterile package from the sterile core, the circulating nurse checks the date on the label under which circumstances?
    A. The package contains mixed media metals.
    B. The package contains a drug.
    C. The package is wrapped in woven fabric.
    D. The package is wrapped in paper.
300. During CO_2 laser surgery of the throat, the endotracheal tube begins to burn. The first action taken to manage the situation is which of the following?
    A. Stop the anesthetic gas.
    B. Pour sterile saline into the mouth.
    C. Decrease the oxygen flow.
    D. Remove the endotracheal tube.

301. What is the meaning of the term *iatrogenic*?
  A. An event happens to a patient randomly
  B. An event happens to a patient as a result of treatment
  C. An event happens to a patient who resists treatment
  D. An event happens to a patient with drug tolerance

302. Laboratory values between male and female patients vary in which of the following results?
  A. Differential
  B. Platelets
  C. Red counts
  D. Blood pH

303. The differential blood value refers to which of the following?
  A. Prothrombin and partial thromboplastin times
  B. Values of the various white cells
  C. Liver enzymes
  D. Electrolytes

304. The patient has a myelodysplastic disease. Which of the blood cell components is measured to monitor the progression of the disease?
  A. White blood cells
  B. Red blood cells
  C. Lymphocytes
  D. Platelets

305. Which of the following laboratory values is cause for alarm?
  A. Potassium 3.7
  B. Calcium 12.6
  C. Glucose 98
  D. Sodium 138

306. The patient arrives in the preoperative holding area with a hematocrit of 50%. What is the significance of this laboratory value?
  A. This value is within normal limits.
  B. The patient has a bleeding disorder.
  C. The patient is anemic.
  D. This value is high.

307. The patient has a white cell count of 18,000. What is the implication of this laboratory value?
  A. The patient has an alcohol dependency.
  B. The patient is diabetic.
  C. The patient may have an infection.
  D. The patient is hyperthermic.

308. The patient is admitted with acute pancreatitis. Evaluation of the patient's laboratory results includes an elevation in which of the following values?
  A. Eosinophils
  B. Amylase
  C. Basophils
  D. Troponins

309. Which of the following potassium values is not within normal limits?
  A. 2.5 mmol/L
  B. 3.7 mmol/L
  C. 4.6 mmol/L
  D. 5.1 mmol/L

310. The diabetic patient has a glucose fingerstick test in the preoperative holding area. Which of the following test results is cause for concern and should be reported to the anesthesia provider and the surgeon?
  A. 82
  B. 94
  C. 100
  D. 225

311. The adult patient's platelet count is 100,000 mm^3. What can this value indicate?
  A. The count is within normal limits.
  B. The count is high.
  C. The count is slightly low.
  D. The count must be repeated to confirm.

312. Which of the following white blood cells measured in the differential may indicate an allergic reaction?
  A. Lymphocytes
  B. Monocytes
  C. Basophils
  D. Eosinophils

313. During the surgical procedure, the anesthesia provider sends blood to the laboratory for a hemoglobin and hematocrit (H&H) value. Which of the following levels is a cause for concern?
  A. Hemoglobin 13, hematocrit 45%
  B. Hemoglobin 10, hematocrit 30%
  C. Hemoglobin 15, hematocrit 40%
  D. Hemoglobin 12, hematocrit 46%

314. Arterial blood gases (ABG) are taken to measure which of the following aspects of the patient's condition?
  A. Oxygen and carbon dioxide values
  B. Status of blood loss
  C. Cerebral perfusion
  D. Peripheral perfusion

315. Which of the following ABG values may indicate metabolic acidosis?
  A. pH 7.25
  B. pH 7.40
  C. $Paco_2$ 48
  D. $Paco_2$ 44

316. Which of the following blood test values indicate a higher risk for blood loss during the surgical procedure?
  A. High hemoglobin and hematocrit (H&H)
  B. Elevated differential
  C. Low electrolytes
  D. Prolonged prothrombin time (PT) and partial thromboplastin time (PTT)

317. The morphology of the patient's red blood cells indicates the presence of nuclei. What does this mean to the patient's physiologic condition?
  A. The patient is healthy.
  B. The patient is utilizing available oxygen.
  C. The red cells cannot carry oxygen.
  D. The red cells are full of CO_2.

318. The patient is jaundiced on arrival to the OR. The circulating nurse checks the laboratory work and assesses the patient. Which laboratory value is commonly elevated for patients with this condition?
    A. Serum sodium
    B. Bilirubin
    C. Platelets
    D. pH

319. The patient has a history of sickle cell disease. The circulating nurse will assess the patient for which of the following during the preoperative assessment?
    A. Painful joints
    B. Difficulty swallowing
    C. Pallor
    D. Hypotension

320. Which of the following drugs adversely affects wound healing?
    A. Diuretic use
    B. Steroid use
    C. Analgesic use
    D. Hormone use

321. The female patient indicates she takes oral contraceptives. The circulating nurse knows that the patient is at risk for which of the following complications?
    A. Hemorrhage
    B. Infertility
    C. Thrombus
    D. Infection

322. The patient has been taking diuretics for several months. The circulating nurse will commonly find which of the following changes in the patient's preoperative laboratory work?
    A. Low hemoglobin and hematocrit
    B. Low electrolytes
    C. High sodium
    D. High potassium

323. The trauma patient arrives unconscious directly to the OR on arrival. The circulating nurse is not able to fully assess the patient. No family is available for questioning. The patient's condition requires anesthesia administration to make the following assumption during intubation?
    A. The patient is expectant and will die in the OR.
    B. The patient will arouse enough before anesthesia is administered.
    C. The patient will need a tracheotomy.
    D. The patient may have a full stomach and will need cricoid pressure.

324. The patient is a victim of assault and has been shot by an unknown assailant. The patient arrives at the OR fully clothed. The circulating nurse helps to preserve potential evidence by which of the following actions?
    A. Cutting out the bullet holes in the clothing and placing the cut pieces into a plastic bag
    B. Rinsing the area with sterile saline before undressing the patient
    C. Leaving the clothing on the patient and cutting open the area around the surgical site
    D. Removing the clothes by cutting along the seams and placing into a paper bag

325. The patient is an infant who had a few sips of water a few hours before surgery. The circulating nurse knows which of the following concerning the infant's preoperative oral intake?
    A. The sips of water will be of no consequence.
    B. The surgery will be cancelled.
    C. The surgery will be delayed for 6 hours.
    D. The patient will have a nasogastric tube inserted before intubation.

The Perioperative Nursing Roles

Role of the Scrub Person as Part of the Sterile Team

Prepares
- Sterile instruments and supplies
- Works in concert with the circulating nurse to set up the operating room (OR)
- Surgeon's specific procedural needs
- Procedure-specific needs
- Hemostatic techniques
- Suture and closure materials

Sterile Technique
- Scrubs, gowns, and gloves using the closed gloving method
- Establishes the sterile field
- Facilitates the surgical procedure
- Anticipates the needs of the sterile team
- Gowns other team members using the open assisted gowning and gloving technique

Adaptability
- Participates in preincision time out
- Remedies any breach of sterile technique

- Requests and prepares material needed by surgeon
- Keeps the sterile field neat and functional

Accountability
- Establishes baseline counts with circulating nurse
- Informs the circulating nurse of items placed inside patient
- Double-checks items dispensed to the sterile field
- Labels all medication containers and delivery devices
- Reports volume of drug administered to patient for documentation by circulating nurse

Safety
- Manages sharps
- Prevents retained foreign objects in the patient
- Reconciles counts and is accountable for items used in the surgical procedure

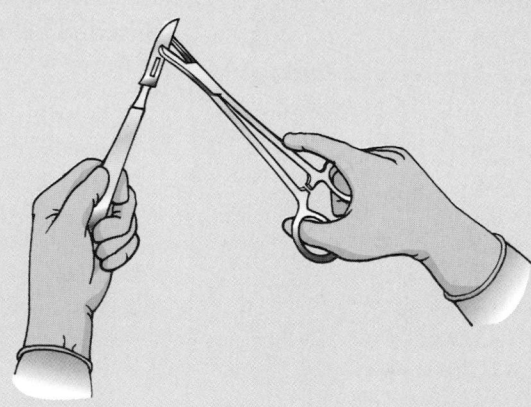

Role of the Circulating Nurse as Part of the Nonsterile Team

Indirect Patient Care
- Assists with OR preparation
- Opens sterile supplies
- Prepares medication for use in OR
- Maintains patient confidentiality
- Communicates with surgical services personnel
- Pretests equipment
- Plans postoperative care
- Initiates discharge planning

Direct Patient Care
- Patient identification
- Patient assessment
- Identifies correct surgical site
- Transfers patient between cart and bed
- Participates in preoperative time out procedure
- Assists the anesthesia provider
- Provides skin antisepsis
- Provides thermoregulation
- Prevents electrosurgical injury
- Collaborates with patient fluid intake and output
- Monitors vital signs as needed
- Provides dressings and drains

Coordinates
- Plans for each member of the sterile team to enter the sterile field
- Positioning, prepping, and draping
- Connection of surgical machinery

- Laboratory tests
- Multidisciplinary teams
- Diagnostic activities
- Emergency response to patient crisis
- Communication with patient's significant others

Anticipates
- Sequence of the procedure
- Needs of the sterile team
- Breaches of sterile technique
- Hemostatic needs
- Radiation (ionizing and nonionizing) protection for sterile team
- Potential for patient's physiologic changes
- Wound class at conclusion of the procedure
- Patient responses to care
- Significant other's response to patient's condition

Accountability
- Participates in time out
- Validates implants
- Documents patient care
- Specimen care and reporting
- Promotes a culture of safety
- Accountability for instruments, sponges, and sharps
- Patient's advocate
- Evaluates patient outcomes
- Provide handoff report to perianesthesia nurse

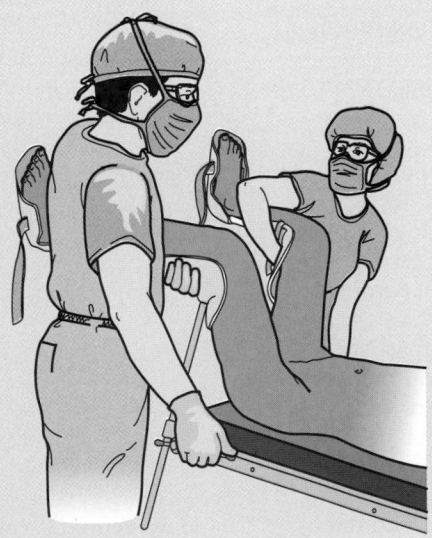

Systematic Activities for the Scrub Person

Baseline Systematic Activity	Systematic Critical Thinking Activity
Room Setup • Plan for patient to enter the room without contaminating the setup. • Plan for position of patient, surgeon, and anesthesia provider.	Determine the position of the surgeon and preference for positioning of the scrub person before setting up table.
Case Cart Contents • Instrument set(s) • Custom pack • Gowns • Sterile towels • Prep supplies • Additional soft goods	Check cart contents. Inspect package integrity. Check for each item listed on case cart sheet. Record preference changes on case cart sheet for computer update.
Items to Have Available • Suture • Sponges • Pack of towels • Gloves • Staplers • Dressing	Have extra preferred suture in the room. Extra sponges may be needed.
Table Setup • Open the main custom drape pack. The outer wrapper is the sterile table drape. • Determine which part of the table will be closest to the draped patient and establish this area as the working end of the table. Sharps and sutures should be opened onto this location. • Open remaining items into a position of function. Inspect package integrity. • Do not open items into closed container system. Edges are unsterile. • Don eyewear. • Open gown and gloves for self before performing hand and arm cleansing. • Don gown and gloves using closed glove procedure. Remember to tie in. • Set up the working end of the table according to position of patient. • Plan to pass off cords in one direction. • Sterile marker and labels are placed on the sterile instrument table near the working end. • Place items once. Do not leave trash on the field.	The surgical site on the patient is the "ground zero" for the establishment of the level of the sterile field. Stack drapes in order of use and place away from main instrument setup area of sterile table. Create towel roll(s) for instrument stringers. Align stringer on the roll with shortest instruments closest to the working end of the table. Instrument ratchets are open on the table and closed on the Mayo stand. Establish baseline: Count instruments, sharps, and sponges with circulating nurse. Plan for exchange of scalpel by no touch technique.
Mayo Stand Setup • Drape the Mayo stand. Cover surface with one unfolded towel to protect from perforation by sharps. A towel roll can be used to organize instruments on the Mayo stand.	Mayo setup: 2 scalpels, 3 scissors (1 curved and 1 straight Mayo and 1 Metzenbaum), 4 curved Crile hemostats, 2 medium pickups, 4 Allis forceps, and 2 small skin retractors (Army-Navy) 2 light handles, suction tubing and suction tip (Yankauer), electrosurgical unit (ESU) pencil and holder, tip cleaner, and sponges
Medication and/or Chemicals on the Sterile Instrument Table • Place medication cups near edge of field. • Validate all medications and solutions with circulating nurse and then apply labels.	Label syringes and administration devices after the solution or medication has been dispensed to the field. Do not label ahead of time because the wrong drug or solution could be poured. Label states name of product and percent.

(Continued)

Systematic Activities for the Scrub Person—cont'd

Baseline Systematic Activity	Systematic Critical Thinking Activity
Irrigation and Fluids on the Sterile Instrument Table • Place basins near edge of sterile field. Label is applied after the solution is poured. • Label all delivery devices.	Normal saline or other solution for irrigation Sterile water for instrumentation
Patient Positioning • Stand clear and remain sterile, because positioning is a nonsterile activity.	Note the presence of safety restraints and padding as the second set of eyes. Drapes and blankets can obscure safety straps.
Team Gowning • Assist team to gown and glove using the open assisted or closed assisted method. • Contaminated gloves are changed using the open method. Circulating nurse will remove contaminated gloves. Scrub person will reglove the individual.	Do not pass any towels or gowns from the sterile field during the procedure. Biologic contamination is present.
Patient Draping • Prep solution must be completely dry. • Patient is draped to establish the level of the sterile surgical field before instrument tables are positioned for use.	Some surgeons use towel clips to secure drapes. Nonperforating styles are preferred. Some surgeons suture or staple specialty drapes in place.
Procedure Start and Flow • Position Mayo stand. • Position sterile instrument table. • Hand off ESU cords, tubing, and cables to circulating nurse. • Apply light handles. • Place two sponges on field adjacent to incision. • Provide scalpel for skin (place skin knife aside on working end immediately after use; disarm and reload as time permits). • Provide ESU for hemostasis (keep in holder when not in use). • Clean the ESU pencil tip. • Keep instrumentation free of debris with moist sponge. • Trade one for one sponges and needles. • Open soiled sponges completely before discarding into sponge bucket.	Initiate time out before skin scalpel is provided. • Correct patient • Correct site • Correct procedure Inform circulating nurse if any uncounted item has been brought into the surgical field. Reconcile all counts by starting at the patient and working toward Mayo stand and then to instrument table. Count sponges and sharps at each cavity within cavity closure. Do closing counts of sponges, sharps, and instruments during surgical site closure. Contain pathology specimen in closed container as much as possible before passing to gloved circulating nurse.
Dressings and Drains • Double-check type of dressing material before circulating nurse dispenses to field. • Dressing is placed over surgical site after incision is cleaned. • Disconnect tubing and cords from field. • Drapes are removed by rolling them off and away from the patient after placement of the surgical site dressing.	Wet sponge followed by dry sponge to clean closed incision. Wound closure strips may be placed over subcuticular closure. Dressing is positioned over cleaned incision before removal of drapes. Skin surrounding the dressing area is cleaned with wet and dry sponges before tape is applied.
Procedure Completion All reusable instruments are opened or disassembled and placed in bins for decontamination in the processing area. Enzyme solution or foam may be applied before transit.	Remove the Bovie tip and place in sharps container. Disarm scalpels. Open all instrument ratchets and box locks, and place in mesh tray.

(Continued)

Systematic Activities for the Scrub Person—cont'd

Room Breakdown	Trash Disposal
• When patient leaves the room, the table can be broken down completely. • Dispose of sharps in sharps container. • Remove light handles. • Case cart is reloaded with used instrument trays and reusable equipment. • Don examination gloves after removing gown and gloves, and washing hands. • Transport the case cart to the processing area.	Dispose of biologic trash in biohazard containers. Dispose of clean trash in regular garbage receptacle. Dispose of linens in hampers. Remove contaminated gown first followed by gloves using peel-off glove-to-glove–skin-to-skin method. Wash hands with soap and water after removing gloves. Clean all case-specific equipment with antiseptic and return to storage.

Systematic Activities for the Circulating Nurse

Baseline Systematic Activity for All Cases	Systematic Patient Care
Patient Assessment and Safety • Assess for patient identity and correct site information concerning the planned procedure; note the presence of correct site markings • Assess physiologic and psychological status • Laboratory work • Current medications and herbals • Allergies and sensitivities • Last intake by mouth • Location of family or significant other	Talk to the patient and determine understanding of the procedure. Observe surgeon's initials on surgical site. Follow facility policy concerning difficult to mark sites. Check the paperwork/chart/computer for consents, tests, and family contact information. Check for x-rays, digital information, or scans for use during the procedure. Consult with anesthesia provider and surgeon for information exchange.
Room Setup • Ensure a clear path for emergency equipment. • Plan for adequate positioning of the anesthesia provider. • Check the OR bed for correct position. • Make sure lights are in working order.	Ensure all necessary positioning aids are available. Plan for entrance of patient without impeding the process of setup or contamination. Plan setup for position of instrument table in relation to surgical field.
Standard Room Equipment • Appropriate OR bed with armboards • Patient transfer device • Sequential compression device • Two intravenous (IV) poles • Patient-warming device • Mayo stand • Instrument table • Prep stand • Monopolar ESU and dispersive electrode • Suction collection apparatus • Platform steps for team	Check equipment (suction and ESU) for proper function. Place equipment in a position of function. Plan for cords and tubing to be passed off in one direction. Avoid having cords and cables as "trip hazards" if lights are lowered for endoscopy or other procedure where the lighting is changed.
Case Cart Contents • Instrument set(s) • Custom pack • Gowns • Sterile towels • Prep supplies • Additional soft goods	Check cart contents. Inspect package integrity. Check for each item listed on case cart sheet. Record preference changes on case cart sheet for computer update.

(Continued)

Systematic Activities for the Circulating Nurse—cont'd

Baseline Systematic Activity for All Cases	Systematic Patient Care
Items to Have Available • Suture • Sponges • Sterile towels • Gloves • Staplers • Dressings	Have a few sizes available. Only open if necessary. Charge only for items used.
Table Setup • Place packs to be opened on clean, dry table surface. • Do not open items into closed container system. Edges are unsterile. • Open adequate gowns and gloves for surgeon and first assistant. • Tie gowns of team. • If blades are opened separately, inform scrub person of location on the field.	Open sterile packs in a position of function. Establish and document baseline: Count instruments, sharps, and sponges with scrub person. Provide additional sterile supplies as needed by scrub person.
Medication and/or Chemicals on the Sterile Field • Obtain medications and/or chemicals for sterile field using patient identification number. • Dispense medications without aerosolization. • Draw up with needle and syringe. Remove needle before delivering drug to field.	Validate medication type and dose with the scrub person. Validate total amount given and administered. Charge only for drugs used on sterile field.
Irrigation on the Sterile Field • Obtain solutions of appropriate temperature for sterile field. • Dispense solutions without aerosolization. Pour in one continuous motion.	Dispense normal saline or other isotonic solution to the field after verifying the date, name, and seal integrity. Do not recap bottles unless saved for nonsterile use. Remaining solution can be used to clean the patient after the dressing is applied and drapes are removed.
Assisting the Anesthesia Provider • Assist with positioning during regional anesthesia. • Stand at patient's side during induction of general anesthesia.	Help anesthesia personnel with IV or intubation if needed. Prepare to apply cricoid pressure as needed during intubation.
Patient Positioning • Don nonsterile gloves. • Position devices as appropriate. • Provide adequate exposure of surgical site. • Apply appropriate safety restraints. • Apply dispersive electrode after patient is positioned. Do not cut or reapply.	The anesthesia provider will indicate when it is safe to start positioning and prepping. The anesthesia provider and surgeon will determine the appropriate safe position for the surgical procedure.
Skin Prep: Determine Patient Potential for Skin Sensitivity • One-step • Two-step	Open and set up appropriate skin prep materials. Alcohol-based preps can be a fire hazard if fumes accumulate under drapes. Expose the surgical site without undue exposure. Protect nontarget areas from pooling. Drapes should not be applied until prep has dried completely.
Procedural Positioning of Equipment and Team • Assist scrub person to move sterile table adjacent to surgical field. • Attach cords, cables, and tubing to appropriate devices. • Place suction canister in direct view of anesthesia provider. • Provide standing platforms/steps as needed.	Scrub person will hand off cords and cables in one direction. Determine machine settings per surgeon. Scrub person will place sterile Mayo stand over sterile field.

(Continued)

Systematic Activities for the Circulating Nurse—cont'd

Procedure Start and Flow	Documentation
• Initiate the time out, verifying the patient name, procedure, and correct site. • Prepare specimens for pathology. • Communicate with family or significant other within acceptable parameters for patient privacy.	• Procedural times and time out • Additional items not in the baseline count added to field or placed in patient • Assure that all implants, scans, and procedure-specific items are present before the procedure is started; validate these items during the time out process and document on the surgical checklist • Handle specimen containers wearing examination gloves • Family updates as appropriate
Dressings and Drains • Dispense dressing materials to sterile field at end of procedure. • Don nonsterile gloves to clean skin edges after patient is undraped. • Tape dressings. Avoid affixing to hairy surface.	One-step prep should not be removed.
Procedure Completion • Reconcile closing count with scrub person. Begin count from surgical field on patient to Mayo stand to instrument table. Sponges in sponge bucket are counted in increments of size and initial packaging amounts. • Prepare handoff report for postprocedural area nursing staff. • Transport patient to postprocedural area with anesthesia provider.	Give handoff report to registered nurse in postprocedural area: • Patient name and age • Allergies or sensitivities • Current procedure and type of anesthesia • Location of incisions, dressings, and drains • Special needs (language, vision, hearing) • Location of family or significant other • Any procedure-specific information • Pertinent comorbidity

1. Why is it important to keep the doors of the operating room (OR) closed?
   A. Because the air pressure gradient is positive inside the room and negative in the hallway to minimize particulate transfer from the hall.
   B. Because the air pressure gradient is negative inside the room and negative in the hallway to keep the airflow equalized.
   C. Because the air pressure gradient is positive inside the room and positive in the hallway to keep the airflow equalized.
   D. Because dust and particulates are contained in the room when the door is closed.

ANS: A
Rationale: The airflow is positive in the room and negative in the hall to minimize particulate transfer from the hall.

2. What is an advantage of steam sterilization?
   A. All instrumentation can be cleaned in less than 4 minutes
   B. It is convenient, inexpensive
   C. Long processing time, expensive
   D. Nontoxic, expensive

ANS: B
Rationale: Steam is the most convenient form of sterilization because it is inexpensive, has faster cycle times, and leaves no residue. Instrumentation must be cleaned properly to remove all residues before sterilization. It is not for use on heat-sensitive items.

3. Relative temperature and humidity of the OR should be maintained between which of the following levels?
   A. 58°F–65°F and 50%–75% humidity
   B. 70°F–85°F and 50%–70% humidity
   C. 60°F–70°F and 30%–70% humidity
   D. 68°F–75°F and 20%–60% humidity

ANS: D
Rationale: Correct temperature and humidity prevent condensation inside the instrument packs to inhibit microbial growth and provide relative normothermia for the patient. Too dry permits static sparks.

4. Which of the following hemostatic agents is derived from beef (bovine) products?
   A. Thrombin
   B. Gelfoam
   C. Surgicel
   D. Oxycel

ANS: A
Rationale: Thrombin is derived from bovine source. The patient may be allergic to beef products. Gelfoam is porcine. Surgicel is plant-based cellulose. Oxycel is from a chemical source.

5. Which pathogen causes Creutzfeldt-Jakob disease (CJD)?
   A. Virus
   B. Bacteria
   C. Prion
   D. Dementia

ANS: C
Rationale: Prions cause CJD and are a nonliving protein. Confirmation is done by a brain tissue biopsy after death (autopsy).

6. Methods for affixing a burn dressing include all of the following except:
   A. Staples
   B. Tape
   C. Sutures
   D. Ties

ANS: B
Rationale: Tape is not used because it can cause additional injury to the surrounding area and disturb healing tissue.

7. Which form of cold high-level disinfection solution may be used for plastics, rubber, and some endoscopes?
   A. Bleach
   B. Isopropyl alcohol
   C. Glutaraldehyde
   D. Cobalt-60

ANS: C
Rationale: Glutaraldehyde (Cidex or Banicide) is a cold solution that provides high-level disinfection.

8. How does Spaulding's classification identify the three levels of patient care items?
   A. Critical, semicritical, noncritical
   B. High, medium, low
   C. Clean, dirty, contaminated
   D. Sterile, clean, dirty

ANS: A
Rationale: The Spaulding's classification of patient care items is critical items (sterile), semicritical items

(high-level disinfection), and noncritical items (intermediate or low disinfection).

9. Which packaging material is best for processing small single instruments?
   A. Peel pack or pouch
   B. Rigid container
   C. Nonwoven blue wrapping material
   D. Custom pack

ANS: A
Rationale: A peel pack or pouch is easy to sterilize, the item is visible for identification, and it can be stored efficiently.

10. Which process is used to determine the total body surface area (TBSA) burned in an adult?
    A. Lund-Browder
    B. Multiply body weight by 9 and divide by 4
    C. Rule of nines
    D. Divide body weight (in kilograms) by height (in centimeters)

ANS: C
Rationale: This process is used for adults. Sections of the body are scored in segments of 9%.

11. LASER plume is best managed by which of the following methods?
    A. Smoke evacuator
    B. Wall-mounted suction
    C. Canister suction with a gauze sponge over the tip
    D. Irrigation of the site to prevent plume accumulation

ANS: A
Rationale: Special suction device that captures the smoke (plume) and filters the biohazardous materials.

12. During a malignant hyperthermia crisis, dantrolene (Dantrium) is reconstituted with which of the following solutions?
    A. Sterile water for injection
    B. Sterile saline for injection
    C. Sterile Ringer's lactate for injection
    D. Sterile dextrose for injection

ANS: A
Rationale: Sterile water is the only diluent that does not interfere with the action of the drug. A large volume without preservative is needed.

13. Epinephrine is commonly added to injectable local anesthetics for which of the following reasons?
    A. Prevents stinging and burning of the tissues
    B. Provides a palpable surgical landmark by plumping up the skin
    C. Dilutes the anesthetic to increase the safety margin of administration
    D. Hemostasis

ANS: D
Rationale: Epinephrine is a vasoconstrictor and minimizes bleeding at the site.

14. Reprocessing of single-use items is regulated by which organization?
    A. US Food and Drug Administration (FDA)
    B. Centers for Disease Control and Prevention (CDC)
    C. Environmental Protection Agency (EPA)
    D. Association for the Advancement of Medical Instrumentation (AAMI)

ANS: A
Rationale: The FDA sets the regulations for the reprocessing of single-use items.

15. Which organization oversees the safety of the workplace and has the authority to fine an institution for breaches of safety guidelines?
    A. The Joint Commission (TJC)
    B. Association for the Advancement of Medical Instrumentation (AAMI)
    C. Occupational Safety and Health Administration (OSHA)
    D. Association of periOperative Registered Nurses (AORN)

ANS: C
Rationale: OSHA is a governmental agency and has legal authority to levy fines for failure to comply with safety.

16. Which endospore is used in the biological indicator for dry heat processing?
    A. *Geobacillus stearothermophilus*
    B. *Bacillus atrophaeus*
    C. *Clostridium perfringens*
    D. *Proteus vulgaris*

ANS: B
Rationale: *Bacillus atrophaeus* is the endospore used for dry heat sterilization.

17. Which of the following is an early sign of malignant hyperthermia (MH)?
    A. Unexplained tachycardia
    B. Trismus
    C. Elevated body temperature
    D. Convulsions

ANS: A
Rationale: The heart rate elevates because oxygen demand initially increases.

18. Bipolar electrosurgery does not require the use of an inactive dispersive electrode for which of the following reasons?
    A. The radiofrequency current passes through the active tip of the forceps to the patient's tissue and returns it to the generator through the inactive tip of the same forceps.
    B. The radiofrequency current passes through the bipolar forceps and disperses into the patient's tissues.
    C. The radiofrequency current is very weak and does not need to return to the generator.

D. The radiofrequency current is applied to tissue only in short bursts and is of no risk for injury to the patient.

ANS: A

Rationale: The current does not pass through the patient's body. The current is applied and returned to the generator via only the location of the tips of the forceps.

19. The Association for the Advancement of Medical Instrumentation (AAMI) recommends that sterile items be stored in a designated area with ventilation and air-conditioning under which conditions?
    A. Humidity >75%, temperature at 75°F
    B. Humidity between 25% and 45%, temperature at 65°F
    C. Humidity between 30% and 70%, temperature <75°F
    D. Humidity between 20% and 50%, temperature <50°F

ANS: C

Rationale: Storage rooms should have a humidity of between 30% and 70% and temperature <75°F. There should also be at least four air exchanges per hour.

20. Which of the following is a malignant hyperthermia trigger?
    A. Nitrous oxide
    B. Halothane
    C. Sodium pentothal
    D. Oxygen

ANS: B

Rationale: All volatile anesthetic gases are malignant hyperthermia triggers.

21. Improper cleaning and processing of eye instrumentation can cause which of the following conditions?
    A. Glaucoma
    B. Cataracts
    C. Toxic anterior segment syndrome (TASS)
    D. Evisceration

ANS: C

Rationale: TASS causes postoperative inflammation from an unknown substance entering the anterior chamber. It can cause a toxic reaction leading to eye damage.

22. The dispersive electrode pad placement during monopolar electrosurgery depends on which of the following for safety?
    A. The electrode is placed over a fleshy area close to the surgical site.
    B. The electrode is cut to fit the area if the patient is smaller than 60 pounds in body weight.
    C. The electrode is repositioned if it becomes lose or fails to stick completely.
    D. The electrode should be applied before the patient is positioned for the procedure.

ANS: A

Rationale: The dispersive electrode is placed over fleshy tissue to equally spread the current and not impede the return to the generator. It must never be cut to size or repositioned. The pad is placed on the patient after final positioning to decrease the risk for shifting or allowing gaps in the conductive surface area.

23. Air exchange in the OR is controlled for atmospheric safety. How many total air exchanges take place per hour in the OR, and how many of these are fresh air from the outside?
    A. 15 total exchanges with 3 fresh air exchanges
    B. 20 total exchanges with 4 fresh air exchanges
    C. 25 total exchanges with 5 fresh air exchanges
    D. 15 total exchanges with 5 fresh air exchanges

ANS: B

Rationale: This is the 2018 recommended practice for air exchanges in the restricted area.

24. When not in use, the safest place for the electrosurgical handpiece is in which of the following?
    A. In the handpiece holder attached to the Mayo stand
    B. In the dominant hand of the first assistant for immediate use
    C. In the small basin at the working end of the sterile instrument table
    D. In the fold of the drape at the edge of the incision

ANS: A

Rationale: The handpiece should be stored in the holder to prevent burns and fires when not in use.

25. Why would intraluminal isopropyl alcohol be used during the processing of an endoscope?
    A. To decrease drying time
    B. To remove any residual bioburden
    C. For sterilization of the channels
    D. As a backup to sterilization

ANS: A

Rationale: Isopropyl alcohol (70%–90%) should be used to rinse the channels of an endoscope to quicken the drying time before storage; follow manufacturer's device instruction for use (IFU).

26. What is the purpose of the inactive dispersive electrode pad attached to the patient's skin during monopolar electrosurgery?
    A. Returns the radiofrequency current from the active electrode to the generator
    B. Grounds the patient
    C. Prevents electrical shock in team members
    D. Eliminates the risk for surgical burns in the patient

ANS: A

Rationale: The purpose of the inactive electrode pad is to return the electrical current to the grounded generator as the current passes through the patient's tissues.

27. Which of the following attire is worn in the unrestricted area of the OR?
    A. Scrub suit and hair cover are required
    B. Cover gown or laboratory coat should be worn over scrub suit
    C. Scrub suit, mask, and hair cover are required
    D. Street clothes

ANS: D

Rationale: No special attire is required in the unrestricted area.

28. Endoscopic use of electrosurgery is safest when which parameter is followed?
    A. The foot pedal is operated by the user of the cautery device.
    B. The foot pedal is operated by the first assistant.
    C. The metallic electrosurgical forceps are used with a mixed composition trocar and sleeve.
    D. The char on the end of the forceps is dipped in sterile saline.

ANS: A

Rationale: Care is taken not to active the cautery unintentionally. Other team members may step on the pedal at the wrong time and cause serious injury. All components should be insulated and of the same material.

29. What safety features should be near the disinfection and sterilization areas in case of exposure?
    A. Safety signs
    B. Eyewash and showers
    C. Extra gloves
    D. Lids for chemicals

ANS: B

Rationale: Eyewash stations and showers should be in the immediate area of the decontamination and sterilization areas in case of exposure.

30. Trendelenburg's position is used for which of the following purposes?
    A. To shift abdominal contents cephalad
    B. To provide a closer working space for general surgical instruments
    C. To provide clear access to the stomach for gastric procedures
    D. To shift the gallbladder into grasping range

ANS: A

Rationale: The lower level of the upper torso causes internal organs to move toward the upper body for exposure of the pelvic organs.

31. Antiseptic solutions used for surgical skin cleansing of the face and ears should not contain which of the following chemicals?
    A. Saline
    B. Chlorhexidine (Hibiclens)
    C. Iodophor (Betadine)
    D. Parachlorometaxylenol (PCMX)

ANS: B

Rationale: Chlorhexidine is toxic to eyes and ears.

32. The patient is positioned for a craniotomy. The anesthesiologist indicates that a venous air embolus is suspected. What immediate actions are taken by the team to alleviate the problem?
    A. The surgery is stopped and the incision closed in rapid succession.
    B. The patient is positioned in reverse Trendelenburg with the left side elevated.
    C. The patient is positioned in steep Trendelenburg's with the right side elevated.
    D. The surgeon packs the surgical site and calls for an x-ray because the air will look darker than the surrounding tissue.

ANS: C

Rationale: The anesthesia provider will pass a right atrial catheter to remove the air embolus from the right atrium.

33. Intestinal stomas are considered contaminated. Which of the following nursing actions is one method for containing and preventing stomal contamination during the surgical procedure for stomal closure?
    A. Cleanse and dry the stoma last and cover with a clear adherent adhesive dressing.
    B. Cleanse the stoma first and cover with a Betadine-saturated gauze sponge.
    C. Prep the skin around the stoma without touching the contaminated intestinal tissue.
    D. Prep the stoma immediately after the incision line and incorporate the surrounding skin of the abdomen.

ANS: B

Rationale: The stoma should be prepped first and covered to prevent the contamination of the primary incision line. Gloves should be changed after cleaning and covering the stoma. Be sure to account for the sponge used for the stomal cover when reconciling the counts.

34. What is the weight limit of instrument trays for sterilization?
    A. No more than 10 pounds
    B. No more than 15 pounds
    C. No more than 25 pounds
    D. No more than 50 pounds

ANS: C

Rationale: Instrument trays, which includes the weight of the tray and the instruments, should not weigh more than 25 pounds. This is for lifting safety and sterilization.

35. Which endospore is used to test steam sterilization, and when is it used?
    A. *Geobacillus stearothermophilus*, every load
    B. *Geobacillus stearothermophilus*, required weekly, every load with implants
    C. *Bacillus atrophaeus*, weekly
    D. *Bacillus atrophaeus*, daily

ANS: B

Rationale: A biologic indicator containing *Geobacillus stearothermophilus* is required weekly. Most facilities use them daily and in all loads with implants.

36. The patient indicates that she uses herbal preparations for brain circulation and memory improvement. What should the perioperative nurse know about herbs used for this reason?
    A. Most herbs used for this reason can affect the patient's clotting mechanisms.
    B. Herbs such as this are purchased over the counter and have no impact on the surgical procedure.
    C. Many herbs are the cause of thrombosis if the patient is immobile for more than 2 hours.
    D. Herbs are essentially harmless if taken in small quantities.

ANS: A

Rationale: Many of these herbs are anticoagulants and can cause intraoperative hemorrhage.

37. Surgical dyes are used to stain tissue during surgery. Which of the following surgical dyes is also used for intraoperative renal diagnostics?
    A. Methylene blue
    B. Brilliant green
    C. Scarlet red
    D. Gentian violet

ANS: A

Rationale: When injected intravenous (IV), the methylene blue dye stains the urine green during excretion. The surgeon and anesthesia provider can monitor urinary output.

38. The anesthesia provider is intubating the patient and indicates that the patient is demonstrating gastric reflux. Which of the following actions is performed by the perioperative nurse to assist with the intubation?
    A. Durant procedure
    B. Valsalva maneuver
    C. Crede maneuver
    D. Cricoid pressure

ANS: D

Rationale: This closes the esophagus during intubation to prevent aspiration of gastric contents.

39. Safe administration of local anesthetics from the sterile field includes which of the following actions of the scrub person?
    A. Labeling the medicine cup and the syringe before the drug is poured
    B. Drawing up the drug as the circulating nurse holds the vial in position for the label to be read by both team members
    C. Removing the needle as soon as the surgeon hands the syringe back
    D. Labeling the medicine cup and the syringe after the drug is poured

ANS: D

Rationale: This is important to prevent the administration of the wrong drug in the wrong dose.

40. What is the purpose of a biologic indicator?
    A. To make sure no microorganisms are left in the sterilizer
    B. To make sure the set temperature was achieved
    C. To document that process parameters were met
    D. To determine the length of time to kill endospores

ANS: C

Rationale: A biologic indicator is a commercially prepared endospore strip or vial placed inside the sterilizer to determine that all parameters of sterilization have taken place. The endospores should be killed if the sterilization process was successful. It is compared with an unprocessed control biologic.

41. The patient is having a gynecologic procedure that will result in several individual specimens of endometrial tissue. What information is important to include on the pathology specimen requisition that will facilitate a correct diagnosis?
    A. Antibiotic use
    B. Last menstrual period date
    C. Marital status
    D. Sexual orientation

ANS: B

Rationale: This is important for the pathologist to know when determining the secretory phases of the endometrium.

42. The patient has had four gallstones removed and the surgeon has ordered these sent to the pathologist for diagnostic testing. The perioperative nurse performs which of the following actions?
    A. The stones would be sent to pathology in a dry cup with a lid.
    B. The stones would be sent to pathology in a cup of 10% formalin with a lid.
    C. The stones would be placed in a cup of Bowen's solution with a lid.
    D. The stones would be placed in a cup of normal saline with a lid.

ANS: A

Rationale: Stones should always be sent dry. Some stones would dissolve if placed in fluid, making diagnosis impossible.

43. How should peel packs or pouches be sterilized and stored?
    A. Plastic side down
    B. Inside of a tray
    C. Paper side down
    D. On their side

ANS: D

Rationale: Peel packs or pouches should be sterilized and stored on their side, front to back. They should not be placed inside trays or placed flat because the plastic side is impermeable for sterilization. They may be heat sealed and a chemical indicator is on the paper side.

44. Which of the following statements is true concerning patients who are having a surgical procedure while positioned in the prone position?
    A. The patient is positioned and prepped, then anesthetized.
    B. The patient is anesthetized in the lateral position and prepped, then rolled onto the abdomen.
    C. The patient is anesthetized on the operating bed, then turned by the team before they perform the prep.
    D. The patient is anesthetized on the transport cart in the supine position.

ANS: D

Rationale: The patient is anesthetized on the cart, then lifted into the prone position for the prep.

45. Reverse Trendelenburg's position is used for which of the following surgical procedures?
    A. Bariatric procedure
    B. LAHV (laparoscopic-assisted vaginal hysterectomy)
    C. Laparoscopic tubal ligation
    D. Spinal fusion

ANS: A

Rationale: Upper internal organs are shifted caudad so the stomach and the diaphragm are more clearly visualized.

46. Which sterilization process would be utilized if instrumentation is possibly contaminated with prions from Creutzfeldt-Jakob disease?
    A. Soak in hypochlorite solution for 1 hour, steam sterilize for 1 hour at 270°F
    B. Soak in hydrogen peroxide for 30 minutes, steam sterilize for 30 minutes at 270°F
    C. Soak in sterile water for 1 hour, steam sterilize for 1 hour at 270°F
    D. Soak in ethylene oxide for 30 minutes, steam sterilize for 18 minutes at 270°F

ANS: A

Rationale: Prions are a nonliving protein and are hard to destroy. Follow facility policy. Instrumentation should be soaked in a hypochlorite solution (bleach) 1:10 or sodium hydroxide solution 40 g for 1 hour, then steam sterilized. The sterilization time will differ depending on the type of steam sterilizer:
    Gravity displacement: 270°F (132°C) for 1 hour.
    Prevacuum: 274°F (134°C) for 18 minutes

47. Placing a supine patient's arms on the armboards can cause nerve damage under what conditions?

    A. Adduction of the arm greater than 10 degrees
    B. Abduction of the arm greater than 90 degrees
    C. Circumduction of the glenoid fossa in a 45-degree circumference
    D. Extension of the shoulder less than 10 degrees

ANS: B

Rationale: Abduction of the arm greater than 90 degrees causes brachial nerve damage by stretching.

48. The patient is in the OR for x-ray contrast studies of the gallbladder. Which of the following is avoided to minimize error in diagnosis?
    A. Shaking the syringe containing the contrast media
    B. Mixing the contrast media with sterile normal saline for injection
    C. Placing the contrast media in a metallic medicine cup on the field
    D. Using room-temperature IV saline as a diluent

ANS: A

Rationale: Shaking the syringe would create bubbles that would show as artifacts on the x-ray.

49. Which of the following drugs is given intraoperatively as a thrombolytic agent?
    A. Heparin
    B. Warfarin
    C. Protamine
    D. Streptokinase

ANS: D

Rationale: Streptokinase is used to break up clots.

50. The patient is having an excisional biopsy of her left breast. The surgeon indicates that the specimen needs to go to pathology for a frozen section. Which of the following can best facilitate the frozen diagnostic process?
    A. Sending the specimen in a cup of saline with a lid
    B. Sending the specimen fresh in a cup with a lid
    C. Sending the specimen fresh in a clamp
    D. Sending the specimen in a cup with a few drops of formalin and a lid

ANS: B

Rationale: Sending the specimen in a cup of saline or formalin can cause problems with the freezing process. A clamp could crush cells.

51. The patient will have a plaster splint applied to the right arm at the end of the case. Which of the following methods is the correct way to prepare a plaster splint?
    A. The plaster bandage is dipped in cool to tepid water immediately before use.
    B. The plaster is soaked in warm water for 10 minutes before use.
    C. The plaster roll is dipped in warm saline so the patient will not become chilled during the application process.
    D. The plaster bandage is allowed to partially dry before application.

ANS: A

Rationale: Plaster has an exothermic effect and can severely burn the patient if warm water is used.

52. Which heated solution provides high-level disinfection (HLD) and sterilization by passing through ultraviolet light and then rinsed with filtered tap water?

A. Ozone
B. Ionizing radiation
C. Peracetic acid
D. Ethylene oxide

ANS: C

Rationale: Peracetic acid is used for heat-sensitive instrumentation. It works by oxidation and does not leave any residue because it is rinsed away. Items are processed and used immediately. This is also known as STERIS.

53. A man aged 29 years is having a right inguinal herniorrhaphy. The surgeon has requested a 1-inch Penrose drain. What information should the circulating nurse know about the use of this drain?
   A. The drain is secured to the patient's skin with a 3-0 nylon suture at the end of the case.
   B. A safety pin is attached to the end of the drain during closure.
   C. A half-inch Penrose drain should be available in case the 1-inch drain is too long.
   D. The drain is used during the procedure only as a retractor and is discarded at the end of the case.

ANS: D

Rationale: It is dipped in sterile saline and used to gently retract the spermatic cord. It becomes part of the count reconciliation at the end of the procedure.

54. Which of the following statements best describes when wound class should be assigned for each surgical procedure according to the Centers for Disease Control and Prevention (CDC)?
   A. Wound class is the basis for the selection of a preoperative antibiotic preparation.
   B. Wound class is assigned at the end of the case as a predictor of the risk for postoperative infection.
   C. Wound class is assigned at the start of the case as a prevention of cross-contamination.
   D. Wound class is determined preoperatively to help the team prepare the correct instrumentation for the procedure.

ANS: B

Rationale: The CDC has determined that assigning wound class based on the conditions of the surgical intervention does reflect the incidence of postoperative infection. The classification is confirmed at the end of the case

55. A surgical procedure involving entrance into a natural body orifice is classified by the Centers for Disease Control and Prevention (CDC) as which of the following?
   A. Class I
   B. Class II
   C. Class III
   D. Class IV

ANS: B

Rationale: Natural body orifices have inherent microorganisms.

56. Which of the following cultures renders inaccurate results when exposed to room air?
   A. Aerobic culture
   B. Tissue culture
   C. Anaerobic culture
   D. Bone marrow culture

ANS: C

Rationale: The microorganisms die when exposed to air. They will not grow for use in diagnosis.

57. Which recommendations should be followed when preparing items for sterilization and disinfection?
   A. Follow facility policy.
   B. Follow manufacturer's instructions for use (IFU).
   C. Follow Universal Protocol.
   D. Follow the Association for the Advancement of Medical Instrumentation (AAMI) guidelines.

ANS: B

Rationale: Processing depends on the IFU and how the item is used in patient care. Items cannot be HLD or sterilized unless proper cleaning practices have been implemented.

58. The shelf life of sterile packages and instrumentation depends on which of the following?
   A. Time
   B. Process
   C. Date
   D. Event

ANS: D

Rationale: With recommended storage, shelf life is event related. Integrity of the package should have been maintained.

59. The surgeon plans to do a cell block and washing of the peritoneal cavity. Which of the following statements is true concerning the performance of this procedure?
   A. The surgeon will instill sterile normal saline into the peritoneal cavity. The solution is aspirated and sent to the laboratory for cancer diagnosis.
   B. The surgeon will instill sterile water into the peritoneal cavity. The solution is aspirated and spun down for fibrin content.
   C. The surgeon will instill sterile normal saline into the peritoneal cavity. The solution is aspirated and sent to the radiology department for measurement of the radioactive assay.
   D. The surgeon will instill sterile normal saline into the peritoneal cavity to remove abscessed tissue. The solution is aspirated and discarded before the primary incision is created.

ANS: A

Rationale: Cell block and washing is done to identify cancer cells.

60. The patient is having a frozen section biopsy under local anesthesia. The surgeon indicates that the specimen is to go directly to the waiting pathologist, who will in turn immediately report the results. Which of the following patient care activities can the

perioperative nurse implement to minimize the patient's stress in this circumstance?
A. Provide a warm blanket.
B. Prevent excess exposure of body parts during the skin prep.
C. Place a sign on the door indicating that the patient is awake.
D. Indicate on the pathology slip that the patient is awake.

ANS: D
Rationale: This signals the pathologist to avoid the use of the intercom for reporting results.

61. A 62-year-old patient is scheduled for a bone marrow biopsy. Which of the following statements is correct concerning this procedure for this patient?
A. The specimen will be taken from either the sternum or the iliac crest.
B. The specimen will be taken from the distal end of the tibia or the femur.
C. The specimen will be obtained after the administration of radio contrast.
D. The specimen will be obtained under fluoroscopy to confirm needle placement.

ANS: A
Rationale: The specimen must be taken from a flat bone to obtain forming cells in an adult.

62. The adult patient is scheduled for a tonsillectomy. Which of the following actions would be appropriate for care of the specimens?
A. The specimens are combined in one cup and covered with saline.
B. The specimens are sent for gross inspection and discarded.
C. The specimens are sent in two separate cups labeled left and right.
D. The specimens are cultured for beta strep.

ANS: C
Rationale: The tonsils need to be sent separately in case cancer is discovered in one or the other. The lymphatic spread of cancer depends on the drainage in the region of the affected organ. The neck and throat drain on separate sides, which is predictive of metastasis.

63. Thrombin is used in the following manner for hemostasis over a large body surface?
A. Thrombin is used as a topical hemostatic agent.
B. Thrombin is mixed with sterile injectable saline and injected slowly over a period of 3 minutes.
C. Thrombin is titrated by the anesthesia provider.
D. Thrombin is used as a component of intraperitoneal irrigation in the event of hemorrhage.

ANS: A
Rationale: Thrombin is only used topically. It is fatal if injected or absorbed into an open vessel.

64. Which of the following is a contraindication for the use of a tourniquet?

A. Infection in the limb
B. Hypertension
C. Geriatric
D. Amputation

ANS: A
Rationale: Never use a tourniquet on an infected limb because a bolus of infectious microbes can be released when the cuff is deflated. This can cause a mycotic aneurysm.

65. Which best describes the definition of sterile?
A. Free from most microorganisms, but not endospores
B. Free from endospores and all microorganisms
C. Free from biofilm
D. Reduction in microorganisms

ANS: B
Rationale: Sterile means that an item is free from all living microorganisms and endospores. A sterile item can be used on nonintact tissue or entry into the vascular system.

66. During carbon dioxide (CO_2) laser use, which of the following safety precautions apply?
A. Green-colored glasses with side shields, covered windows, and locked doors
B. Clear plastic or glass eyewear with side shields, no shiny surfaces, and moist drapes around the surgical site
C. Orange-yellow–colored glasses with side shields, covered windows, and a fiber splitter
D. Specialized contact lenses and eye-caps on the telescope, covered windows, and a metallic handpiece

ANS: B
Rationale: CO_2 lasers do not penetrate glass or plastic. The laser will bounce off shiny surfaces and ricochet around the room until the energy is absorbed. It is a thermal laser, so it can start a fire in dry drapes and sponges.

67. Which of the following is a porcine hemostatic agent?
A. Avitene
B. Surgicel
C. Gelfoam
D. Epinephrine

ANS: C
Rationale: Gelfoam is porcine, Avitene is collagen, Surgicel is cellulose, and epinephrine is produced synthetically.

68. For what purpose is a Bowie-Dick test performed?
A. Confirms the air vacuum is working
B. Removes debris from the sterilizer
C. Confirms sterility
D. Measures internal air pressure

ANS: A
Rationale: The Bowie-Dick test confirms the air pump or vacuum is functioning properly to remove air in the prevacuum sterilizer. The test is required weekly, but is recommended daily before sterilization of the first load.

69. Which of the following methods is appropriate for prevention of wrong site surgery according to The Joint Commission?
    A. The site is initialed by the surgeon and validated by the perioperative nurse.
    B. The site is identified by the perioperative nurse and initialed by the patient.
    C. The site is identified by the patient and initialed by the perioperative nurse.
    D. The site is identified by the perioperative nurse and initialed by a second nurse as validation.

ANS: A
Rationale: The Joint Commission states the surgeon must mark the site in conjunction with the patient.

70. Appropriate sterile attire consists of which of the following?
    A. Scrub suit, gloves, cap, and mask
    B. Gown, gloves, cap, mask, and eyewear
    C. Scrub suit, cap, and mask
    D. Cover gown, shoe covers, and mask

ANS: B
Rationale: Sterile attire is worn when scrubbed for a surgical procedure.

71. Venous pooling in the patient's pelvis is most pronounced in which of the following positions?
    A. Seated
    B. Prone
    C. Lateral
    D. Lithotomy

ANS: A
Rationale: The pelvis accumulates venous blood when seated.

72. Which of the following is a necessary component of a fire or explosion?
    A. Nitrogen
    B. Oxygen
    C. Hydrogen
    D. Ether

ANS: B
Rationale: Oxygen is part of the required fire triangle of oxygen, fuel, and ignition.

73. What are the three most important factors to remember concerning the safety of the team in the presence of ionizing radiation?
    A. Age of the x-ray machine, shielding, time
    B. Time, shielding, age of the x-ray machine
    C. Time, shielding, distance
    D. Bone penetration, shielding, distance

ANS: C
Rationale: Main protection points are based on removing the risk for exposure to x-ray.

74. Which chemical processing method produces a gas or vapor to sterilize sensitive items by low-temperature oxidation?
    A. Peracetic acid
    B. Isopropyl alcohol

C. Hydrogen peroxide
D. Ionizing radiation

ANS: C
Rationale: Hydrogen peroxide produces a gas or vapor that sterilizes sensitive items at a low temperature (130°F, or less than 55°C), such as wrappers, envelopes, or items with lumens. It is a nontoxic method. It is also known as STERRAD.

75. Standard Precautions applies to which of the following?
    A. Blood
    B. All body fluids, secretions, and excretions except sweat, regardless of whether they contain visible blood
    C. Mucous membranes and nonintact skin
    D. All of the above

ANS: D
Rationale: All biologic materials from the patient are potential contaminants.

76. Critical items are processed to which degree for patient use according to the Spaulding's classification of the importance of patient care items?
    A. Disinfected
    B. Sterile
    C. Aseptic
    D. Decontaminated

ANS: B
Rationale: Critical items enter or contact the vascular system of the body. The risk for infection is high if the items are not sterile.

77. Sterility of a packaged item is in question if:
    A. A peel pack was used for a metal object.
    B. The tape on the outer wrapper has more than three stripes.
    C. A stain is seen on the lower end of the wrapper.
    D. The item is sequentially wrapped.

ANS: C
Rationale: All stains on the packaging are suspicious. The item inside is considered contaminated.

78. Which of the following is not one of the four elements of malpractice?
    A. Abandonment
    B. Duty
    C. Causation
    D. Damages

ANS: A
Rationale: The four elements of malpractice are duty, breach of duty, causation, and damages.

79. The standard acronym RACE is used in the event of fire in the OR or other patient care areas. Which of the following represents what the acronym stands for?
    A. Remove patients. Activate alarm. Close doors. Extinguish the fire.
    B. Rescue patients. Activate alarm. Contain fire. Evacuate.

C. Remove fuel source. Activate alarm. Cover burned areas. Exit the area.

D. Recover patient belongings. Activate alarm. Call for help. Evacuate.

ANS: B

Rationale: Organized behaviors during a fire feature life-saving activities in an orderly manner.

80. In which situation can immediate-use steam sterilization (IUSS) be applied?
    A. To flash a tray for faster turnover time
    B. To sterilize implants
    C. In emergency situations
    D. It should never be used

ANS: C

Rationale: IUSS should be used only in emergency situations with a biologic and chemical indicator. It should not be used for convenience or implants.

81. The process of sterilization can best be described as which of the following?
    A. A physical or chemical process rendering an item free from all microbial life and endospores
    B. Use of a steam sterilizer
    C. Decontamination rendering an item safe to handle with bare hands
    D. Chemical process rendering an item free from all microorganisms

ANS: A

Rationale: Sterilization is the physical or chemical process by which an item is processed to destroy all microorganisms and endospores.

82. Which of the following gloving methods is appropriate for inserting a Foley catheter?
    A. Closed gloving
    B. Open assisted gloving
    C. Closed assisted gloving
    D. Open gloving

ANS: D

Rationale: Open gloving does not require the donning of a gown as in wearing appropriate attire for entering the sterile field. Items A to C require a sterile gown.

83. When prepping a patient for a perineal and abdominal surgical approach, which of the following areas should be prepped first?
    A. Perineum
    B. Umbilicus
    C. Lower abdomen
    D. Midline abdomen

ANS: A

Rationale: Prepping the perineum first prevents splashes and aerosolization of perineal contaminants.

84. Which of the following retains its own blood supply?
    A. Allograft
    B. Xenograft
    C. Free flap
    D. Pedicle flap

ANS: D

Rationale: Pedicle flaps retain attachment to the donor site of origin. The other choices are avascular.

85. Which of the following best describes the function of the argon beam coagulator?
    A. Monopolar coagulation
    B. Vasoconstriction caused by gas
    C. Mini flame thrower
    D. Bipolar coagulation

ANS: A

Rationale: Argon beam coagulation is a form of monopolar cautery.

86. Heparin does which of the following?
    A. Promotes clots
    B. Prevents clots
    C. Dissolves clots
    D. Mobilizes clots

ANS: B

Rationale: Prevents clots, but cannot dissolve clots.

87. Which of the following is a passive drain?
    A. Hemovac
    B. Penrose
    C. Jackson-Pratt
    D. Sump

ANS: B

Rationale: Penrose drains do not use a vacuum device to aid drainage.

88. Sellick's maneuver is also known as which of the following?
    A. Cricoid pressure
    B. Intubation
    C. Extubation
    D. None of these

ANS: A

Rationale: Stabilization of the cricoid process during intubation.

89. In an ileorectal anastomosis where the stapler is introduced through the rectum, how are the two round specimens labeled when removed from the internal circular stapler?
    A. Together with a suture around the distal specimen
    B. Separately as two specimens marked distal and proximal
    C. Together with a suture around the proximal specimen
    D. None of these

ANS: B

Rationale: Separating the two specimens allows the pathologist to examine distal and proximal tissue condition for clear margins of anastomosis.

90. Where should used surgical instrumentation cleaning begin?
    A. After the case
    B. In the processing department

C. At point of use
D. Wiped before handing up to the sterile field
ANS: C
Rationale: Instrumentation should be cleaned at the point of use. Instruments on the sterile field should be wiped with sterile water to prevent corrosion by saline. Enzymatic cleaners can be used before transport to the processing department.

91. Which two organ systems are closely observed when the patient has low blood pressure?
A. Cardiac and renal
B. Neurologic and respiratory
C. Endocrine and integument
D. Musculoskeletal and digestive
ANS: A
Rationale: The heart rate and output influence renal function in support of the patient's blood pressure.

92. A chemical trigger for malignant hyperthermia is which of the following?
A. Intravenous narcotics
B. Nitrous oxide
C. Nondepolarizing muscle relaxants
D. Depolarizing muscle relaxants
ANS: D
Rationale: Depolarizing muscle relaxants trigger malignant hyperthermia.

93. What is the drug of choice for reversal of hypnotic and sedative drugs?
A. Epinephrine
B. Atropine
C. Heparin
D. Narcan
ANS: D
Rationale: Narcan is the universal reversal drug for depressant medications.

94. Laparoscopic surgical cases require instrument, sponge, and sharps counts for which of the following reasons?
A. The case can convert to open very quickly.
B. The instruments can slip into the puncture site.
C. The sets can easily get mixed together.
D. Replacement parts are very expensive.
ANS: A
Rationale: Different instrument sets are used if a laparoscopic procedure necessitates opening the abdomen. Confusion can ensue if the items used in one case are confused with another. The counts can be incorrect.

95. The timed cycle for wrapped instruments processed in a gravity displacement sterilizer should be?
A. 240°F (115. 6°C) exposure for 5 minutes
B. 250°F (121°C) exposure for 10 minutes
C. 270°F (132°C) exposure for 25 minutes
D. 275°F (135°C) exposure for 10 minutes
ANS: D

Rationale: Wrapped or packaged items are recommended to be sterilized at 275°F (135°C) for an exposure time of 10 minutes.

96. Dry heat is a form of sterilization used for what type of items?
A. Retractors
B. Sponges
C. Talc or glass
D. Implants
ANS: C
Rationale: Dry heat is commonly used for items that cannot be exposed to moisture, such as oil, foil packages, talc, glass jars, tubes, and delicate metal instruments. Dry heat is a longer process because the hot air must circulate to destroy any microorganisms. A *Bacillus atrophaeus* biologic is required for dry heat.

97. Which of the following is true concerning carbon dioxide gas (CO_2) used during inflation for laparoscopy?
A. Is sterile
B. Is warm
C. Contains particulate
D. Is delivered as a fluid to the patient
ANS: C
Rationale: Particles are present inside the gas tanks. Inline filters are used to remove the material before the gas is delivered to the patient.

98. Epinephrine has which effect on the patient's physiology?
A. Increases heart rate
B. Decreases heart rate
C. Dilates blood vessels
D. None of these apply
ANS: A
Rationale: Epinephrine increases the patient's heart rate.

99. Compartment syndrome is treated by which of the following methods?
A. ACE wrap
B. Fascial incisions
C. Plaster casting
D. Amputation
ANS: B
Rationale: Linear incisions are made in the patient's fascia to release pressure caused by accumulation of blood and fluids.

100. Which of the following is included in the restricted area?
A. Storage areas for sterile supplies used in the OR
B. Preoperative holding area
C. Operating room director's office
D. Dressing rooms
ANS: A

Rationale: Appropriate attire is required in the sterile storage areas. The other selections do not have a special attire requirement.

101. Which stage of general anesthesia can lead to patient death?
    A. I
    B. II
    C. III
    D. IV
ANS: D
Rationale: The IV stage of anesthesia can cause loss of control of the patient's vital signs.

102. Fluid bottles may be recapped and reused under what conditions?
    A. If the fluid is to be warmed
    B. If the bottle is sterile
    C. If the pourer is wearing gloves
    D. Fluid bottles may not be recapped and reused
ANS: D
Rationale: Once the bottle is uncapped and poured, the lip of the bottle is considered unsterile.

103. Contrast medium used during a surgical procedure:
    A. Is administered only by anesthesia personnel.
    B. Enhances visualization during diagnostic imaging procedures.
    C. Is tinted for easy identification.
    D. Is used only in full strength.
ANS: B
Rationale: Contrast medium is used to visualized structures during x-ray.

104. Skin that is taken from an unburned area of a patient and used as a transplant is referred to as which of the following?
    A. Autograft
    B. Homograft
    C. Heterograft
    D. Allograft
ANS: A
Rationale: Autograft material is taken from the patient's body.

105. Which of the following general inhalation anesthetics is not a malignant hyperthermia trigger?
    A. Nitrous oxide
    B. Halothane
    C. Forane
    D. Enflurane
ANS: A
Rationale: Nitrous oxide is not a volatile anesthetic.

106. When sterilizing a wrapped instrument in a pre-vacuum sterilizer, what is the appropriate temperature setting and exposure time?
    A. 250°F (121°C) for 30 minutes
    B. 250°F (121°C) for 45 minutes
    C. 270°F (132°C) for 4 hours
    D. 270°F (132°C) for 4 minutes

ANS: D
Rationale: Prevacuum sterilization is a high-powered system. Sterilization times are shorter with high temperatures around 270°F (132°C) and pressure of 27 psi (pounds per square inch). A completed cycle including drying time can be under 30 minutes.

107. Which is not true about endospores?
    A. They persist on a semicritical item.
    B. They persist on a sterile item.
    C. They persist after high-level disinfection.
    D. They persist after intermediate-level disinfection.
ANS: B
Rationale: Sterile items are considered free of endospore contamination.

108. Tumescence is performed before which of the following surgical procedures?
    A. Blepharoplasty
    B. Mentoplasty
    C. Liposuction
    D. Rhytidoplasty
ANS: C
Rationale: Tumescence is used to instill fluids into a fatty layer for liposuction.

109. Bier block anesthesia uses which of the following techniques?
    A. Double tourniquet
    B. Single tourniquet
    C. Elevated head of the operating bed
    D. Cricoid pressure
ANS: A
Rationale: Tourniquets are inflated and deflated in succession as part of the regional anesthetic process.

110. Manufacturers commonly use which low-temperature sterilization process using oxygen and water for plastics, metal, and heat-sensitive items?
    A. Radiation
    B. Ozone
    C. Dry heat
    D. Glutaraldehyde
ANS: B
Rationale: Ozone uses oxygen and water to sterilize items by oxidation. It is a process that takes about 5 hours. It requires a *Geobacillus stearothermophilus* biological indicator.

111. An abnormal filmy attachment of two surfaces or structures that are normally separate is which of the following?
    A. Hemorrhage
    B. Adhesion
    C. Herniation
    D. Fistula
ANS: B
Rationale: Adhesions occur when tissues adhere to each other.

112. The scrub nurse establishes the sterile field by first performing which of the following actions?
    A. Gowning and gloving with the open technique
    B. Gowning and gloving with the closed technique
    C. Gowning and gloving with the assisted open technique
    D. Gowning and gloving with the assisted closed technique

ANS: B
Rationale: The sterile field should be established using the closed gowning and gloving technique.

113. Semicritical items are processed to which degree for patient use?
    A. Decontaminated
    B. Sterile
    C. Disinfected
    D. Aseptic

ANS: C
Rationale: Semicritical items are not sterile, only disinfected to a high or intermediate level.

114. Which statement(s) is/are true about sterile persons as they move about in the sterile field?
    A. Pass back to back
    B. Pass face to face
    C. Both of these
    D. None of these

ANS: C
Rationale: The back is not considered sterile, and team members can pass each other in that orientation. Two sterile front areas can pass facing each other.

115. Counting sponges, sharps, and instruments at the end of the surgical procedure should be performed in which order?
    A. Mayo stand, incision, table, and off-field sponge receptacle
    B. Off-field sponge receptacle, table, Mayo stand, and incision
    C. Table, Mayo stand, incision, and off-field sponge receptacle
    D. Incision, Mayo stand, table, and off-field sponge receptacle

ANS: D
Rationale: Starting the count at the incision and working through the Mayo stand, instrument table, and off-field sponge receptacle allows the surgeon to proceed with the closure process.

116. Bier, spinal, and epidural blocks are common types of which form of anesthesia?
    A. Local infiltration
    B. MAC
    C. General anesthesia
    D. Regional anesthesia

ANS: D
Rationale: Regional anesthesia targets specific areas of the body and is administered by an anesthesia provider.

117. Eyewear worn as protection during LASER use is determined by which of the following?
    A. Thickness
    B. Color
    C. Optical density
    D. Composition

ANS: C
Rationale: The formulation of the glass density protects the wearer's eyes from LASER light waves.

118. Why should instrumentation taken from a steam sterilizer not be placed on a cold surface?
    A. It may cool to fast.
    B. It may create fog.
    C. Moisture may develop, causing contamination.
    D. It could melt the surface.

ANS: C
Rationale: Hot items should be placed on a wire rack for cooling to prevent condensation, which can cause strike-through contamination.

119. The toxic level of lidocaine used as a local anesthetic for an average adult is which of the following doses?
    A. 20 mg
    B. 200 mg
    C. 100 mg
    D. 125 mg

ANS: B
Rationale: Typical local infiltration should not exceed 4 mg/kg. The average adult limit is 200 mg.

120. Which of the following is true regarding the actions of heparin?
    A. It is used to prevent clots.
    B. It is used to break down clots.
    C. It is used to encourage coagulation.
    D. None of these answers apply.

ANS: A
Rationale: Heparin minimizes the risk for an embolus.

121. Which of the following is used as a topical solution for coagulation at the surgical site?
    A. Heparin
    B. Surgicel
    C. Gelfoam
    D. Thrombin

ANS: D
Rationale: Thrombin is the only solution used topically for coagulation. It is never injected.

122. Informed consent is obtained by which of the following surgical team members?
    A. Perioperative nurse
    B. Surgeon
    C. Nurse practitioner
    D. First assistant

ANS: B
Rationale: Only the person performing the procedure can obtain informed consent.

123. Atropine is administered preoperatively to control which of the following physiologic properties?
    A. Lower blood pressure
    B. Decrease secretions
    C. Prevent vomiting
    D. None of these apply

ANS: B

Rationale: Decreasing secretions minimizes the risk for aspiration.

124. "Balanced anesthesia" refers to the maintenance of which stage of anesthesia?
    A. Stage I
    B. Stage II
    C. Stage III
    D. Stage IV

ANS: C

Rationale: The patient's physiology is under safe pharmacologic control at stage III.

125. Bacteria forms a protective mechanism known as an endospore that is best destroyed by which process?
    A. Precleaning
    B. Steam under pressure
    C. High-level disinfection
    D. Decontamination

ANS: B

Rationale: Steam under pressure permits full penetration of the endospore capsule when chemicals cannot effect a kill.

126. Which chemical used for sterilization can be toxic and requires special personal protective equipment (PPE)?
    A. Ethylene oxide
    B. Peracetic acid
    C. Ozone
    D. Hydrogen peroxide

ANS: A

Rationale: Ethylene oxide is flammable and toxic, and requires special PPE and monitoring badge. Employee records must be kept for 30 years because it is carcinogenic.

127. How should metal basin sets be sterilized?
    A. Individually
    B. Face down
    C. Face up
    D. On the side, slight lean forward

ANS: D

Rationale: Metal basins should be placed on the side with a slight lean forward so the steam can contact the whole surface. Sets should be separated by wicking material to prevent moisture buildup.

128. Saline solution should not be used to clean stainless-steel instruments because of which of the following reasons?
    A. Saline will bond with the instrument at a chemical level.
    B. The salt will pit the stainless-steel finish on the instruments.

C. It may not be available.
    D. It is expensive.

ANS: B

Rationale: Saline is corrosive because of the salt content.

129. What is the process that ensures that all microorganisms including endospores are killed?
    A. High-level disinfection
    B. Asepsis
    C. Enzymatic action
    D. Sterilization

ANS: D

Rationale: Sterilization takes microorganisms to the lowest possible level.

130. A wound expected to heal by primary intention is considered to be which of the following?
    A. Packed wound
    B. Draining incision
    C. Sutured incision
    D. Complicated wound

ANS: C

Rationale: Primary closure is a simple wound that is not packed.

131. Chemical indicators can be placed on the outside and inside of packages. There are different classes. Where is a class 1 indictor placed?
    A. Inside a ridged container
    B. Inside a peel pack
    C. On the outside of all packaging and containers
    D. Inside drapes

ANS: C

Rationale: A class 1 chemical indicator is placed on the outside of all packages and containers before sterilization. The indicator will change color after processing for identification. An example is tape.

132. The safety belt is not used in which of these positions?
    A. Kraske
    B. Supine
    C. Lithotomy
    D. Prone

ANS: C

Rationale: A safety belt over the abdomen can increase intraabdominal pressure when the legs are in lithotomy position. The stirrups minimize the risk for falls.

133. Which person is responsible for the independent actions of the surgical technologist at the sterile field?
    A. Surgeon
    B. Circulator
    C. Surgical technologist
    D. Charge nurse

ANS: C

Rationale: All personnel performing independent actions are responsible for self-behaviors.

134. Reverse Trendelenburg's position requires which of the following OR bed attachments?
    A. Shoulder support and pads for the ear
    B. Footboard and thigh strap
    C. Two armboards and adhesive tape
    D. Allen stirrups and four towels

ANS: B
Rationale: The upper body is elevated and the footboard decreases the downward shift.

135. Which method of commercial sterilization uses a radioactive isotope?
    A. Cobalt-60
    B. Cobalt-49
    C. Cobalt blue
    D. Cobalt ion

ANS: A
Rationale: Cobalt-60 is the radioactive method of sterilization. Thermal and chemical rays are responsible for the destruction of microorganisms. It is a commercial FDA-approved sterilization method. It can take between 10 and 20 hours. Chemical indictors are placed on the outside of the items and biologic indicators on the inside.

136. Noncritical items should be processed in this manner according to Spaulding's theory of the importance of patient care items?
    A. Have been autoclaved for 3 minutes or more
    B. Have not been sterilized, but high-level disinfected
    C. Have only one wrapper instead of two
    D. Have no need to be sterile at any time

ANS: D
Rationale: Noncritical items are not sterile or processed in any special manner.

137. The lithotomy position is accomplished by which of the following?
    A. Holding both ankles up so the knees remain straight during the transition
    B. Frog-legging the patient to externally rotate the hip joints first so they will move freely
    C. Raising the legs into stirrups one at a time so the blood pressure remains stable
    D. Two people raising the legs up into stirrups at the same time

ANS: D
Rationale: There is no evidence that raising one leg at a time is beneficial to the patient's physiology.

138. If adult response to drug therapy is considered the norm, pediatric patients are observed for which difference in response?
    A. There is no variance in response
    B. Unusual responses to some drugs
    C. None of these apply
    D. Decreased responses to some drugs

ANS: B
Rationale: Pediatric patients need different dosages than adults.

139. The presence of food or fluid in the stomach during surgery increases the danger to which body system?
    A. Surgical site
    B. Digestive system
    C. Respiratory system
    D. Urinary tract

ANS: C
Rationale: Aspiration is a risk.

140. The pediatric patient's mother accompanies him to the OR. She begins to cry as she sees her child go under anesthesia. Why is she having this reaction?
    A. The environment is strange.
    B. The sleep state resembles death.
    C. Her child looks very small and helpless.
    D. All of these apply.

ANS: D
Rationale: Parents frequently have an emotional reaction when their child looks helpless. A transporter should be available to escort the parent to the surgical waiting room.

141. The formation of which toxic product can be formed if the preparation and acration is not done correctly when using ethylene oxide?
    A. Ethylene peroxide
    B. Ethylene glycol
    C. Ethylene dioxide
    D. Ethylene chloride

ANS: B
Rationale: Ethylene glycol is a toxic residual formed with EO (ethylene oxide) gas and water. It can cause hemolysis of red blood cells if it comes in contact with tissue. Special instrument preparation includes using forced air to clear items with lumens and tubes. Aeration is also a necessary part of processing to remove any residual gas.

142. What is the purpose of chemical sterilization indicators?
    A. Verification that the item is sterile
    B. Indicates the parameters of sterilization were complete
    C. Placed in implant trays to verify sterilization
    D. Determines that the item was packaged correctly

ANS: B
Rationale: Chemical sterilization indicators (CIs) are used on the outside and inside of all sterilized items. Outside indicators may change color to identify processed items from unprocessed items. Indicators placed inside of packages and trays indicate that the parameters of sterilization have taken place, such as time and recommended temperature. Chemical indicators range from class 1 to class 6 CIs. Each CI has its recommended uses for monitoring the type of sterilization parameters.

They do not guarantee sterilization. They are also used along with biological indicators.

143. The pediatric patient is being prepped for a femur fracture. You notice that there are several round, burnlike sores at the base of the patient's buttocks. What is your first action?
    A. Bring this to the attention of the surgeon.
    B. Observe that this may be an abuse situation and you should mind you own business.
    C. Rest assured that someone else will follow up on this finding and complete your sterile setup.
    D. It is probably caused by incontinence and not a concern at this time.

ANS: A

Rationale: The injury to the child could be an indicator of abuse and must be reported.

144. How many vials of dantrolene should be stocked to stabilize a patient during a malignant hyperthermia crisis?
    A. 10
    B. 12
    C. 22
    D. 36

ANS: D

Rationale: The 36 vials may be needed to stabilize the 70-kg patient. More is also used when the patient goes to the postanesthesia care unit (PACU).

145. Pediatric intubation requires which of the following considerations?
    A. Cuffed endotracheal tubes from birth
    B. Uncuffed endotracheal tubes after the age of 8 years
    C. Uncuffed endotracheal tubes before the age of 8 years
    D. No special considerations

ANS: C

Rationale: The pharyngeal tissue younger than the age of 8 years cannot tolerate a cuffed endotracheal tube.

146. The pathogenic material responsible for Spongiform encephalopathy is predominately found in which tissue?
    A. Neurologic
    B. Muscle
    C. Bone
    D. Blood

ANS: A

Rationale: Neurologic tissue is affected by prion diseases.

147. The surgeon wants to measure the urine produced by each kidney. Which of the following drainage devices would the nurse prepare?
    A. Foley catheter
    B. Urethral catheter
    C. Ureteral catheter
    D. None of these

ANS: C

Rationale: The urine is measured via each individual ureter from each kidney.

148. When inspecting a rigid container before opening, the nurse notices the plastic breakaway locks are missing. What action should be taken?
    A. Open the lid slowly toward the body.
    B. If the lid is tight, use it.
    C. Consider the tray unsterile.
    D. Check the indicator inside.

ANS: C

Rationale: The tray should be considered unsterile and sent back to the sterile processing department. The breakaway locks are placed to make sure the tray has not been tampered with. An external chemical indicator should also be on the outside of the container and inspected before opening.

149. In 2018, the Spaulding's classification regarding endoscopes and instrumentation processing changed. How did the processing recommendation change?
    A. An endoscope and instrumentation should be processed in a steam sterilizer.
    B. An endoscope and instrumentation should be processed with dry heat.
    C. An endoscope and instrumentation should be ozone processed.
    D. An endoscope and instrumentation should be sterile.

ANS: D

Rationale: In 2018, a modification to the Spaulding's classification was made by scientific studies, recommending that all endoscopes and instrumentation should be sterile. Studies showed that some microorganisms are resistant to HLD chemicals. Sterile instrumentation introduced through an HLD endoscope can cause transfer of resistant microorganisms to a sterile cavity. (*AORN guidelines for perioperative practice*, 2018, p. 830–833.)

150. A pregnant patient is demonstrating hypotension when placed in the supine position. The surgical team positioning the patient can provide hemodynamic support by performing which of the following actions?
    A. Place the patient in reverse Trendelenburg's position.
    B. Place the patient in low Trendelenburg's position.
    C. Elevate the patient's left hip.
    D. Elevate the patient's right hip.

ANS: D

Rationale: Elevating the right hip displaces the enlarged uterus from the vena cava, allowing venous return to the heart and lungs.

151. Which of the following drugs is used to counteract heparin?
    A. Thrombin
    B. Mannitol

C. Protamine

D. Atropine

ANS: C

Rationale: Protamine is an anticoagulant used to halt the effects of heparin.

152. Sterile saline is safe to use for irrigation at which of the following temperatures?

A. 104°F

B. 108°F

C. 115°F

D. 120°F

ANS: A

Rationale: Irrigation at a temperature higher than 104°F may be harmful to the patient.

153. The circulating nurse records the lot number for implants when used in a patient for which of the following reasons?

A. To ensure that the correct implant was used

B. To track the implant in the event of a recall

C. To record the implant use for inventory replacement

D. To confirm the implant was safe for use

ANS: B

Rationale: The lot number is used when a defect is discovered in a particular batch of implants.

154. What is the purpose of the Surgical Care Improvement Project (SCIP)?

A. To prevent positioning injuries

B. To prevent wrong site surgery

C. To prevent pressure injuries

D. To prevent surgical site infection

ANS: D

Rationale: The Centers for Medicare and Medicaid Services (CMS) will not reimburse facilities for preventable surgical infections.

155. Universal Protocol requires which of the following for every patient having a surgical procedure?

A. Time out and the use of a checklist

B. Patient's signature on the OR record

C. Surgeon's signature on verbal orders

D. None of the above

ANS: A

Rationale: Time out and the use of a checklist is a universal form of patient safety and protection.

156. Which of the following is considered a "never event" by the Centers for Medicare and Medicaid Services (CMS) and is not reimbursable?

A. Delayed arousal from anesthesia

B. Retained surgical items (RSIs)

C. Wound class III

D. Resolved incorrect count

ANS: B

Rationale: When counting protocol is followed, the accountability for items used in surgery prevents items from being left in patient's bodies.

157. Bacterial secretions that persist on infected surfaces and resist antibiotic therapy are referred to as which of the following?

A. Primary secretions

B. Differential exudate

C. Transudate

D. Biofilm

ANS: D

Rationale: Biofilm is a complex layering of mucus produced by bacteria that is difficult to penetrate and kill.

158. When should the processing of a flexible endoscope begin?

A. At the point of use, within 4 hours

B. At the point of use, within 1 hour

C. At the point of use, within 3 hours

D. At the point of use, when time permits

ANS: B

Rationale: Flexible endoscopes should be flushed with water and wiped down with an enzymatic cleaner as soon as the procedure is complete. Endoscopes should be transported to the processing area in a biohazard container placed horizontally. Processing should begin within 1 hour of use to prevent the drying of any bioburden.

159. When a surgical count is incorrect, the first action by the circulating nurse should be which of the following?

A. Call x-ray.

B. Inform the surgeon.

C. Check the trash bin.

D. Notify the supervisor.

ANS: B

Rationale: Informing the surgeon is the best action and allows the surgical site to be searched.

160. A patient experiencing local anesthetic systemic toxicity (LAST) will exhibit which of the following symptoms as a first indicator of a reaction?

A. Numbness of the lips and tongue

B. Bradycardia

C. Sleepiness

D. Hallucinations

ANS: A

Rationale: Neurologic symptoms associated with facial sensation are commonly the first signs.

161. A pressure injury assessment does not include which of the following?

A. Age

B. Use of handheld retractors

C. Body mass index (BMI)

D. Nutrition status

ANS: B

Physical attributes of the patient are assessed preoperatively. Intraoperative use of retractors is not assessed at this time.

162. What is the purpose of documenting every load number and parameters after sterilization or processing?
    A. To make sure the correct instruments are in the tray
    B. To keep records in case there is a recall or sterilization failure
    C. To make sure all the instruments are returned
    D. To keep track of loaner trays

ANS: B
Rationale: Documentation of all processing activities is recorded in case a sterilization device is defective or there is a recall. Each load has a lot number for tracking. All physical, chemical, and biologic parameters are documented. Some systems have a printout for recording, and other systems are computerized.

163. Noise and extraneous commotion should be avoided during which of the following activities?
    A. Phase III of anesthesia
    B. Patient positioning
    C. Emergence from anesthesia
    D. Patient prepping

ANS: C
Rationale: The patient is at risk for airway compromise caused by excitation as he or she emerges from anesthesia.

164. Incapacitated patients need assistance to move from the transport cart to the operating bed. How many personnel are required to move this patient from one surface to another?
    A. 2
    B. 3
    C. 4
    D. 6

ANS: C
Rationale: For safety, four personnel are needed to guide the head, feet/legs, sending side, and receiving side.

165. Which of the following organizations set the standard for reporting of sentinel events?
    A. AAMI (Association for the Advancement of Medical Instrumentation)
    B. NIOSH (National Institute for Occupational Safety and Health)
    C. TJC (The Joint Commission)
    D. APIC (Association for Professionals in Infection Control and Epidemiology)

ANS: C
Rationale: TJC established the requirement of reporting sentinel events in concert with accreditation of healthcare organizations.

166. When placing the patient in the supine position, where should the safety belt be secured?
    A. Over the thighs, 2 inches above the knees
    B. Over the abdomen at the level of the iliac crest
    C. Over the anterior tibia, 2 inches below the knees
    D. Over the chest, below the axillary line

ANS: A
Rationale: Over the thighs above the knees provides the greatest control over the largest flexion muscles of the legs.

167. The Perioperative Nursing Data Set (PNDS) is the standardized language that captures nursing care data in the perioperative environment. Which of the following defines data associated with the PNDS?
    A. Nursing process
    B. Domains that frame the nursing diagnosis
    C. Documentation of nursing intervention
    D. Identification of desired outcomes

ANS: B
Rationale: The PNDS is subdivided into domains that capture the nursing process in perioperative patient care.

168. National Patient Safety Goals (NPSGs) are established by which professional organization to promote patient safety in the healthcare environment?
    A. ANA
    B. AORN
    C. CDC
    D. TJC

ANS: D
Rationale: The Joint Commission sets the standard for healthcare facilities and the safety of patients.

169. Patients who report a sensitivity to shellfish are likely allergic to which of the following substances?
    A. Iodine
    B. Fish protein
    C. Prep solution
    D. Chlorhexidine

ANS: B
Rationale: Iodine allergy is extremely rare. Allergy or sensitivity to shellfish is associated with fish protein.

170. Patients positioned in steep Trendelenburg's position are at risk for which of the following complications?
    A. Cerebral edema
    B. Intestinal ischemia
    C. Urinary retention
    D. Foot drop

ANS: A
Rationale: Positional compromise in steep Trendelenburg position is associated with cerebral edema.

171. Comorbidities associated with immediate postoperative complications include which of the following conditions?
    A. Allergies and sensitivities
    B. Previous surgical incisions
    C. Cardiorespiratory disease
    D. Urinary tract infection

ANS: C
Rationale: Critical body systems (cardiac and respiratory) are essential to life.

172. Patient privacy is protected by laws enacted by the Department of Health and Human Services (HHS) branch of the federal government. Which of the following protects the patient's healthcare information?
    A. CDC
    B. FDA
    C. OSHA
    D. HIPAA

ANS: D
Rationale: HIPAA is the Healthcare Insurance Portability and Accountability Act.

173. Implants should be sterilized with a biologic and which class chemical indicator?
    A. Class 2
    B. Class 3
    C. Class 4
    D. Class 5

ANS: D
Rationale: A class 5 indicator verifies that parameters such as time, temperature, and steam requirements were attained.

174. Medication given by the anesthesia provider to decrease intraocular pressure during cataract surgery is which of the following?
    A. Mannitol
    B. Benzodiazepine
    C. Diazepam
    D. Fentanyl

ANS: A
Rationale: Mannitol is a diuretic.

175. Select the best method for transporting contaminated instruments to the processing area?
    A. Instruments soaking in saline in a red bin, inside a case cart
    B. Instruments soaking in sterile water, inside a case cart
    C. Back table covered with a drape
    D. Instruments sprayed with an enzymatic cleaner, sharps secured, placed in a closed cart

ANS: D
Rationale: Dirty or contaminated instruments should be kept moist with sterile water or sprayed with an enzymatic cleaner. They should not be cleaned with saline because it can cause corrosion. Placing instruments in excess fluid could cause spillage on the way to the processing area. All contaminated instrumentation should be confined in a closed cart.

176. Which of the following communicable diseases is spread by direct contact?
    A. Mumps
    B. Measles
    C. Hepatitis C
    D. Tuberculosis

ANS: C

Rationale: Hepatitis C requires direct contact with contaminated blood.

177. The patient with a DNR (do not resuscitate) order on file is coming to the OR for placement of a central line. The circulating nurse knows which of the following statements is false?
    A. The patient is having a palliative procedure.
    B. The DNR order is always suspended when a patient comes to the OR.
    C. The patient wants to have the central line inserted to prolong comfort.
    D. The patient wants to make autonomous end-of-life care decisions.

ANS: B
Rationale: DNR orders are not always suspended when the patient goes to the OR. The patient may be having a palliative procedure, but may still want no resuscitation if a natural death (AND) happens during the procedure. Documentation between the patient and the surgeon should be clear before the procedure starts.

178. The female patient has body piercings. What is the best, understandable explanation the circulating nurse can give to the patient for removing the piercings before the surgical procedure?
    A. The piercings are unattractive.
    B. The piercings will reflect the OR lights, causing distortion of the field.
    C. The piercings could interfere with the electrosurgical device (ESU) used during the procedure.
    D. The piercing could be lost during the procedure.

ANS: C
Rationale: The patient may not understand all the reasons for removing piercings; however, the patient is likely to understand the explanation that the ESU is necessary for a successful surgical procedure and will be more compliant about removing them.

179. After the lid of a rigid container is opened, what is the next step for validating correct processing parameters?
    A. Hold the container so the scrub nurse can reach the sterile handles.
    B. Place the lid under the opened tray.
    C. Inspect the filters in the lid.
    D. Take the count sheet out of the tray.

ANS: C
Rationale: The filters should be removed and checked for moisture. If the filter is damp, the instruments are not considered sterile.

180. The patient has donated blood in advance of his scheduled surgical procedure. The circulating knows which of the following is true concerning the use of his blood?

A. The blood is for autologous use only.
B. The blood can be used for other patients.
C. The blood has been typed and cross-matched.
D. The blood has been frozen for storage.

ANS: A

Rationale: The blood cannot be used for anyone else and has not been typed and cross-matched to another patient. The blood is only stored fresh.

181. A complication of overheating the patient during the procedure is which of the following?
    A. The surgical procedure will be extended in time.
    B. The patient can lose undetectable fluids through sweat.
    C. The instrumentation will become slippery.
    D. The monitoring devices will not record the vital signs accurately.

ANS: B

Rationale: The patient will sweat under the drapes, losing fluids that are difficult to assess. This can lead to a fluid deficit in a compromised patient.

182. One feature of the SCIP (Surgical Care Improvement Project) is preoperative administration of antibiotics as appropriate. Which of the following best describes this aspect of the SCIP protocol?
    A. Routine antibiotic administration the night before surgery
    B. Vancomycin administration 2 hours before the incision
    C. Addition of an antibiotic to all irrigation solutions
    D. Administration of Benadryl before antibiotic use to minimize the risk for allergic reaction

ANS: B

Rationale: If antibiotics are required, routine antibiotics are given 1 hour before incision. Vancomycin, if necessary, can be given up to 2 hours before incision.

183. The patient has signed a declination for the use of blood during surgery for religious reasons. The circulating nurse knows that hypovolemia can be treated by which of the following interventions without violating the patient's wishes?
    A. Plasma infusion
    B. Packed cell infusion
    C. Crystalloid infusion
    D. Vasoconstrictor infusion

ANS: C

Rationale: Crystalloids contain no blood products and can be used to expand the vascular compartment.

184. Which is the proper way to mark an instrument for identification?
    A. Place a colored sticker on the handle before sterilization.
    B. Engrave a name on the handle.
    C. Have a number laser etched on the instrument.
    D. Carve the instrument name on it.

ANS: C

Rationale: Identification numbers or codes should be laser etched on the instrument. The finish should be smooth to prevent trapping of microorganisms.

185. Select the correct statement regarding the handling of loaner trays.
    A. Loaner instruments should be delivered to the processing department, inspected, and sterilized.
    B. Loaner instruments can be used if they are unopened and sterile.
    C. Loaner instruments can be sterilized in the delivered containers.
    D. Loaner instruments can be brought in by a vendor and flashed.

ANS: A

Rationale: Loaner instruments should be requested several days before a scheduled case. They should follow facility policy. They should be brought to the processing department for decontamination, cleaning, inspection, and sterilization. Following a procedure, they should be decontaminated and given back to the vendor clean and complete.

186. Which of the following is acceptable for use as a prep in the vagina if the patient has a Betadine sensitivity?
    A. Chlorhexidine in saline
    B. Alcohol in saline
    C. Iodine in saline
    D. Baby shampoo in saline

ANS: D

Rationale: No other cleansing solution is safe for vaginal prep. Baby shampoo diluted in saline offers cleansing of the area without the risk of harming the mucosa.

187. The patient is having a cataract extraction under local anesthesia. During the procedure the patient will have a nasal cannula for oxygen. What risk is apparent to the circulating nurse as the patient is draped?
    A. The patient could suffocate.
    B. The nasal cannula can cause oxygen to accumulate under the drape, causing a fire.
    C. The surgical field could be obscured by the drape.
    D. The drape is too short to protect the surgical site.

ANS: B

Rationale: Oxygen is part of the fire triangle and supports a fire in the event of an ignition source. Oxygen can accumulate under the drape, posing a fire hazard.

188. The surgical procedure requires the use of lead protection because of ionizing radiation used during the procedure. The circulating nurse knows which of the following is true concerning the use and care of lead aprons?
    A. After use, the aprons are folded and stored in the closet.

B. After use, the aprons are sent to the instrument processing area.

C. After use, the aprons are hung on hooks to prevent creases and breaks in the lead lining.

D. After use, the aprons are stored in the radiologist's locker.

ANS: C

Rationale: Protective lead aprons must never be folded, to minimize the risk for fracturing the integrity of the lead protection. The aprons should be hung on hooks to keep them intact.

189. The electrosurgical unit (ESU) is alarming intermittently. The circulating nurse's first action should be which of the following?
    A. Check the integrity of the dispersive return electrode.
    B. Call the biomed department.
    C. Turn off the power to the ESU.
    D. Turn up the power to increase the current.

ANS: A

Rationale: The first action is to check the dispersive return electrode. The ESU is designed to block the current from the generator if the return electrode is not intact.

190. Which of the following statements is the correct way to handle incoming supplies for storage?
    A. Check the inventory list and place the shipping carton in the designated spot in the sterile core.
    B. Label the shipping carton and stack it on the floor near the substerile room.
    C. Remove all items from the shipping carton and place them in the sterile core.
    D. Place the shipping carton under the sink in the substerile room.

ANS: C

Rationale: All incoming supplies should be removed from the original containers. Outside containers and cardboard can bring in insects and contaminants. Closed cabinets or storage rooms that are environmentally controlled are recommended. Items should not be stored under sinks, where they can get wet or contaminated.

191. The patient is having a total thyroidectomy and parathyroidectomy. What is the physiologic risk to the patient postoperatively when the thyroid and the parathyroid glands are removed?
    A. Unattractive scarring at the neckline
    B. Aversion to iodized salt
    C. Convulsions caused by calcium release
    D. Torticollis associated with adhesions

ANS: C

Rationale: Calcium regulation is interrupted when the thyroid gland and parathyroids are removed. The patient could go into a "thyroid crisis."

192. The surgeon is using a tourniquet for the surgical procedure. The circulating nurse should do which of the following actions as the procedure progresses?

A. Decrease the inflation pressure every 15 minutes.

B. Inform the surgeon when inflation time has reached 1 hour.

C. Increase the inflation pressure every 15 minutes.

D. Inform the surgeon when inflation time has reached 2 hours.

ANS: B

Rationale: Tissue ischemia can cause damage when prolonged inflation time is not monitored. The circulating nurse should inform the surgeon when 1 hour has been reached and every 15 minutes thereafter.

193. The patient is known to be HIV-positive. What precautions should the circulating nurse take to prevent transmission to the surgical team?
    A. Use only disposable supplies for the procedure.
    B. Request extra personnel for patient positioning.
    C. Wear double gloves for the prep.
    D. Proceed with the room preparation as with any other case.

ANS: D

Rationale: All surgical cases should proceed with the same precautions, and every patient should be treated in the same manner.

194. The circulating nurse observes that the patient has a dry ulcer on the anterior surface of his right leg. The leg appears pale, white, and hairless. This observation indicates which of the following conditions exists in the patient's leg?
    A. The patient has impaired arterial circulation in the right leg.
    B. The patient has serious heart disease.
    C. The patient has a form of cancer in the leg.
    D. The patient has an injury to the ileo-inguinal canal on the right.

ANS: A

Rationale: Impaired arterial circulation causes the tissue to become ischemic and pale. Ulcers are dry, and the skin is shiny and hairless because of lack of circulation.

195. Which wound class will be assigned at the end of the surgical procedure when bile leaks into the abdomen during a cholecystectomy?
    A. Class I
    B. Class II
    C. Class III
    D. Class IV

ANS: C

Rationale: Gastrointestinal spillage is a contamination factor. Wound class is based on the risk for postoperative infection.

196. Large, powered instruments such as drills and saws may contain which of the following that may not be sterile?
    A. Saw blade
    B. Drill bit
    C. Battery
    D. Reamer

ANS: C

Rationale: Some large, powered equipment may contain batteries that are not sterile. The batteries are placed into the equipment by the circulating nurse as the scrub nurse holds the device open. A sterile shield is used to keep the equipment from getting contaminated. The batteries are removed from the equipment after the procedure and wiped down with a cleaning solution and charged.

197. The surgeon indicates that he or she will be seated for the surgical procedure. The circulating nurse prepares the room for which of the following scenarios?
    A. Seats for the surgeon and first assistant
    B. Seats for all the sterile team members
    C. Seat for the surgeon only
    D. Seat for the surgeon and the scrub person

ANS: B

Rationale: If the procedure will be performed by a seated surgeon, the entire team must be seated.

198. The intended surgical procedure on the patient's arm will be performed on a hand table attached to the operating bed. How is the patient's arm positioned on the hand table?
    A. The arm is extended 45 degrees onto the hand table.
    B. The arm is circumducted to protect the glenoid fossa.
    C. The arm is abducted 90 degrees onto the table.
    D. The arm is pronated on the table.

ANS: C

Rationale: The arm is abducted only 90 degrees onto the table. The pronation or supination of the hand will depend on the intended procedure.

199. The abdominal prep boundaries for an abdominal aortic aneurysm procedure are outlined as which of the following?
    A. Begin at the incision line and prep to the periphery.
    B. Begin at the nipple line and prep to the pubis.
    C. Begin with the umbilicus followed by the incision line to the periphery.
    D. Begin with the periphery moving toward the incision line.

ANS: C

Rationale: The umbilicus is prepped first followed by the incision line to the periphery.

200. The abdominal skin has been prepped with an alcohol-based prep. What steps minimize the hazard associated with using this type of prep?
    A. Allow the solution to dry completely before draping.
    B. Dry the surface with a sterile towel before applying drapes.
    C. Allow the solution to pool in the umbilicus to prevent infection.
    D. Cover the prepped area with a fenestrated drape to hasten drying.

ANS: A

Rationale: The alcohol-based prep solution is flammable and must be dry to prevent the accumulation of combustible vapors under the drapes.

201. If a single-use item is reprocessed, what information must be included on the package label?
    A. The reprocessed date and time
    B. The facility where it was reprocessed
    C. Manufacturer's name, lot number, number of times the item was reprocessed
    D. How the item was reprocessed, name of the person who processed it

ANS: C

Rationale: The reprocessed item should contain the manufacturer's name, lot number, and times the item was reprocessed. Critical items are not recommended for reprocessing. All reprocessed items must be tracked. Patients have the right to know if reprocessed items were used during their procedure.

202. The circulating nurse communicates with the post-operative care nurse at the conclusion of the surgical procedure. The communication during this phase of care is referred to as which of the following?
    A. Postoperative report
    B. Hand-over report
    C. Exchange of assessment
    D. Perioperative data exchange

ANS: B

Rationale: The hand-over report is a standardized method of communicating information concerning the patient's condition and care in the operating room.

203. Surgical site closure is defined by three methods employed to promote healing. The approach used for chronic wounds where the skin edges cannot approximate is referred to as which of the following?
    A. Packed wound
    B. Primary closure
    C. Secondary closure
    D. Tertiary closure

ANS: C

Rationale: Secondary closure is used when the wound healing is promoted from the wound bed up to the surface. No suturing is possible. The wound may need periodic debridement.

204. The abdominal surgical incision site is verified by the patient and the perioperative nurse during the preoperative assessment. Visual confirmation is denoted by which of the following indicators?
    A. The surgeon's initials on the site
    B. The X on the skin

C. The patient points to the area

D. The sticker placed over the organ

ANS: A

Rationale: The surgeon should initial the site with indelible ink as confirmation of the surgical site. Only the person performing the procedure should mark the surgical site.

205. Dantrolene will be administered to a patient during a malignant hyperthermia crisis starting at which dose?

A. 25 mg/hour

B. 25 mg/L

C. 2.5 mg/kg

D. 25 mL/hour

ANS: C

Rationale: The starting dose of dantrolene is 2.5 mg/kg and may be increased to 10 mg/kg as needed.

206. A necessary retractor is accidently dropped on the floor. What action can the circulating nurse take?

A. Wash the retractor in a designated sink, then flash the retractor in a prevacuum sterilizer for 3 minutes at 270°F.

B. Clean the retractor in the scrub sink and flash it in the prevacuum sterilizer for 4 minutes at 270°F.

C. Spray the retractor with enzymatic cleaner, then flash it in the prevacuum sterilizer for 3 minutes at 270°F.

D. Wipe it with alcohol and return it to the sterile field.

ANS: A

Rationale: Immediate-use steam sterilization (IUSS) can be used for emergency situations. The item should be cleaned in a designated area. Dirty or contaminated items should not be cleaned in scrub sinks. Metal and nonporous heat-stable items can be autoclaved for 3 minutes at 270°F. Items that are porous or have tape, lumens, or contain plastic or rubber should be autoclaved at 10 minutes at 270°F. Any item with a tube or lumen should be flushed with water and sterilized while wet.

207. Instrumentation placed in a washer-decontaminator goes through which phases?

A. Rinsing, sterilization

B. Prerinse, wash, rinse, steam, heat

C. Prerinse, wash, sterilization

D. Prerinse, wash, dry, sterilization

ANS: B

Rationale: The washer-decontaminator first prerinses the instrumentation with cold water to remove any bioburden, washes with a detergent, and rinses the detergent, then uses steam and heat. This process enables the instruments to be safely handled, but not sterile for patient use.

208. The boundaries of the surgical scrub include which areas of the hands and arms?

A. Nails, hands, and arms to the mid-forearm

B. Nails, hands, and arms to 2 inches above elbows

C. Nails, hands, and arms to the antecubital fossae

D. Nails, hands, and arms to the axilla

ANS: B

Rationale: The nails, hands, and arms above the elbows is the best scrub for aseptic cleaning.

209. The first assistant is using sponges during electrosurgical use for hemostasis. What consideration for patient safety is the primary concern during this process?

A. A sponge could be left in the patient

B. The sponge could ignite if not moistened

C. The sponge count could be incorrect

D. The sponge could be too small to be effective

ANS: B

Rationale: A dry sponge in contact with the electrosurgical tip can ignite, causing a fire.

210. Minimizing the risk for particulate in the surgical site prevents adhesions. The use of sponges can generate lint that can enter the patient. How can the scrub nurse minimize the dispersal of lint in the patient?

A. Moisten the sponges by dipping them into the irrigation basin.

B. Moisten the sponges by placing them in the irrigation basin before the solution is poured.

C. Moisten the sponges by using the Asepto syringe before handing to the field.

D. Moisten the sponges by wringing them out over the irrigation basin before use.

ANS: C

Rationale: Moisten the sponges using the Asepto to prevent the lint from floating in the irrigation basin.

211. The patient is scheduled for a surgical procedure of the right leg. The surgeon plans to use a tourniquet but declines at the last minute because of which of the following contraindications?

A. History of deep vein thrombosis (DVT)

B. Anticoagulation therapy

C. Diabetes

D. Obesity

ANS: A

Rationale: The patient is at risk for repeated DVT if the circulation is occluded for a long period for the procedure.

212. The patient is having CO_2 laser excision of human papillomavirus (HPV) of the uterine cervix under local anesthesia. The circulating nurse protects the patient from the contaminated plume by which of the following methods?

A. Placing drapes over the patient's face
B. Placing a laser mask over the patient's nose and mouth
C. Placing extra drapes over the abdomen
D. Placing an oxygen cannula in the patient's nose

ANS: B
Rationale: The patient should not be allowed to breathe the HPV-laden plume.

213. The surgeon wants to visualize the patency of the patient's fallopian tubes during a laparoscopic procedure. The circulating nurse should prepare and instill which of the following as directed during the procedure?
A. Contrast media mixed with sterile saline via a uterine cannula
B. Monsel's solution mixed with sterile saline via a uterine cannula
C. Methylene blue dye mixed with sterile saline via a uterine cannula
D. Acetic acid solution mixed with sterile saline via uterine cannula

ANS: C
Rationale: Instillation of methylene blue solution through the uterine cannula allows the surgeon to observe patency of the fallopian tubes through the laparoscope.

214. The patient will have fluoroscopy for a closed reduction during the surgical procedure. The circulating nurse will provide which of the following for the patient's protection during the use of ionizing radiation?
A. Lead shields for the gonads, thyroid, and abdomen
B. Additional drapes as protection from contamination
C. Radiolucent arm boards
D. Dosimeter on the patient's gown

ANS: A
Rationale: Exposed areas not part of the surgical procedure should be protected from ionizing radiation.

215. Which of the following bacteria form endospores that are resistant to sterilization?
A. Staphylococcus
B. Streptococcus
C. Clostridia
D. Spirochetes

ANS: C
Rationale: The only bacterial species that form endospores are clostridia and bacillus.

216. The patient is in lithotomy in sling stirrups. Which nerve group is at risk from this position?
A. Femoral
B. Peroneal
C. Inguinal
D. Tibial

ANS: B
Rationale: The peroneal nerve is easily injured by the upright posts of the stirrups.

217. The patient has a swollen, red leg with a weeping, anterior tibial ulcer. This observation by the circulating nurse indicates which of the following conditions?
A. Alcoholism
B. Diabetes
C. Crohn's disease
D. Venous return complications

ANS: D
Rationale: The signs exhibited by the patient indicate a venous return problem. The cause could be an injury; it is not always a comorbid condition until diagnosed.

218. CNOR is the designated credential used when officially certified. What is the significance of these initials?
A. It means certified operating room nurse.
B. It means certified perioperative nurse.
C. It is an acronym.
D. It is a permanent credential.

ANS: B
Rationale: Nurses who work in patient care areas where invasive procedures are performed are eligible for the credential, not only the OR. It must be renewed.

219. Patient assessment by the circulating nurse begins with which of the following activities?
A. Patient identification by name and date of birth
B. Checking the patient's wristband
C. Reading the charted notes
D. Confirming the signature on the consent form

ANS: A
Rationale: The nurse should always confirm the patient's identity before proceeding with an assessment.

220. The scrub nurse needs to change a contaminated glove during the surgical procedure. The circulating nurse, wearing examination gloves, removes the contaminated glove for the scrub nurse. Which method is appropriate for the scrub nurse to don a new sterile glove?
A. Closed gloving
B. Open gloving
C. Closed assisted gloving
D. Double gloving

ANS: B
Rationale: Closed methods involve pulling the contaminated cuff back over the hand. Open gloving is the most appropriate method the nurse can use to reapply a sterile glove.

221. A sterile team member needs to change both the contaminated gown and gloves. Which of the following actions is the best approach to reestablish the sterile attire?
A. Remove the gown before removing the gloves.

B. Untie the gown and open new gloves on the back table.

C. Remove gloves followed by the gown.

D. Remove the gloves, then the gown, and rescrub.

ANS: A

Rationale: The gown comes off first followed by the gloves. A new sterile attire set can be applied without rescrubbing.

222. The circulating nurse manages metallic forensic evidence using which of the following methods?

A. The metallic specimen is taken to the laboratory in a metal basin.

B. The metallic specimen is placed in a plastic cup with saline.

C. The metallic specimen is placed in a dry plastic cup.

D. The metallic specimen is given directly to the supervisor.

ANS: C

Rationale: The metallic specimen is placed in a dry plastic cup. The metal piece should not be placed in a metal container that could change the markings on the surface. The facility in cooperation with the local authorities will have a "chain of custody" protocol.

223. Autologous tissue is taken for reuse by the patient at a later date. The circulating nurse should consider the following best practice when storing the patient's tissue according to facility policy?

A. The container is placed in a plastic bag.

B. The container is labeled with the patient's name and date.

C. The container is immersed in dry ice.

D. The container is filled with sterile water.

ANS: B

Rationale: The facility will have specific policies about the storage of autologous tissue. The circulating nurse must label the tissue container immediately before placing in storage.

224. The surgeon requests Gelfoam during an open spinal surgery. What property concerning this hemostatic agent should the circulating nurse understand for this type of procedure?

A. Gelfoam should not be retained in confined spaces.

B. Gelfoam is only used dry.

C. Gelfoam is available only in a powdered form.

D. Gelfoam should be left in place for hemostasis.

ANS: A

Rationale: Gelfoam swells up to 45 times its weight and would cause compression in the spinal canal if enclosed.

225. The patient is scheduled for a surgical procedure using magnetic resonance imaging (MRI). The preoperative nurse should assess the patient for which of following?

A. Allergy to iodine

B. Implanted metallic devices

C. History of hiatal hernia

D. Sensitivity to general anesthesia

ANS: B

Rationale: Metallic devices other than titanium will react by attraction to the MRI.

226. An adolescent male is reluctant to remove his underwear and don a gown for surgery. The preoperative nurse should take which of the following actions?

A. Instruct him to completely undress despite his protests.

B. Call the main desk and have his parents brought to the preoperative area.

C. Allow him to wear the gown over his underwear and inform the circulating nurse.

D. Call the main desk and cancel the surgical procedure.

ANS: C

Rationale: Allow him to wear the gown over his underwear. They can be removed in the operating.

227. The fire marshal is inspecting the surgical suite. The resulting report indicates which of the following is a violation of safety?

A. Shelving is 12 inches above the floor

B. Shelving is 6 inches from the wall

C. Shelving is layered 24 inches apart

D. Shelving is 10 inches from the ceiling

ANS: D

Rationale: The ceiling and upper shelving space must be 18 inches to permit room for the sprinkler system to be effective in the event of a fire.

228. Anesthesia personnel check the gas machine before each surgical procedure. The circulating nurse should understand which of the following concerning waste anesthetic gas?

A. The gas is recirculated through the machine.

B. The exhaled gas from the patient is evacuated via the scavenger capture hose.

C. The machine does not lose gas into the room air.

D. The need for excess gas capture has been eliminated by the use of a microprocessor.

ANS: B

Rationale: The purple hose at the rear of the gas machine evacuates exhaled waste gases from the patient.

229. Which of the following is true about prion contamination?

A. Prions are transferred via droplets.

B. Prions are killed via steam under pressure.

C. Prions can multiply on inanimate surfaces.

D. Prions are not living and cannot be killed.

ANS: D

Rationale: Prions are not alive and cannot multiply. Because they are proteins, they are transferred via direct contact.

230. A capacitative return electrode has which of the following characteristics?
    A. Is positioned under the patient's full body length
    B. Attaches to two limbs
    C. Is only used with bipolar electrosurgery
    D. Is only used with argon beam coagulators

ANS: A

Rationale: A capacitative return electrode does not attach to the patient. It is placed under the patient. It is used with all forms of monopolar surgery. Bipolar docs not use a return electrode.

231. What is the primary hazard associated with surgery of the head and neck?
    A. Retained surgical items
    B. Tissue damage from radiation can distort the surgical planes
    C. Fire is an extreme risk when electrosurgery (ESU) is used near or around the airway
    D. Loss of airway control

ANS: C

Rationale: Ignition caused by ESU in the presence of oxygen is a dire risk in head and neck surgery.

232. The surgeon requested biologic fibrin sealant. The circulating nurse knows the following about the prepacked delivery unit?
    A. The product is kept on ice until used.
    B. The product is supplied in two syringes.
    C. The product is mixed with 50-mL platelets.
    D. The product is preheated before use.

ANS: B

Rationale: The product arrives in two syringes that are mixed simultaneously when applied to tissue.

233. The patient received a packed cell transfusion in the emergency department before arriving in the OR. The circulating nurse assesses the patient and suspects a transfusion reaction. What signs have aroused the nurse's suspicion?
    A. The patient has an elevated body temperature greater than the admitting baseline
    B. The patient is unconscious
    C. The patient seems confused
    D. The patient is complaining of thirst

ANS: A

Rationale: A rising body temperature is an early sign of transfusion reaction. The temperature change is immediately reported to the surgeon and the anesthesia provider.

234. The patient is jaundiced and scheduled for a cholecystectomy. Which of the following conditions can present during the surgical procedure?
    A. Incontinence of the bladder
    B. Hypertension
    C. Hypoglycemia
    D. Impaired coagulation

ANS: D

Rationale: Liver disease can cause problems with blood clotting factors that can lead to hemorrhage.

235. The female patient is having an abdominal surgical procedure that is anticipated to last 4 or more hours. Which set of steps is appropriate for the surgical prep?
    A. Prep the abdomen, the perineum, then insert the Foley using a fresh prep setup.
    B. Prep the perineum, the abdomen, then insert the Foley using a fresh prep setup.
    C. Prep the perineum, insert the Foley, then prep the abdomen using a fresh prep setup.
    D. Prep the abdomen, insert the Foley, and then prep the perineum using one prep setup.

ANS: C

Rationale: The perineum and the Foley insertion should be done before the abdomen to minimize the risk for perineal splash to a freshly prepped abdomen. After prepping the perineum, a second kit and gloves are used for the abdomen.

236. Vaccination for communicable diseases is recommended for all healthcare workers. Which of the following diseases is also known as rubella and is spread through droplet transmission?
    A. Chickenpox
    B. Mumps
    C. German measles
    D. Small pox

ANS: C

Rationale: Rubella is a viral disease known as German measles. Viral diseases are difficult to treat and easier to prevent.

237. The patient is having a toe amputation for gangrene. The circulating nurse knows the following is true concerning gangrene?
    A. Gangrene is caused by a virus.
    B. Gangrene is caused by a form of clostridia.
    C. Gangrene is caused by ischemia.
    D. Gangrene is caused by cross-contamination.

ANS: B

Rationale: Gangrene is caused by clostridia, which is a bacterium that forms endospores.

238. The surgeon requests 1 ounce of a pharmacologic solution. The circulating nurse dispenses how much solution to the scrub nurse's medicine cup?
    A. 30 mL
    B. 20 mL
    C. 15 mL
    D. 10 mL

ANS: A

Rationale: 30 mL equals 1 ounce.

239. The patient has a fractured femur. Which of the following is a potential life-threatening complication?

A. Air embolus
B. Fat embolus
C. Ileo-inguinal compression
D. Foot drop

ANS: B
Rationale: Fat can be released into the vascular system from the patient's bone marrow and embolize.

240. The patient is undergoing cataract removal surgery. The surgeon has requested medication to dilate the patient's pupils. The circulating nurse will provide which of the following eye drops for the surgeon's use?
A. Miotic drops
B. Mydriatic drops
C. Fluorescein drops
D. Viscoelastic drops

ANS: B
Rationale: Mydriatic drops are cycloplegic medications that dilate the pupil.

241. The surgeon injects the uterus with Pitressin during a hysterectomy. What is the purpose of this drug?
A. Vasodilation
B. Hormone suppression
C. Hypertension control
D. Vasoconstriction

ANS: D
Rationale: Injection of a vasoconstrictor decreases the risk for blood loss during surgery.

242. Which of the following hemostatic agents is only used dry?
A. Gelfoam
B. Thrombin
C. Avitene
D. Silver nitrate

ANS: C
Rationale: When used as a sponge or powder, the fibrin in the patient's blood forms a gel-like hemostatic barrier.

243. The surgeon has requested cultures of the patient's open wound before an incision and drainage of an abscess. Which of the following is the best action of the circulating nurse?
A. Culture the open wound before the site is prepped.
B. Culture the wound after the site is prepped.
C. Culture the wound after the abscess is opened.
D. Culture the site before primary closure.

ANS: A
Rationale: Culturing the open areas of the wound before the prep prevents the antiseptic from altering the results.

244. The patient has a deep laceration over the eyebrow. What does the circulating nurse know about preparing the patient's injury?
A. The eyebrow is shaved.
B. The eyelashes are trimmed.
C. The eyebrow is not shaved.
D. The eyelashes are coated with gel.

ANS: C
Rationale: Eyebrows are not shaved because they may not grow back.

245. Which nerve is at risk during parotid gland surgery?
A. Mastoid
B. Facial
C. Auricular
D. Hypoglossal

ANS: B
Rationale: The facial nerve is located within the parotid gland.

246. The patient is having a split-thickness skin graft (STSG). The surgeon plans to expand the graft to cover more of the denuded area. Which process will the surgeon likely use to cover a large area with a small tissue sample?
A. Free-hand graft
B. Dermatome
C. Mesher
D. Braithwaite blade

ANS: C
Rationale: A mesher is used to cut slits in the STSG to cause it to expand over a larger area.

247. The pediatric patient is having a cheiloplasty. The circulating nurse knows that this surgical procedure corrects which of the following congenital conditions?
A. Cleft palate
B. Baby bottle teeth
C. Microtia
D. Cleft lip

ANS: D
Rationale: The lip failed to fuse during gestation.

248. The patient is scheduled for a Bristow procedure. What position will be used for the patient's surgical procedure?
A. Beach chair semi-Fowler's
B. Supine with extra padding under the surgical site
C. Lateral, with the surgical site elevated
D. Prone, with the arms on armboards

ANS: A
Rationale: The beach chair position enables the free motion of the shoulder.

249. The patient has a parathyroidectomy during a thyroidectomy. The parathyroid glands are saved for physiologic use by which of the following methods?
A. Flash frozen for further studies
B. Cut into small pieces and implanted in the patient's forearm
C. Preserved in Bowen's solution
D. Chilled in sterile saline for 2 hours after removal

ANS: B
Rationale: The cut-up gland segments are implanted into the muscle. They begin to function in calcium regulation after a few weeks.

250. The surgeon plans to use a postoperative suprapubic catheter. The circulating nurse knows which of the following is true about the use of this catheter?
    A. The patient will have a total cystectomy as part of the procedure.
    B. A urostomy will be created using the patient's ureters.
    C. Fluid is instilled into the bladder and the catheter is inserted in the lower abdomen.
    D. The catheter will be inserted using a nephroscope.

ANS: C

Rationale: The bladder and trigone will remain intact. The suprapubic catheter is a temporary urinary drainage device as an alternative to a Foley.

251. Which of the following drugs will be given by the anesthesia provider to reverse the effects of a nondepolarizing muscle relaxant?
    A. Neostigmine
    B. Narcan
    C. Tracrium
    D. Pavulon

ANS: A

Rationale: Neostigmine is a cholinergic that reverses the effect of nondepolarizing muscle relaxants.

252. During setup for the surgical procedure, when is the best time for the circulating nurse to open and dispense the dressings to the sterile field?
    A. After the initial count
    B. After the time out
    C. After the incision is made
    D. After the final closing count

ANS: D

Rationale: Dispensing the dressings after the final count prevents error by not accidently counting the dressing material into the counting process.

253. The World Health Organization (WHO) is in place for which of the following purposes?
    A. To set health standards in the United States
    B. To promote universal health and wellness
    C. To enforce health standards in third world countries
    D. To globally monitor surgical practice

ANS: B

Rationale: WHO promotes health and wellness throughout the world.

254. The surgeon requests a flat plate of the abdomen before the surgical procedure. What is a flat plate?
    A. A flat plate is an x-ray that uses nonionic contrast.
    B. A flat plate is an x-ray that uses ionic contrast.
    C. A flat plate is also known as a KUB (kidneys, ureters, and bladder) x-ray without contrast.
    D. A flat plate is also known as a KUB x-ray with contrast.

ANS: C

Rationale: A flat plate (KUB) is done before surgery on select patients without contrast as a scout film to detect select internal structures.

255. The circulating nurse is weighing sponges to estimate blood loss. The scale is balanced to account for extraneous weight of materials and irrigation. Which of the following is correct for estimating blood loss?
    A. 1 g = 1 mL
    B. 2 g = 1 mL
    C. 0.5 g = 1 mL
    D. 1.5 g = 1 mL

ANS: A

Rationale: After balancing (Tare) the scale, the remaining weight is the blood.

256. The circulating nurse adds a pack of hemostats to the sterile field at the request of the scrub nurse. Before delivering the instruments to the field, the circulating nurse does which of the following?
    A. Records the date and time of sterilization
    B. Asks the scrub nurse to count the number of hemostats currently present on the sterile field
    C. Inspects the package for integrity
    D. Records the number of hemostats being given to the scrub nurse

ANS: C

Rationale: The package must be intact before delivery to the sterile field. Counting of the contents takes place after delivery. Sterility is event related.

257. The circulating nurse prepares chest rolls for the patient's prone procedure. The placement is necessary for which reason?
    A. To elevate the spine for visualization of the surgical site
    B. To decrease pressure on the vena cava
    C. To protect the patient's genitalia
    D. To relieve the respiratory system

ANS: B

Rationale: The vena cava is relatively low pressure. Pressure from body weight causes increased venous pressure and changes the hemodynamic status of the patient.

258. When should the patient's prep begin?
    A. Immediately after positioning
    B. After gowning and gloving
    C. After the anesthesia provider indicates the patient is stable
    D. As soon as the setup is completed by the scrub nurse

ANS: C

Rationale: External stimulation caused by prepping could precipitate a physiologic decline if the anesthesia is not in full effect.

259. The patient is having a laminectomy. Where should the dispersive return electrode be positioned on the patient's body?
    A. On the patient's posterior thigh
    B. On the patient's biceps
    C. On the patient's gastrocnemius
    D. On the patient's chest

ANS: A
Rationale: The electrode should be placed on the fleshy part close to the surgical site.

260. During the initial sponge count, the packaged number of the contents is wrong. What should the circulating nurse do to minimize error in the final count?
    A. Document the number and continue the count.
    B. Isolate the pack of sponges in a plastic bag and place it on the circulator's desk.
    C. Throw the pack of sponges in the clean trash bin for recycling.
    D. Add an additional sponge to make the count correct.

ANS: B
Rationale: The incorrect sponges should be removed from the field and isolated in a bag, not tossed into trash. Any packaging material should be saved in the event the pack's lot of processed sponges contain errors.

261. The patient is admitted directly from the emergency department. The emergency procedure begins as soon as the patient is placed on the OR bed. An initial count was not performed. At the conclusion of the surgical procedure, what should the circulating nurse do?
    A. Attempt to count as the procedure proceeds.
    B. Do not add any extra sponges to the sterile field.
    C. Add only 10 sponges at a time to the sterile field.
    D. Request an x-ray when the procedure is complete.

ANS: D
Rationale: Although trying to count during the chaos of the emergency sounds logical, the best action would be to request an x-ray at the end of the procedure.

262. The pediatric patient is going to postanesthesia care unit (PACU) after a tonsillectomy. The best position for the child during transport is which of the following?
    A. In high Fowler's position
    B. Supine
    C. On the left side
    D. Seated

ANS: C
Rationale: The left-side positioning allows drainage from the mouth to minimize the risk for aspiration of blood.

263. The C-arm will be used for the orthopedic extremity procedure. What can the circulating nurse do to protect the patient?
    A. Place lead shielding over the patient.
    B. Place lead shielding under the patient.
    C. Place lead shielding over the patient's thyroid.
    D. Place lead gonad shield over the patient's groin.

ANS: B
Rationale: The x-ray is delivered from below the patient. Protection must be underneath.

264. During an abdominal aortic aneurysm repair surgery, the surgeon may ask the circulating nurse to perform which action?
    A. Periodically check bilateral pedal pulses on the patient.
    B. Call the family to give updates every 15 minutes.
    C. Pour warm sterile saline into the surgical site.
    D. Inflate the tourniquet over the thighs.

ANS: A
Rationale: The surgeon wants to know the status of the circulation in the lower legs.

265. The patient has been to x-ray for a needle localization biopsy. The circulating nurse performs the prep with the following in mind?
    A. The wire is removed immediately before the prep and discarded in the sharps box.
    B. The wire must remain in situ for accurate diagnosis.
    C. The wire can be bent to the medial side of the chest wall to facilitate the prep.
    D. The wire is not sterile and could contaminate the prepped area.

ANS: B
Rationale: The wire marks the area and depth of the biopsy and is critical for diagnosis.

266. The patient is in lithotomy. The circulating nurse knows that hypotension can be minimized by which of the following actions?
    A. One leg at a time is removed from the stirrups and placed on the OR bed.
    B. Both legs are removed from the stirrups by two personnel and slowly lowered to the OR bed.
    C. The stirrups are lowered to the level of the OR bed before moving the legs to the OR bed.
    D. The patient is frog-legged before placing the legs on the OR bed.

ANS: B
Rationale: Both legs are removed from the stirrups simultaneously. There is no evidence-based research to demonstrate that one leg at a time benefits the patient in any way.

267. Which type of local anesthesia is appropriate for a circumcision?
    A. 1% lidocaine plain
    B. 0.25% Marcaine with Wydase
    C. 1 % lidocaine with epinephrine
    D. 2 % Pontocaine plain

ANS: A

Rationale: Additives can cause vasoconstriction, which in turn can cause ischemic necrosis.

268. Which of the following measures should the circulating nurse follow when the patient is in the prone position?
    A. Ask the transporter to stand by for the specimen delivery.
    B. Position the crash cart near the door.
    C. A transport cart should be immediately available in case of the need to place the patient supine during an emergency.
    D. Provide a headlamp for the surgeon.

ANS: C

Rationale: A transport cart should be immediately available for repositioning the patient in an emergency.

269. The patient is positioned supine with arms tucked in at the sides. Which of the following is the appropriate method of securing the arms with a drawsheet?
    A. The drawsheet extends over the elbows and is tucked under the mattress.
    B. The drawsheet encases the hands and forearms and is tucked under the mattress.
    C. The drawsheet cases the hands and forearms and is fan folded next to the patient.
    D. The drawsheet extends over the elbows and is tucked under the patient.

ANS: D

Rationale: The drawsheet should only be tucked under the patient to minimize the amount of strain on the patient's shoulders.

270. The patient will have a Foley inserted before the skin prep. The circulating nurse does which of the following before catheterizing the patient?
    A. Asks the patient to void in the preoperative area
    B. Pretests the Foley balloon
    C. Positions the patient and prepares the Foley insertion supplies
    D. Gowns and gloves using the closed gloving technique

ANS: C

Rationale: Position and prepare the supplies first. Never pretest the Foley balloon according the manufacturer. Balloons are pretested at the factory and are folded to minimize urethral trauma. Pretesting the balloons causes the folds to refold incorrectly and can cause excoriation of the urethra.

271. The surgeon instructs the circulating nurse to label the specimen as a bezoar. What is this?
    A. An ingested hairball
    B. A staghorn stone

C. A tumor from the small intestine
D. A thyroglossal duct cyst

ANS: A

Rationale: This is hair intentionally ingested by the patient. It accumulates in the digestive tract.

272. Which of the following practices decrease the risk for biologic exposure during a needlestick?
    A. Rinsing the gloves with betadine
    B. Double gloving
    C. Using an alcohol-based hand hygiene product
    D. Using a brush method scrub for the first scrub of the day

ANS: B

Rationale: Double gloving causes much of the biologic matter to remain on the outside of the glove if perforated.

273. Which of the following is the most common cause of surgical site infection?
    A. *Streptococcus*
    B. *Escherichia coli*
    C. *Staphylococcus aureus*
    D. *Pseudomonas*

ANS: C

Rationale: *S. aureus* is the most common surgical site infection.

274. The patient has a wound infection scheduled for debridement. The defect cannot be sutured at the initial procedure but is planned for a few days later. What closure method will be used?
    A. Primary closure
    B. Secondary intention
    C. Retention sutures
    D. Delayed primary closure

ANS: D

Rationale: Delayed primary closure is commonly used when the incision boundaries are debrided and cleaned before primary closure.

275. The surgeon requests antibiotic irrigation in sterile saline. The circulating nurse prepares the medication in which manner?
    A. Draws the medication into a syringe and expresses the drug into the irrigation basin through the needle
    B. Draws the medication into a syringe and expresses the drug into the bottle of sterile saline before pouring to the sterile field
    C. Pops the top of the vial and pours the drug into the sterile irrigation basin on the sterile field
    D. Draws the medication into a syringe, removes the needle, and expresses the drug into the irrigation basin

ANS: D

Rationale: The best method is to draw the drug into a syringe, remove the needle, and express the medication into the irrigation basin on the field. This method prevents aerosolization of the drug.

276. The OR is equipped with laminar airflow. The circulating nurse knows that the purpose of this airflow is which of the following?
    A. Provides ultra-clean filtered air for the sterile field
    B. Removes particulate from the sterile field
    C. Maintains the patient's body temperature
    D. Sterilizes air before it reaches the sterile field

ANS: A
Rationale: Although the air is filtered, it is never sterile. The patient's body temperature is monitored because the air is not warmed and could cause hypothermia.

277. A potential complication associated with prone position is which of the following?
    A. Epistaxis
    B. Ocular ischemia
    C. Deafness
    D. Torticollis

ANS: B
Rationale: Intraocular pressure can cause ischemia, leading to blindness.

278. The anesthesia provider uses capnography to monitor the patient. Which of the following parameters is observed using this method?
    A. Carbon dioxide
    B. Oxygen
    C. Lactic acid
    D. Acidosis

ANS: A
Rationale: Carbon dioxide is the waste production of metabolism. Any excess would signal a problem with the respiratory system.

279. Which of the following methods is unsafe for delivering medications to the sterile field?
    A. Pouring irrigation solution into a basin on the sterile field.
    B. The circulating nurse draws the drug into a syringe before dispensing to the medicine cup.
    C. The circulating nurse holds the vial while the scrub nurse pierces and withdraws the drug.
    D. The circulating nurse dispenses the presterilized glass ampule to the sterile field.

ANS: C
Rationale: The risk for an avoidable needlestick is high when someone else holds the vial.

280. When positioning a patient, which of the following does not provide a pressure reduction surface?
    A. Gel pad
    B. Towel roll
    C. Egg crate foam
    D. Memory foam mattress

ANS: B
Rationale: Towel and blanket rolls do not alternate pressure once body weight is applied. The rolls compress and remain compressed.

281. Which of the following is correct for positioning the supine patient's legs?
    A. Flex the knees 5–10 degrees on a pillow.
    B. Place a safety strap over the tibia.
    C. Maintain the heels in contact with the bed.
    D. Flex the bed at the knee.

ANS: A
Rationale: Flexing the knees relieves stress on the lower back.

282. Which of the following is not a method of preventing hypothermia in the patient?
    A. Place a forced air warming drape over the patient.
    B. Place a blanket from the warming cabinet over the patient.
    C. Place a warming blanket under the patient.
    D. Pour warm irrigation into the scrub nurse's sterile basin.

ANS: C
Rationale: Do not put a warming blanket under the patient. Continuous pressure from the patient's body weight does not permit redistribution of heated contact and could cause heat to accumulate in one spot, causing a burn.

283. The legs of a patient in a seated position should be arranged in which manner?
    A. Frog-legged
    B. Knees flexed 30 degrees
    C. Straight
    D. Abducted 10 degrees

ANS: B
Rationale: Flexion of the knees relieves pressure on the patient's lower back and prevents the patient from sliding downward on the OR bed.

284. Which of the following is a potential source of pressure injury during positioning?
    A. Peripheral IV
    B. Implanted pacemaker device
    C. Dentures
    D. Artificial nails

ANS: B
Rationale: Pressure originating under the skin can cause subsurface pressure injury when the patient is positioned with device bearing the patient's weight.

285. The patient is positioned laterally. Which of the following considerations is the best position for the legs?
    A. The upper leg is straight.
    B. The lower leg is straight.
    C. The upper leg is flexed.
    D. The lower leg is elevated.

ANS: A
Rationale: The upper leg is straight and the lower leg is flexed. A pillow is placed between the knees.

286. When using kidney braces in the lateral position, which of the following is the correct placement?
    A. The shorter brace is placed anterior.
    B. The shorter brace is placed adjacent to the longer brace.
    C. The longer brace is placed anterior.
    D. The longer brace is placed posterior.

ANS: C
Rationale: When using kidney braces, the longer brace is placed anterior and the shorter brace is placed posterior against the lumber spine.

287. Which of the following best describes the padding under the patient in a lateral position?
    A. A chest roll under the thorax from axilla to iliac crest
    B. A blanket roll under the thorax above the diaphragm
    C. An axillary roll under the thorax at the level of the seventh to ninth rib
    D. A gel pad under the patient's neck above the clavicle

ANS: C
Rationale: The axillary roll relieves pressure from the patient's body weight on the shoulder. A chest roll would elevate the patient's body on a lateral plane, causing the sacral to extremity weight distribution to be disproportionate. The position could be unstable.

288. When the patient is prone, the arm boards should be in which position related to the patient's body?
    A. Even with the patient's chest
    B. Slightly lower than the patient's chest
    C. Even with the OR bed
    D. Angled greater than 45 degrees to the patient's body

ANS: B
Rationale: The arm boards should be slightly lower than the patient's chest to minimize stress on the patient's shoulders and upper thorax.

289. The surgeon requests bilateral ureteral stent placement before performing an abdominal hysterectomy. What is the rationale for this additional procedure?
    A. Identification of the ureters during dissection
    B. Instillation of antibiotic irrigation
    C. Urinary measurement intraoperatively
    D. Injection of methylene blue

ANS: A
Rationale: The stents provide a tactile and visual outline of the ureters during dissection.

290. During an emergency in the OR, which of the following assessment notations facilitates prompt treatment of the patient's crisis?
    A. Notation of the chronologic age of the patient
    B. Notation of the location of the waiting family
    C. Notation of the patient's religion
    D. Notation of the patient's weight in kilograms (kg)

ANS: D
Rationale: Emergency drugs are calculated using the patient's weight in kilograms. The patient's weight in kilograms is more reliable than the chronologic age.

291. The patient has a penicillin allergy. Which of the following antibiotics is safe for use with this patient?
    A. Ampicillin
    B. Ciprofloxacin
    C. Amoxicillin
    D. Ticarcillin

ANS: B
Rationale: Ciprofloxacin is a quinolone and is safe for use. The other choices are related beta-lactams.

292. When transporting a patient with chest tubes, which of the following is appropriate for managing the tubes during transport to the PACU?
    A. Clamp the tubes.
    B. Disconnect the tubing.
    C. Keep the drainage receptacle below the chest.
    D. Drain the water from the collection unit.

ANS: C
Rationale: Keeping the drainage receptacle below the level of the chest facilitates drainage.

293. Administration of large quantities of fluids during an emergency surgical procedure requires which of the following access lines?
    A. Central line
    B. Arterial line
    C. Additional peripheral line
    D. Arteriovenous shunt

ANS: A
Rationale: A central line enters the venous system at a large chest vein and can accommodate a large volume of fluid delivery.

294. The patient has thoracic outlet syndrome. Which of the following surgical procedures is performed to alleviate the patient's symptoms?
    A. Resection of the clavicle
    B. Resection of the first rib
    C. Resection of the anterior mediastinum
    D. Resection of the cervical nerve plexus

ANS: B
Rationale: The first rib is the cause of the nerve compression and it is removed.

295. The patient is having a rhytidectomy. Which procedure is performed on the patient?
    A. Microdermabrasion
    B. Laser resurfacing
    C. Blepharoplasty
    D. Face lift

ANS: D
Rationale: Rhytids are wrinkles. A face lift diminishes the wrinkles of the face.

296. Precautions when using polymethylmethacrylate (PMMA) for the team include which of the following?
    A. Avoid wearing contact lenses.
    B. Avoid bright lights.
    C. Avoid moving about in the sterile field.
    D. Avoid glove changes.

ANS: A

Rationale: The FDA warns that the fumes of the PMMA can bond with gas-permeable contact lenses and cause damage.

297. The surgeon is performing an embolectomy. Which device will be requested for the completion of the surgical procedure?
    A. Guidewire
    B. A 20-cc syringe
    C. Fogarty catheter
    D. A swivel knife

ANS: C

Rationale: A Fogarty catheter is passed into the vessel, inflated, and withdrawn to remove the clot.

298. The surgeon is performing a rhinoplasty. Which of the following drugs is drawn into the syringe for hemostasis?
    A. Thrombin
    B. Afrin
    C. Lidocaine with epinephrine
    D. Epinephrine

ANS: C

Rationale: Lidocaine with epinephrine is used for hemostasis.

299. When obtaining a sterile package from the sterile core, the circulating nurse checks the date on the label under which circumstances?
    A. The package contains mixed media metals.
    B. The package contains a drug.
    C. The package is wrapped in woven fabric.
    D. The package is wrapped in paper.

ANS: B

Rationale: The dates are important when the package contains an unstable element, such as a drug. Other packs are considered sterile unless the integrity is compromised (event related).

300. During CO_2 laser surgery of the throat, the endotracheal tube begins to burn. The first action taken to manage the situation is which of the following?
    A. Stop the anesthetic gas.
    B. Pour sterile saline into the mouth.
    C. Decrease the oxygen flow.
    D. Remove the endotracheal tube.

ANS: D

Rationale: The burning endotracheal tube is removed, then replaced immediately with a smaller tube for oxygenation.

301. What is the meaning of the term *iatrogenic*?
    A. An event happens to a patient randomly
    B. An event happens to a patient as a result of treatment
    C. An event happens to a patient who resists treatment
    D. An event happens to a patient with drug tolerance

ANS: B

Rationale: Iatrogenic injury happens as a direct result of treatment (i.e., positioning, drug administration, or other event in the care of healthcare providers).

302. Laboratory values between male and female patients vary in which of the following results?
    A. Differential
    B. Platelets
    C. Red counts
    D. Blood pH

ANS: C

Rationale: Female patients have a slightly lower red cell count and may have a lower hemoglobin and hematocrit value.

303. The differential blood value refers to which of the following?
    A. Prothrombin and partial thromboplastin times
    B. Values of the various white cells
    C. Liver enzymes
    D. Electrolytes

ANS: B

Rationale: The differential is the value of each of the five types of white blood cells.

304. The patient has a myeloplastic disease. Which of the blood cell components is measured to monitor the progression of the disease?
    A. White blood cells
    B. Red blood cells
    C. Lymphocytes
    D. Platelets

ANS: D

Rationale: Myeloplastic disease affects the bone marrow and the development of platelets. Platelets decrease in circulating numbers. The patient has a deficient clotting mechanism.

305. Which of the following laboratory values is cause for alarm?
    A. Potassium 3.7
    B. Calcium 12.6
    C. Glucose 98
    D. Sodium 138

ANS: B

Rationale: The calcium is elevated and should be reported to the anesthesia provider and surgeon.

306. The patient arrives in the preoperative holding area with a hematocrit of 50%. What is the significance of this laboratory value?
    A. This value is within normal limits.
    B. The patient has a bleeding disorder.
    C. The patient is anemic.
    D. This value is high.

ANS: A
Rationale: This value is within normal limits and no cause for concern.

307. The patient has a white cell count of 18,000. What is the implication of this laboratory value?
    A. The patient has an alcohol dependency.
    B. The patient is diabetic.
    C. The patient may have an infection.
    D. The patient is hyperthermic.
ANS: C
Rationale: The patient may have an infection, either localized or systemic.

308. The patient is admitted with acute pancreatitis. Evaluation of the patient's laboratory results includes an elevation in which of the following values?
    A. Eosinophils
    B. Amylase
    C. Basophils
    D. Troponins
ANS: B
Rationale: Amylase is an enzyme that is associated with the pancreas.

309. Which of the following potassium values is not within normal limits?
    A. 2.5 mmol/L
    B. 3.7 mmol/L
    C. 4.6 mmol/L
    D. 5.1 mmol/L
ANS: A
Rationale: 3.7–5.1 mmol/L potassium is the normal value.

310. The diabetic patient has a fingerstick test in the preoperative holding area. Which of the following test results is cause for concern and should be reported to the anesthesia provider and the surgeon?
    A. 82
    B. 94
    C. 100
    D. 225
ANS: D
Rationale: Blood glucose greater than 100 is considered abnormal. The patient may need regular insulin before the surgical procedure and a repeat fingerstick. It also may indicate that the patient has consumed food before arriving at the facility.

311. The adult patient's platelet count is 100,000 mm^3. What can this value indicate?
    A. The count is within normal limits.
    B. The count is high.
    C. The count is slightly low.
    D. The count must be repeated to confirm.
ANS: C
Rationale: The platelet count should be between 150,000 and 400,000. The count is slightly low and may indicate that the patient may have blood loss during the surgical procedure.

312. Which of the following white blood cells measured in the differential may indicate an allergic reaction?
    A. Lymphocytes
    B. Monocytes
    C. Basophils
    D. Eosinophils
ANS: D
Rationale: Eosinophils indicate an inflammation, such as an allergic reaction. They are short-lived white cells formed in the bone marrow that respond in the presence of inflammation.

313. During the surgical procedure, the anesthesia provider sends blood to the laboratory for a hemoglobin and hematocrit (H&H) value. Which of the following levels is a cause for concern?
    A. Hemoglobin 13, hematocrit 45%
    B. Hemoglobin 10, hematocrit 30%
    C. Hemoglobin 15, hematocrit 40%
    D. Hemoglobin 12, hematocrit 46%
ANS: B
Rationale: The H&H is somewhat low and will likely require a repeat test if additional blood loss happens as the surgical procedure progresses. Blood replacement is not indicated at this point, but volume expansion is employed.

314. Arterial blood gases (ABG) are taken to measure which of the following aspects of the patient's condition?
    A. Oxygen and carbon dioxide values
    B. Status of blood loss
    C. Cerebral perfusion
    D. Peripheral perfusion
ANS: A
Rationale: The levels of oxygen and carbon dioxide in the arterial blood are indicators of the respiratory efficiency.

315. Which of the following ABG values may indicate metabolic acidosis?
    A. pH 7.25
    B. pH 7.40
    C. $Paco_2$ 48
    D. $Paco_2$ 44
ANS: A
Rationale: A low pH indicates acidosis. Normal blood pH is 7.35–7.45.

316. Which of the following blood test values indicate a higher risk for blood loss during the surgical procedure?
    A. High hemoglobin and hematocrit (H&H)
    B. Elevated differential
    C. Low electrolytes
    D. Prolonged prothrombin time (PT) and partial thromboplastin time (PTT)
ANS: D
Rationale: The PT and PTT are indicators of clotting times. Prolonged times indicate a clotting disorder and the potential for bleeding during the surgical procedure.

317. The morphology of the patient's red blood cells indicates the presence of nuclei. What does this mean to the patient's physiologic condition?
    A. The patient is healthy.
    B. The patient is utilizing available oxygen.
    C. The red cells cannot carry oxygen.
    D. The red cells are full of CO_2.

ANS: C
Rationale: The patient's red blood cells cannot carry oxygen if a nucleus is present. These red cells are immature and do not support the patient's physiology.

318. The patient is jaundiced on arrival to the OR. The circulating nurse checks the laboratory work and assesses the patient. Which laboratory value is commonly elevated for patients with this condition?
    A. Serum sodium
    B. Bilirubin
    C. Platelets
    D. pH

ANS: B
Rationale: Hemoglobin is released when the red blood cells break down (hemolysis) and enter the circulatory system. It is common in hepatitis and gallbladder disease.

319. The patient has a history of sickle cell disease. The circulating nurse will assess the patient for which of the following during the preoperative assessment?
    A. Painful joints
    B. Difficulty swallowing
    C. Pallor
    D. Hypotension

ANS: A
Rationale: A patient with sickle cell disease may exhibit pain in the joints if a sickle cell crisis is starting.

320. Which of the following drugs adversely affects wound healing?
    A. Diuretic use
    B. Steroid use
    C. Analgesic use
    D. Hormone use

ANS: B
Rationale: Steroids reduce the inflammatory response necessary for healing.

321. The female patient indicates she takes oral contraceptives. The circulating nurse knows that the patient is at risk for which of the following complications?
    A. Hemorrhage
    B. Infertility
    C. Thrombus
    D. Infection

ANS: C
Rationale: Contraceptives increase the risk of blood clots

322. The patient has been taking diuretics for several months. The circulating nurse will commonly find which of the following changes in the patient's preoperative laboratory work?
    A. Low hemoglobin and hematocrit
    B. Low electrolytes
    C. High sodium
    D. High potassium

ANS: B
Rationale: Diuretics cause a decrease in electrolytes such as sodium and potassium.

323. The trauma patient arrives unconscious directly to the OR on arrival. The circulating nurse is not able to fully assess the patient. No family is available for questioning. The patient's condition requires anesthesia administration to make the following assumption during intubation?
    A. The patient is expectant and will die in the OR.
    B. The patient will arouse enough before anesthesia is administered.
    C. The patient will need a tracheotomy.
    D. The patient may have a full stomach and will need cricoid pressure.

ANS: D
Rationale: All trauma patients are considered to have a full stomach since it may not be possible to ask about the last meal.

324. The patient is a victim of assault and has been shot by an unknown assailant. The patient arrives at the OR fully clothed. The circulating nurse helps to preserve potential evidence by which of the following actions?
    A. Cutting out the bullet holes in the clothing and placing the cut pieces into a plastic bag
    B. Rinsing the area with sterile saline before undressing the patient
    C. Leaving the clothing on the patient and cutting open the area around the surgical site
    D. Removing the clothes by cutting along the seams and placing into a paper bag

ANS: D
Rationale: Preservation of evidence is critical. The clothes are cut along the seams and placed in a paper bag. Placing in plastic could destroy evidence.

325. The patient is an infant who had a few sips of water a few hours before surgery. The circulating nurse knows which of the following concerning the infant's preoperative oral intake?
    A. The sips of water will be of no consequence.
    B. The surgery will be cancelled.
    C. The surgery will be delayed for 6 hours.
    D. The patient will have a nasogastric tube inserted before intubation.

ANS: A
Rationale: A few sips of water to take preoperative medication is generally not an issue. Many surgeons have the patient take oral medications the morning of surgery.

Index

Note: Page numbers followed by *f* indicate figures, *t* indicate tables, and *b* indicate boxes.